WHICH? MEDICINE

WHICH? MEDICINE

Rosalind Grant MRPharmS

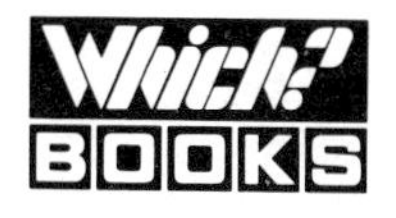

Consumers' Association
and Hodder & Stoughton

Which? Books are commissioned and researched by The Association for Consumer Research and published by Consumers' Association, 2 Marylebone Road, London NW1 4DF, and Hodder & Stoughton, 47 Bedford Square, London WC1B 3DP.

Typographic design by Dick Vine
Cover design by Paul Saunders
Cover photography by John Parker

Acknowledgements to:
The members of the editorial board and advisory council of *Drug and Therapeutics Bulletin* and other medical advisers who helped with this book; University College Hospital pharmacy; *The Medicines You Take* by D R Laurence and J W Black (Croom Helm)

First edition August 1992, reprinted October 1992

British Library Cataloguing in Publication Data
Grant, Rosalind
'Which?' Medicine
I. Title
615.1

ISBN 0-340-55920-9

Thanks for choosing this book . . .

If you find it useful we'd like to hear from you. Even if it doesn't do the job you were expecting, we'd still like to know. Then we can take your comments into account when preparing similar titles or, indeed, the next edition of the book. Address your letter to the Publishing Manager at Consumers' Association, FREEPOST, 2 Marylebone Road, London NW1 4DF.

We look forward to hearing from you.

Typeset by Wyvern Typesetting Limited, Bristol
Printed and bound in Great Britain by Richard Clay Ltd, Bungay, Suffolk

CONTENTS

FOREWORD

By Dr Andrew Herxheimer MB, FRCP, founding Editor of **Drug and Therapeutics Bulletin**

Which? Medicine is a natural extension of *Drug and Therapeutics Bulletin*, Consumers' Association's fortnightly publication for medical professionals. For thirty years the *Bulletin* has addressed patients indirectly – through doctors, pharmacists and journalists – but now this book has been developed from the *Bulletin* to present information about medicines directly to them in easily understandable language.

During those thirty years *Drug and Therapeutics Bulletin* has been a unique source of advice for doctors on prescribing. It has looked critically at the broadest span of drugs, both established and newly introduced, and has campaigned for the simplest and best practice in prescribing. It has never been afraid of being controversial, and was one of the main advocates of a limited list of drugs long before the Government finally brought one on to the statute book in 1985.

Some doctors in the past have been justly criticised for keeping the patient at arm's length, for expecting him or her to shut up and keep taking the medicine; but younger doctors, especially, recognise the value of better-informed patients who question the quality of their care and who make it their business to know what is going on in their bodies. Better communication between doctors and patients, and pharmacists and customers leads to better relationships, better care and better outcomes.

This book gives you the background knowledge for having a good, enlightening conversation with a doctor or pharmacist, and tells you the most important things about particular medicines. I hope it will help you have better consultations, and will guide you between times.

INTRODUCTION

Nowadays good health is the expected norm, even a right. Illness is generally accompanied by the assumption that a medicine will ease the symptoms or effect a cure. In Britain the use of medicines is extensive, particularly by the growing population of people over 65, who receive almost half of all prescriptions.

The reasons people take so many medicines are complex: the desire to take something to make you feel better is deep-rooted, like the sense that eating will overcome hunger, and a prescription often seems the most satisfactory outcome of a consultation for both patient and doctor. The pressure to search for a medicinal cure for every problem, whether or not it is appropriate, is increased by the high media profile of drugs and vigorous marketing by manufacturers.

But how much do you know about the medicine you take? What is in it? How is it supposed to help you? How will it affect your body? Does it have any unwanted effects? If you are to participate effectively in your own health care, you need the answers to these questions and many more besides, but until recently only minimal information has been available to the consumer.

• *IGNORANCE ABOUT MEDICINES*

Imagine a situation. Your doctor writes out a prescription and hands it to you as you leave the surgery, assuming that you will have no difficulty in following the instructions on the label. Later, the pharmacist supplying the medicine says nothing because he or she does not know what the doctor has told you and in any case is not necessarily able to tell from the prescription what the medicine is for. The only help you have is the label on the bottle and your own common sense.

The situation is far from imaginary. In Britain it has been common for many years, even though doctors and pharmacists should tell you about the medicines you take. As a consumer you are most vulnerable when you cannot exercise an informed choice about the products you use. You need to know how to get access to information about the products, which product is safest and most reliable, how to use it and what to do if something goes wrong. Lack of information can be dangerous, and the dangers are not restricted to prescription medicines:

In January 1989 a woman died from liver failure after taking too much paracetamol to treat flu. She simply didn't know that she was putting herself in danger.

Throughout the course of Christmas Day she tried to fight off flu to cook lunch, taking ordinary paracetamol tablets and several paracetamol-based drugs, among which were combination cold medicines. It is possible that she may have had some alcohol, too.

After lunch, feeling ill, she gave up and went to bed, taking two further paracetamol. She then became seriously ill and later died in hospital.

(Case quoted in *Which?*, February 1992)

This is just one of a number of cases where people have taken too much of a medicine without understanding the consequences.

● *MEDICINES SOLD OVER THE COUNTER*

Unlike many other commodities that can be bought medicines have to be regulated because they have the potential to do harm as well as good. Access to prescription medicines is controlled by doctors and other health professionals.

Some medicines for minor ailments can be bought over the counter in pharmacies or from other retail outlets; *Which? Medicine* includes many of them. Generic names (see pages 10 and 14) are given prominence as it has not been possible to list all brands. Although vast numbers of products are available, in fact the range of medicines is limited. For example, the many branded pain-relievers all contain one or more of the four analgesics that can be sold over the counter – paracetamol, aspirin, codeine and ibuprofen.

Successive governments have encouraged consumers to treat minor self-limiting ailments (ones which clear up with time, such as coughs and colds) by buying a medicine rather than seeing a doctor, and during the past decade some medicines which were previously on prescription only have been made available in pharmacies with the pharmacist's guidance. Loperamide (brand names Imodium; Arret) has been added to the range of treatments for diarrhoea and hydrocortisone cream or ointment can now be bought over the counter for treating a limited range of skin problems such as swelling and redness after an insect bite. Other preparations are becoming available, including treatments for vaginal thrush.

● *INFORMATION INITIATIVES*

After many years of debate and research some progress has been made in providing consumers with detailed instructions for taking medicines. Manufacturers have started to include information leaflets with packaged products: around 40 per cent of branded products now come in manufacturers' original packs rather than in brown bottles carrying only the pharmacist's label.

The progress in supplying information for consumers will accelerate as the new European Directive on the labelling of medicines comes into force in January 1994. All medicines, both those on prescription and products sold over the counter, will have to comply with comprehensive labelling requirements. There will also be clear, easy-to-understand package leaflets produced by manufacturers, but these will not include, for example, comparitive information about a group of similar drugs. *Which? Medicine* has no ties to government or industry and supplies independent information that places individual drugs in a wider context – the key to choice.

Consumers' Association campaigns on a wide range of freedom of information issues. It is currently backing a bill to change the law that prohibits disclosure of information about why medicines are licensed and why some are withdrawn. This is an important step towards letting the public know just how safe medicines are.

● *SAFETY*

Taking a medicine to effect a cure seems a simple part of everyday life, but swallowing a tablet is just the beginning of a complex biochemical process which may affect your body in many ways. The intention of this guide is to put the use of medicines into perspective. Many medicines are unlikely to cause serious unwanted effects and not everyone is at risk from those which do, but medicine-taking is not without hazard. Given information you can address this issue and ask your doctor or pharmacist questions about treatment.

Major scares about medicines and the adverse effects of drugs continue to hit the headlines, one being triazolam (brand name Halcion), the benzodiazepine sleeping tablet. Injury from medicines does happen, but many accidents are preventable. If your doctor follows this list of basic duties problems with drug treatment will be kept to a minimum. The checklist has been adapted from an article published in *Drug and Therapeutics Bulletin*.

1. **Restricting the use of drugs** Has your doctor taken a proper decision that drug therapy is warranted? Is there another possible way of treating you? Would the best thing (for mild symptoms) be just to wait and see?

2. **Making a careful choice** of an appropriate drug and dosage. Has your doctor taken into account your own needs and how susceptible you may be to unwanted effects? And the balance of likely risks and benefits of any drug? And the alternative drugs available?

3. **Consultation and consent** Has your doctor consulted you about the treatment that is proposed? Do you understand it? Have you given your informed consent to treatment?

4. **Explanation** A doctor should explain to you how a course of treatment will be given, and what your role in that course of treatment is going to be. Do you know?

5. **Prescription and recording** Your doctor should prescribe with care, and should make sure a record of the prescription is kept.

6. **Supervision** While you are on a course of drugs, the doctor who prescribed them should be looking out for any developments or changes, and altering or adapting the treatment if need be.

7. **Ending drug therapy** when it is no longer needed.

8. **Keeping within the law** as it relates to prescribing and using medicines.

Be an active patient

Before you take a medicine you should at the very least know broadly how it will act in the body and how it will help. You have a right to control what happens in your own body and should do so for the sake of your own safety and well-being. *Which? Medicine* provides the information you need to make informed choices about the medicines you use, whether prescribed or bought over the counter, and to use them well. It goes beyond individual information leaflets by discussing the medicines in the context of the diseases they are used to treat, by comparing and evaluating different treatments and by spelling out the risks and benefits. It will promote active discussion with health professionals and answer questions you forgot or were embarrassed to ask, or that did not occur to you while you were in the surgery.

Use generic names

The *generic*, or non-proprietary, name of a medicine is the name of the active ingredient. Several different brands can contain the same active ingredient and non-proprietary versions of many medicines are made, too. Doctors are encouraged to prescribe generically because generic versions are just as effective and usually cheaper than brands. While the cost to the NHS of medicines is of secondary importance to consumers you should always know the generic name of any medicine you are taking to avoid confusion and duplication. Read the ingredients of any branded products you buy for the same reasons.

Review your medicines

Review your medicines regularly with your doctor, especially if you take medicines routinely. Sort out which you still need to take, which you need to take only occasionally and whether there are any you can stop. It is best to take as few medicines as necessary and at the lowest dose that is effective in order to minimise the risks of unwanted effects and interactions between the medicines.

Demand information

Make sure you get answers to any questions you have. You will find worksheets at the back of the book to help you record details about your medicines and each has a list of questions your doctor and pharmacist should answer every time you get a prescription. You have a duty to learn something about what is wrong with you if you are to make the most of treatment and health professionals have a duty to give you information; become active partners in your health care.

HOW TO USE *WHICH? MEDICINE*

Which? Medicine is concerned with explaining medicine use and the relative merits of different treatments; it does not offer extensive information about all of the thousands of medicines available in Britain, nor is it a dictionary of medicines.

It contains detailed profiles of 80 of the most commonly used drugs (see page 15). Most drug profiles are representative of a particular 'family' of medicines, so that one drug serves as a model for that type of medicinal product. For example, there are over 18 anti-arthritis drugs, most of which are chemically related and have similar effects. One detailed profile of a drug from this class has been compiled and the remaining products listed. Notes on many more preparations are included throughout the text where the drug treatment of specific conditions is reviewed, but it has not been possible to look at all the medicines available in Britain – there are around 6,000.

The opening section introduces medicines on a broad scale – how they work, what the risks are, how they are made and licensed and, most important of all, how best to use them. This is essential reading for anyone who is interested in taking an active and informed approach to using medicines. *Which? Medicine* contains a lot of information about the body and its disorders. Finding out about your body is an important step towards being in control of your health – don't wait until you fall ill.

Each chapter in the second part of the book looks at a particular body system and the medicines developed for the disorders that affect that group of organs.

These sections broadly follow the classification used by the *British National Formulary (BNF)*, a comprehensive handbook for doctors and pharmacists describing the uses, unwanted effects and interactions of the majority of drugs used in Britain. It is produced twice-yearly by the British Medical Association and the Royal Pharmaceutical Society of Great Britain.

You can use *Which? Medicine* to look up a drug you have been prescribed – there's an index of generic and brand names at the back to help you find the relevant section quickly. Remind yourself of what the doctor said, find out more about your illness and make sure you're happy with the consultation. Discuss any doubts or further questions with your doctor. Better still, use this book before a prescription is written or to help choose a medicine bought over the counter. Ask the questions listed on the medicines worksheets (see 'How to improve your use of medicines') and raise any points mentioned in the relevant drug profile. Read about your condition and discuss treatment with your doctor or pharmacist; do not start a course of treatment until you feel fully informed about it.

● *HOW YOU CAN HELP YOURSELF*

Medicines may relieve symptoms, provide comfort and cure, but you can also take other measures to help yourself. Many sections include common-sense suggestions for helping yourself to take an active part in overcoming illness or disorder. For people with long-term conditions, there may be a self-help group.

Ideas in the 'How you can help yourself' sections do not replace taking a medicine if drug treatment is needed, but are intended to supplement treatment so you can do everything possible to help your health. Some illnesses can be managed without drug treatment, for example by careful control of diet.

● *EVALUATION OF MEDICINES*

Wherever possible the book gives an indication of the medicines which are preferred and those that are considered a poor choice. This selection is based on recommendations made in the *Drug and Therapeutics Bulletin* and other sources of independent information such as the *BNF*. These recommendations are based on many years of doctors' and pharmacists' experience of medicine use and information gathered from clinical trials of drugs.

Words used in this book

The words medicine and drug are used interchangeably, although strictly speaking a **drug** is a chemical substance and the active ingredient of a medicine, while a **medicine** contains a drug and other substances (inactive ingredients) which help to deliver the drug to the body. It is more important to remember that a medicine is not necessarily a liquid and that the word drug does not necessarily mean an illicit substance such as heroin.

Medical terms have been explained wherever possible throughout the book and you also will find a glossary in the reference section at the back.

DRUG NAMES

At the start of a drug's life in the laboratory, it is given a **chemical name** and a research number. Later in its development the drug is given a **generic name** – its official medical name, also called the approved name or non-proprietary name – according to World Health Organization principles.

Get to know the generic name of any medicine prescribed for you, because this can reduce confusion and duplication. One week you might be prescribed **diclofenac**, a drug for pain relief and reducing inflammation, and later see another doctor, perhaps at a hospital clinic, who prescribes you **Voltarol**, a brand name of diclofenac. You now have two supplies of the same medicine with different names and may end up taking double the dose without realising.

You should also find out the active ingredients of any preparations you buy over the counter by looking at the information on the packaging. It is easy to buy apparently different cold remedies which turn out to have the same pain-relieving ingredient. Taking several medicines together can mean taking an excessively high dose of one drug; in extreme cases this has led to death.

Generic names, particularly for newer drugs, tend to be standard throughout the world wherever international agreements can be reached. This helps when you travel to other countries, although you will find some differences, especially with older drugs. For example, paracetamol is known as acetaminophen in the USA.

The **brand name** is chosen by the manufacturer alone, intended to be easily pronounced, remembered and written. There may be several brands of the same generic substance, each produced by a different company. The names may bear no resemblance to the generic name.

- ☐ **chemical name** 1-isopropylamino-3-*p*-(2-methoxyethyl) phenoxypropan-2-ol
- ☐ **generic name** metoprolol
- ☐ **brand names** Lopresor; Betaloc

In *Which? Medicine* generic names are given in **bold** type before brand names in order to help you to become familiar with the active ingredient(s) of your medicine. A branded product may contain two or three active ingredients, but you cannot tell this from the name on the label. Furthermore, some medicines that doctors prescribe can also be bought over the counter, but as the

NHS does not pay for over-the-counter products, these preparations have two brand names, one for NHS prescriptions and one for sale over the counter. For example, loperamide has the brand name Imodium on prescription, but is sold over the counter as Arret. Using the generic name helps you to know the medicine you are taking and avoids confusion and duplication.

● *DRUG CLASSES*

All drugs are given a legal category to control how they can be supplied to the public. You may see the abbreviations on the packaging.

Prescription-only medicines (POM) can be obtained only with a doctor's prescription. Most medicines fall into this category because of the complexity of deciding when they should be used and their potential for harm if used improperly.

Medicines sold over the counter are split into two categories. **Pharmacy medicines (P)** may be sold only in a pharmacy and the sale must be supervised by the pharmacist – for example, antihistamines for the relief of hay fever symptoms. **General sale list medicines (GSL)** are sold in other stores, such as supermarkets, as well as pharmacies.

Drugs are also classified according to what they do, in groups such as antidepressants or antacids. These categories can include several families of drugs.

● ▼ *'BLACK TRIANGLE' MEDICINES*

All new prescription medicines are marked with an inverted black triangle (▼) in the *BNF* and other reference books, as well as in advertisements. The triangle is a device alerting doctors to report any suspected adverse reaction to the new medicine to the Committee on Safety of Medicines.

Reading the drug profiles

Each profile begins with the name of the generic drug, followed by a list of the products which contain it. The list is split into prescription and non-prescription products and any products considered a poor choice are listed separately. If there are no headings the products are all prescription-only. A brief description of the drug's uses and how it works follows.

In the lists of drug names, drugs which manufacturers produce under generic name are shown in **BOLD CAPITAL LETTERS**, while drugs produced under the manufacturers' own brand names are in

ORDINARY CAPITALS. Names in **SMALL BOLD CAPITALS** underneath the brand names of similar preparations show what the active ingredient is. The different formulations – tablets, capsules, liquids, etc. – are given too. For example, in the profile of cimetidine, a drug used to heal ulcers, you will see:

CIMETIDINE – Tablets	This is a generic drug available under its own name.
DYSPAMET – Chewable tablets, liquid	This is one manufacturer's product which contains cimetidine.
AXID — Capsules **NIZATIDINE**	Nizatidine is similar in action to cimetidine, so it is included in the same profile; Axid is the brand name of a product (currently the only one) which contains nizatidine.

Before you use this medicine

This section lists what you should tell your doctor or pharmacist when he or she is proposing the medicine as a treatment. You may not be a suitable candidate for treatment because of allergies or other conditions you have. Some medicines are unsuitable for pregnant women.

How to use this medicine

Your doctor or pharmacist should give specific instructions for using a medicine – this will act as a reminder and also gives information about typical use of the medicine and any special storage instructions. **Over 65** details any special instructions for older people, who are more sensitive to the effects of many drugs.

Interactions with other medicines

Medicines interact in many ways. The effects of two drugs may combine usefully but often they will disrupt or modify each other's action in a way which means your treatment must be adjusted in some way. This section lists only the important interactions; tell your doctor or pharmacist if you are using any prescription or over-the-counter preparations.

Unwanted effects

Reading a list of a medicine's unwanted effects can be an unnerving experience. You may wonder whether the drug will really cause all these problems as well as making you better. But you should be aware of the range of unwanted effects so that you can take action if a serious effect occurs. Your doctor or pharmacist can help put the benefits and risks in perspective.

Similar preparations

Many drugs are part of a family of preparations which all work in a similar way. The drug profile applies broadly to all the members of the family listed here; your doctor or pharmacist will be able to tell you about the minor differences and some are mentioned in the text preceding and following the profile.

What isn't in *Which? Medicine*

Medicines that are used mainly in hospital have not been included – for example general anaesthetics, some antibiotics and specialised children's medicines which are usually started in hospital – nor have treatments for cancer or HIV. Other areas not covered include wound dressings, appliances, vaccines and immunological products.

There is little mention of exact dosages because these vary so much depending on who is being treated and for what. Drug abuse is not discussed except with reference to drugs normally used for a medical purpose. Alternative treatments are beyond the scope of this book, although some, particularly relaxation techniques, have a bearing on the 'How you can help yourself' sections.

HOW TO IMPROVE YOUR USE OF MEDICINES

During the last thirty years, many potent medicines have been developed. Patients have received these medicines, often quite passively, with very little information about how the medicine should work in the body and what to do if adverse effects occur. Many doctors suspected that if patients were told about unwanted effects they would not take their medicines. Up until 1972, medicines were labelled merely as 'The Tablets' or 'The Mixture'. Instructions were often limited to 'One tablet to be taken three times a day' or 'One tablespoonful to be taken four times daily'.

In the early '70s doctors and pharmacists began to realise that high-street goods came with better instructions than life-saving medicines. Since then there has been much discussion about what patients should be told, and who should tell them. Research has shown that patients want more information about their medicines. Doctors now realise that if they explain what they expect a medicine to do, both the wanted and the unwanted effects, then a patient is more likely to take a medicine correctly. As a patient, you have a right to such information, and it should now be provided routinely.

A report published in *Which?* magazine in 1991 of a survey of 292 outpatients making a first visit to a specialist found that nearly one in four were not given any information unless they asked for it. One in five left the clinic without a clear understanding of their medical condition and the treatment needed. Nearly half of those surveyed would have liked information leaflets or contact addresses so that they could find out more about their condition, but just one in ten received this type of information. One in five did not ask any questions at all: 63 per cent assumed that they would be told everything they needed to know without asking; 38 per cent thought that their GP would have told them; and 35 per cent said that there did not seem to be enough time for questions.

The message from this survey is that we assume that we will be told about the medical condition and necessary treatment, but not enough information is given and what is given is not always clear. You have a right to know about your health and all aspects of treatment, but that right implies responsibility. Use your doctor to seek information and advice, and if questions are not answered to your satisfaction, obtain a second opinion. To improve the service your doctor gives you and your use of medicines, consider the following:

☐ **take an active part in understanding the illness and its treatment**
☐ **assume nothing**
☐ **ask questions**
☐ **become a full partner with the doctor in managing your illness and in medicine-taking.**

Only you can feel and experience a painful condition or an illness; try to be as accurate as you can in describing what is wrong with you or where it hurts and how long you have had the complaint. This will improve the accuracy of the diagnosis and choice of treatment.

The questions in the Box over the page are relevant when you buy or are prescribed any medicine. You will find a copy of the list on the back of the medicines worksheets at the back of this book. The sheets can be cut out so that you can take one with you to the doctor and jot down the answers to the questions. If you take a medicine every day you should know the answers to most of the questions.

Compliance

Doctors and pharmacists talk about patients *complying* with treatment and define compliance as the extent to which a person's behaviour coincides with medical or health advice.

Compliance is not a one-way process, however, as it involves you, your doctor and your pharmacist. It is the quality of the relationship between you and them that will help you to understand and follow recommendations to take a particular medicine or pursue a special diet. There must be mutual respect and understanding between you and your doctor; treatment is an activity shared by both of you in which you should comply with the needs of each other.

● *REVIEW YOUR MEDICINES*

If you have to take a number of medicines each day and your doctor has not reviewed them recently, here are some suggestions for re-assessing your medicine-taking. You need to have as simple a treatment plan as possible, particularly if you are over 65.

Make an appointment to see your doctor. Collect all the medicines, both prescribed and those bought over the counter, that you are taking at present or have taken within the last month. Using a medicines worksheet from the back of this book, list the medicines. Recording your medicines under the headings

20 QUESTIONS TO ASK ABOUT YOUR PRESCRIPTION

Before the prescription is written

☐ Is there an alternative to treatment with medicines for my condition?
☐ How can I help myself apart from taking the medicine?
☐ What kind of medicine is it?
☐ How will it help me?
☐ How important is it to take this medicine?
☐ Is this a new medicine? If so, what advantages does the new medicine have over older products?

Before the consultation ends

☐ How and when should I take the medicine?
☐ How can I tell if it is working?
☐ For how long should I take the medicine?
☐ What may happen if I do not take it?
☐ What should I do if I miss a dose?
☐ Is the medicine likely to have any unwanted effects? If so, how serious might they be?
☐ What should I do if unwanted effects occur?
☐ Will I need to see you again?
☐ What will you need to know from me then?

When the prescription is dispensed

☐ Can I take other medicines with it?
☐ Are there any foods or drinks I should avoid?
☐ Can I drive a car after taking the medicine?
☐ Where should I keep it?
☐ What should I do with any leftover medicine?

described on pages 22 to 24 will help you and your doctor to see exactly what you take every day as well as the preparations that you take occasionally. Your doctor should never prescribe a medicine or renew a prescription for an old one without knowing exactly which medicines you are taking.

Your local pharmacist can help you fill in the medicines worksheet. Many pharmacies can now hold records of your medicines on computer (patient medication records). If you go to the same pharmacy each time to have your prescriptions dispensed, the pharmacist can, with your permission, list the medicines you take on the pharmacy computer. Each time you have a prescription dispensed the pharmacist can look at your records to check dosages and directions and the risk of drug interactions. Some pharmacists can also record over-the-counter medicines that you buy and alert you to any potential interactions with your prescribed medicines.

Medicines in nursing homes

If you look after an elderly person, for example someone who is confused, you might like to get the doctor, pharmacist or member of the nursing home staff to complete the medicines worksheet. Ask if you can discuss the medicines, finding out what each one is for and why it is being taken. Patients in nursing homes are particularly vulnerable to over-use of medicines. It is important to find out if all the medicines are really necessary. For elderly people, in particular, stopping a medicine can be more beneficial than starting one.

● *REPEAT PRESCRIBING*

Repeat prescribing is the re-writing of a previous prescription without the doctor seeing you for a consultation. Surveys have shown that elderly people and women have a high proportion of repeat prescriptions. Prescriptions most commonly repeated without seeing the doctor are for medicines for rheumatic complaints, nervous and sleeping disorders, oral contraceptives and medicines for conditions which require long-term treatment, such as thyroid disease and high blood pressure. Repeat prescribing may save you time and is certainly convenient for older people who cannot or may prefer not to travel to the surgery. It saves both you and your doctor time.

However, some patients prefer not to see their doctors too often and vice versa, possibly a reflection on the quality of the doctor–patient relationship. Each time a repeat prescription is issued an opportunity to review treatment is lost. Although some diseases and their treatments may not change much over the years, the doctor is less likely to find out if the medicine is acting properly, or if there are adverse effects or interactions. Medicines may be continued for longer than necessary and repeat prescriptions may lead to over-prescribing.

The medicines worksheets

The medicines worksheets at the back of this book will help you record details of the medicines you take, whether you are reviewing existing treatment or starting the first course of a new medi-

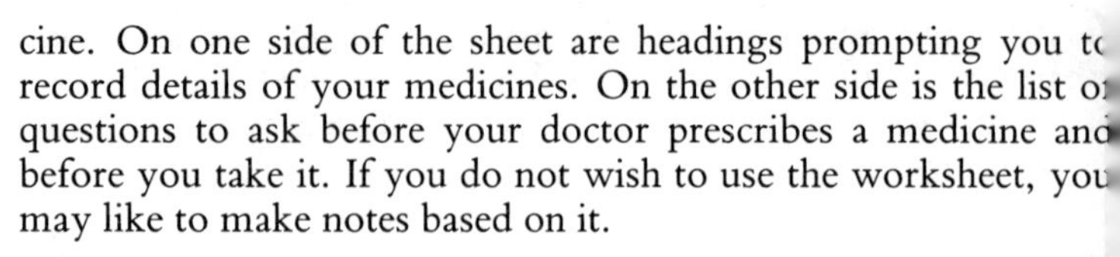

cine. On one side of the sheet are headings prompting you to record details of your medicines. On the other side is the list of questions to ask before your doctor prescribes a medicine and before you take it. If you do not wish to use the worksheet, you may like to make notes based on it.

☐ **Name of the medicine** List the generic and brand name as both are commonly used, and record over-the-counter medicines, including herbal or homoeopathic remedies. The approximate daily amount of tea and coffee (for caffeine) and the quantity of alcohol and tobacco you consume should also be noted. This information is important as it will help you to avoid drug interactions.

☐ **Date started** Recording the date you start taking the medicine may help you later to put any unwanted effects into a pattern.

☐ **Why prescribed** Make sure you understand why the doctor is prescribing each medicine or altering your prescription and make a brief note. For example, 'diuretics – to get rid of the body's extra water'.

☐ **How taken** Record the dose that you take each time, how many times a day and at what time of day. For example, one 500mg tablet, three times a day before breakfast, lunch and supper. Always check whether you should take your medicine before, with or after meals as this timing is critical for the absorption of some drugs.
Dose It is important to note the exact dose rather than just the number of tablets as a drug may be made in different strengths.
Times per day Taking medicines three, four or more times a day is difficult to remember, especially if the routine involves more than four different drugs. Ask your doctor to make the routine as simple as possible. Many manufacturers have incorporated drugs into modified-release preparations so that you need to take only one dose a day. However, a treatment may be seriously disrupted if you forget that one dose. Taking a medicine twice a day may be easier to remember and it may not matter quite as much if you forget one dose out of the two for the day.
When Wherever possible, medicine taking should be linked with daily activities, such as mealtimes or at bedtime when you brush your teeth. When a medicine must be taken four times a day, be sure you understand what the doctor intends. Generally, four times daily means during your waking hours rather than spread over the full 24 hours, but you should always check this with the doctor or pharmacist and work out a convenient routine for taking your medicine.

☐ **How long for** Always find out how long your doctor intends you to take the medicine and record the length of time. When

AIDS TO MEDICINE-TAKING

Many medicines are now supplied in the manufacturers' original packs and many of these are in monthly calendar packs with the days of the week marked. This helps you to see whether you have taken your daily dose. If you have to take more than one or two medicines a day, a daily dose organiser may help to remind you to take your medicine. An alarm set to remind you when to take a medicine can also be useful.

A medicines organiser is a device which has compartments for each medicine and the times of day it must be taken. Pharmacists can supply and fill these boxes, some of which can take a week's supply of medicines or longer; Braille labels are available with some systems. Organisers are now in use in some nursing homes where the supply of medicines to individual patients needs careful control.

should there be a review to gauge the success or failure of treatment? Drug treatment should be for as short a time as possible unless there is evidence that the medicine must be taken for a long time or for lifetime problems such as diabetes or high blood pressure.

□ **Problems to watch out for** Here you can summarise possible unwanted effects. It is particularly important for you to know about these effects in order to be able to recognise them and report them to your doctor. If you have your suspicions about a medicine's unwanted effects, you can always check with a pharmacist to see whether you should return to your doctor or not.

Some medicines very rarely cause an allergic reaction which calls for urgent medical help. You can use the medicine's worksheet to record any drugs which have caused allergic reactions in the past. You must tell your doctor if you are allergic to any medicines.

Other unwanted effects may be less dramatic, but contact your doctor if you are concerned. Some unwanted effects fade in severity as you continue to take the medicine and your doctor should tell you if this is the case.

Include interactions with other medicines, food or alcohol. List any food or medicines that you should avoid when starting a medicine. Always tell your doctor if you are already taking a medicine, whether bought over the counter or prescribed.

□ **How are you taking the medicine?** Be honest with your doctor and say whether or not you are taking the medicine and how often. You should not feel bad about stopping treatment, even if you did not have a strong reason to stop. If you cannot tolerate the drug, say so; perhaps a lower dose could be tried. Not telling your doctor about treatment problems can lead to mistaken conclusions about dosages and which drugs work.

☐ **Any new problems?** Once you have started a medicine you should assume that any worsening of your condition is an unwanted effect of the medicine until proved otherwise. A recent study showed that as many as one in ten unwanted effects is not picked up because patients do not realise that they might experience them. Friends and relatives often notice change where you may not. Older people are more likely to blame many of their problems on old age rather than on drug effects. If you look after an older person it is especially important to think about unwanted effects of drugs and to talk to the doctor about your concerns.

☐ **Is the medicine working?** If not, ask your doctor what should be done.

Where to find information

You may get spoken information about a medicine when you see your doctor, from the practice nurse and from the pharmacist. Written information is provided on the label of the medicine and you may also receive an information leaflet, either in the manufacturer's pack or from the pharmacist.

● *FROM YOUR DOCTOR AT THE TIME THE PRESCRIPTION IS WRITTEN*

Your doctor can give you all the information you need about your medicines although it can be difficult to communicate properly or to make time for it. Writing and giving a prescription to a patient is only part of the consultation and sometimes the doctor appears too busy to talk about the medicines being prescribed. Anxiety about your illness may cloud what you remember of what the doctor says about the diagnosis and the type of illness and what tests, investigations and treatment will be necessary. Studies have shown that many people remember the diagnosis, the tests needed and when to return to the doctor, but not the explanations of the illness and the instructions for treatment.

Doctors sometimes use unfamiliar technical terms. If you have your own ideas about illnesses these may differ from the doctor's, but you may fit the doctor's explanation into your own framework of ideas. Although it is very important that you should understand what the doctor is saying, many people who do not understand hesitate to ask. You can use the medicines worksheet to prompt questions – they can help put you and the doctor on the same wavelength.

● *FROM PRACTICE OR SPECIALIST NURSES*

Many GPs employ practice nurses who assist in running clinics such as those for diabetics, asthmatics, people with high blood pressure and people with weight problems. Nurses who specialise in the management of long-term illnesses such as diabetes can, for example, demonstrate how to use insulin and tell you what you need to know about your medicines. In future, district nurses, midwives and health visitors will be trained and able to prescribe certain medicines and dressings.

● *FROM THE PHARMACIST*

When the pharmacist dispenses your prescription the medicine will be labelled with directions for use. Every time you take a dose of medicine read the label to double-check that you are following instructions carefully and that you have not picked up the wrong medicine. The label should tell you:

☐ the name of the medicine – either generic or brand name, sometimes both
☐ the form of the medicine – tablets, capsules, mixture or ointment, etc.
☐ the strength of the medicine – how much of the active ingredient is in each tablet or in a 5ml spoonful
☐ the dose – how much medicine to take or use each time
☐ the frequency – how often to use the medicine
☐ how to take the medicine – for example with meals or after meals
☐ your name
☐ the name and address of the pharmacy
☐ the date the medicine was dispensed
☐ special storage instructions
☐ to keep the medicine out of the reach of children.

For medicines used on the body rather than taken into the body the words 'for external use only' must appear. There are many other cautionary and advisory instructions which now appear. For example, 'Dissolve or mix with water before taking' or 'Warning. May cause drowsiness. If affected do not drive or operate machinery. Avoid alcoholic drink'. Although the wording of these labels has been carefully thought out, labels can sometimes be confusing. Check with the pharmacist if you are unclear.

Some drugs are used to treat more than one condition, but the prescription does not tell the pharmacist what you are being treated for; it gives only the details about the medicine and the instructions for use. If you discuss your treatment with the pharmacist, you may need to say what the medicine is for so that you can put your treatment in context. A number of pharmacies now have a room or an area where you can speak to the pharmacist privately.

The pharmacist will always include on the label whatever instructions the doctor has given on the prescription. Labels bearing 'As before' or 'Take as directed' are still common but doctors should give specific instructions for each medicine on each occasion, even for repeat prescriptions. Labels on medicines, especially those dispensed in brown bottles, should have precise details of the contents and instructions for use. Mistakes in the amount of medicine to be taken can occur when patients transfer from home to hospital and vice versa. Although you may have the same treatment for years and know the instructions well, it is good practice to have these recorded on the label. Ask the pharmacist to put the instructions on the label if they do not appear on the prescription form.

All labels on medicines dispensed by pharmacists must be typed or mechanically printed. Many labels are generated using a computer and most should be readable. However, some patients, for instance those whose first language is not English, may not read and understand instructions with medicines. Some foreign-language labels or leaflets are available. For the partially sighted, some labels can be printed in larger print size and for the blind some labels are available in Braille.

Some pharmacists can now print information leaflets from their computers and you may be given these when your medicine is dispensed. This will help to fill the gap where manufacturers are slow to provide medicines in packs with information leaflets.

● *PATIENT INFORMATION LEAFLETS*

Although the labelling of dispensed medicines has greatly improved over the last ten years, there is no room to give all the relevant information. Patient information leaflets (PILs) have been developed so that now you can find out what the medicine is, how it can help you, how to use it and what the possible unwanted effects are. In addition, most of the information given on the label will also be included in the leaflet. The leaflets are not intended to take the place of explanation given to you by your doctor or pharmacist, but to remind you of what has been said. The information on the leaflet should also enable you to discuss your treatment and ask questions. Each leaflet should have the following information:

☐ name and class of medicine
☐ what is in the medicine
☐ how to obtain the medicine – on prescription or over the counter
☐ how the medicine works
☐ important points to note before taking the medicine – precautions and warnings about interactions
☐ how to take the medicine
☐ what might happen while you are taking the medicine – unwanted effects
☐ what to do if an overdose is taken
☐ storing the medicine
☐ what to do if you stop the medicine
☐ who makes the medicine – the product licence holder.

Pharmaceutical companies have the task of providing leaflets with their products and must comply with the EC directive on labelling and patient information by 1994. Many medicines supplied in manufacturers' packs rather than brown bottles now have patient information leaflets. With original packs the pharmacist does not need to count or pour medicines from a larger bottle to a smaller one. This type of dispensing disappeared long ago in most European countries, but Britain has been slow to transfer to supplying medicines in packs. Eventually patient information leaflets produced by member companies of the Association of the British Pharmaceutical Industry (ABPI) will be compiled into a compendium for doctors, pharmacists and other health workers. The compendium will also be available in the reference section of the public libraries and for sale to the public.

The pharmaceutical industry will be responsible for providing and presenting patient information for the products it sells. Although leaflets must not advertise prescription medicines, there are concerns that the information will be biased or selectively presented. Guidelines for producing the leaflets do not yet include standard ways to present information. Companies are free to design and produce leaflets in any style so long as they include the core information.

WHAT MEDICINES DO

Nature provides a wealth of chemicals in plants, fungi, animals, bacteria and even minerals. Ancient civilisations used many remedies, particularly those derived from plants, and some of these are still in use today, especially in China, where 1,700 herbal remedies remain popular from a catalogue of over 5,000 plants. Many substances were used crudely: for instance, mercury used as a treatment for syphilis in the sixteenth century would have been quite harmful to the body as well as to the micro-organism causing the disease. Advances in chemistry through the nineteenth century led to a better understanding of the structure of chemicals and eventually to the understanding of a relationship between a chemical substance and its specific effects on the body (*pharmacology*). Early this century, the idea developed that chemicals could kill disease-causing organisms without seriously hurting the human body and scientists have been learning to achieve ever greater precision with drugs ever since. However, the 'magic bullet', a medicine that can deal with the disease without affecting the body in any way, has never been found.

Five uses of medicines

• *TO PREVENT*

Thanks to the efforts of some far-sighted Victorians, much of the improvement in health this century has come from better nutrition, sewage and rubbish disposal and cleaner drinking water, which have greatly reduced people's susceptibility and exposure to many diseases. *Vaccines* further improve public health by protection against specific diseases. A vaccine contains a tiny amount of a substance which usually causes the disease. Your body responds to it by making *antibodies* for that particular disease; these are chemicals made by special white blood cells to combat invading organisms. You are then immune to the disease: if you subsequently come into contact with it, your body will recognise it and produce antibodies to kill the disease-causing organism.

The use of vaccines to prevent killer diseases, such as diphtheria, tetanus and polio, has revolutionised medicine. Doctors qualifying today will rarely see these diseases, and they will never see smallpox because it has been entirely eradicated from the world.

Other examples of preventive medicine include *antimalarial* tablets, *antiseptics* used to keep wounds clean and *antibiotics* used to prevent serious infections that can complicate surgical operations. Oral contraceptives alter the balance of sex hormones in a woman's body to prevent pregnancy.

● *TO CURE*

Medicines are used, sometimes with dramatic effect, to cure diseases caused by microscopic organisms (*micro-organisms*) which get into the body and start infection. These micro-organisms – *bacteria*, *fungi*, *viruses* and *protozoa* – are parasites which live off healthy body cells, multiply and eventually cause disease in the body. Once this pattern of disease was understood in the late nineteenth century, researchers looked for chemicals to kill invading micro-organisms without harming the *host*, the human body.

An antibacterial drug destroys invading bacteria either by stopping their multiplication or by destroying bacterial cells, allowing the body to return to health.

● *TO ADD TO BODY CHEMICALS*

Medicines are sometimes used to increase quantities of the body's own chemicals, such as *hormones*, which are vital for the proper working of the body. The pancreas makes insulin, the hormone responsible for regulating the breakdown of sugar. If the insulin supply fails or does not work correctly, you become diabetic and may then need a daily supply of externally manufactured insulin.

● *TO RELIEVE SYMPTOMS*

Headache, an upset stomach, raised temperature, skin rashes, sneezing and cough are all signs that you are not well. Often these symptoms indicate an illness which is *self-limiting* – that is, your body will get better of its own accord in time. You may take a medicine such as an *analgesic* or a *decongestant* to relieve the symptoms and perhaps a day or two resting in bed – you are the best person to judge your treatment. If you do not start feeling better after a few days and your symptoms do not improve, you must decide whether to see your doctor.

● *TO CONTROL DISEASE STATES*

Some diseases are long-term (*chronic*) conditions and do not get better; they are not self-limiting. The disease may have phases when it is either more or less active, such as rheumatoid arthritis, or you may have the condition all the time, such as raised blood pressure (*hypertension*). A disease can be kept under control by the continuous or intermittent use of a medicine to maintain health, but without achieving a cure.

How medicines work

• *THE STRUCTURE OF THE BODY*

The body is a collection of millions of microscopic units called *cells*. Each type of cell has a distinct job to do. For example, red blood cells carry oxygen around the body, while nerve cells send messages of pain and feeling to the brain. Cells group together to form *tissues*, such as skin and muscle. Groups of tissues form *organs*, for example the heart, lungs, liver and stomach. Groups of organs which work together are called *systems*. The heart, arteries and veins together form the *cardiovascular* system, which keeps blood flowing round your body. To keep the systems, organs and tissues working together, the body has chemicals which act as messengers: for instance, a nerve cell produces a chemical called a *neurotransmitter*, which is part of the chain taking messages from the brain and nerves to muscles.

When you take a medicine, the drug reaches the bloodstream and is then carried to all parts of the body. A non-selective drug is likely to cause many unwanted effects, although these are not necessarily troublesome. A selective drug works on the part of the body where its action is wanted and is effective at a lower dose so there are fewer unwanted effects.

• *CELL INTERFERENCE*

Some drugs work by interfering with the workings of the cell, either on the cell's surface or within it. It is thought that there are special sites on the cell called *receptors* into which the body's own chemicals lock to produce specific effects. A cell has different types of receptors so that different effects can be produced, depending on which chemical has arrived at the cell.

A drug can increase the cell's activity by adding to one of the body's chemicals or decrease activity by blocking receptors to prevent the body's chemicals from working. A drug which enhances cellular activity is called an *agonist* and a drug which dampens the activity down an *antagonist*. For example, the hormones adrenaline and noradrenaline produced by the body's adrenal gland prepare the body for 'flight or fight' when it is challenged in some way. Adrenaline stimulates certain cells by locking into receptors called *adrenoceptors* to prepare the body to defend itself from an unpleasant external event. Beta blockers are antagonists which block beta adrenoceptors, dampening down the stimulating effect of the hormones and slowing the heartbeat. They are used to lower high blood pressure and to treat various other heart disorders, such as angina.

● *REPLACEMENT OF A BODY CHEMICAL*

When the body's glands produce adequate amounts of hormones, the body works well and you feel healthy. If for some reason one of your glands fails to produce sufficient quantities of a hormone, you become ill. If a gland fails gradually you may not realise why you feel under the weather, but there may be a dramatic episode with the immediate loss of hormonal control, such as the onset of diabetes mellitus in a young person when the body's supply of insulin fails suddenly. Regular supplies of insulin from an external source enable a diabetic person to lead a normal active life.

● *OVERCOMING DIETARY DEFICIENCY*

Food supplies the body with other chemicals such as vitamins and minerals. If you lack a particular vitamin for a long period, you suffer from a deficiency disease. Sailors used to suffer from scurvy on long voyages until it was realised that lack of vitamin C caused their symptoms. Lack of vitamin B results in beri-beri, a disease rife during times of famine in Third World countries. Taking an external source of vitamin C or B, respectively, cures these diseases. Only small amounts of vitamins and minerals are needed each day to maintain good health and a balanced diet with plenty of protein, fruit and vegetables usually supplies them.

● *ACTION ON AN INVADING ORGANISM*

Many illnesses are caused by micro-organisms – bacteria, protozoa, viruses and fungi – often referred to as 'germs'. There are micro-organisms around us everywhere and a few can cause harm if they get into the body and overwhelm its defences. Micro-organisms can enter the body through a variety of routes, principally the skin, mouth, nose, vagina and rectum, but also the eyes and ears. Medicines used to combat these infections disrupt the micro-organism, either by killing its cells or by stopping it multiplying.

Entering the body

• *MEDICINES BY MOUTH*

In Britain medicines are most commonly taken by mouth (the oral route). The medicine (either as a tablet, capsule or liquid) passes down the gullet, through the stomach to the intestines, where it is absorbed into the bloodstream. A tablet or capsule contains a measured and therefore consistent dose of the drug. A liquid contains many doses and each time you need a dose you have to measure it yourself. Tablets and capsules are convenient to take and to carry around, but some people – children, for example – find them difficult to swallow.

Most tablets are designed to disintegrate in the stomach and to release the drug for absorption in the small intestine. These tablets should be swallowed with a tumblerful of water. Other tablets may need to be chewed before swallowing or dispersed in water. The activity of some drugs is destroyed by the gastric juices in the stomach, so tablets containing these drugs are covered with a special film called *enteric coating*, to stop the medicine breaking down before it has passed through the stomach.

Some medicines taken by mouth dissolve there – either under the tongue (sub-lingual tablets or spray) or between the cheek and teeth (buccal tablets). These medicines release drugs in the mouth which can be absorbed directly into the bloodstream without passing through the stomach and intestines. These drugs get into the body quickly and are useful when rapid action is needed, for example for pain relief in an attack of angina.

A capsule contains the drug in a hard or soft gelatin shell. The shell breaks open after it has been swallowed to release the contents. Capsules are cylindrical shaped to make them easier to swallow than tablets and can mask an unpleasant-tasting drug. *Modified-release* capsules contain tiny pellets that gradually release a drug.

Many medicines have to be taken three or four times a day to maintain the desired effect. Some can be mixed with ingredients which prolong or even out their activity. By varying these ingredients, the manufacturer can change the rate or the place at which the drug is released from the preparation into the intestine and thus affect absorption into the bloodstream. Taking the medicine once or twice a day is usually more convenient than three or four times daily. Tablets and capsules in *sustained-release* or *controlled-release* form are all types of modified-release products. They may not look different from an ordinary tablet or capsule, but you should know whether you are taking a modified-release product and understand a few points about them.

☐ Do not break or cut the medicine, unless told to do so.
☐ Do not chew or hold the medicine in the mouth.
☐ Take the medicine after a meal with a full glass of water.
☐ Do not worry if you notice the remains of a tablet or capsule in your stool – the drug will have been absorbed.

● *THE RECTAL ROUTE*

A drug can reach the body's systems from the rectum when given by suppository or rectal solution (*enema*). This method avoids the stomach's digestive juices and is also useful if a person is too sick to take a medicine by mouth.

Drugs are also used for their local effect in the rectum to soothe painful piles or as enemas for ulcerative colitis.

● *INJECTIONS*

Giving a medicine by injection (*parenteral* administration – implying not by the mouth or rectum) allows the drug to get into the body without passing through the stomach where it may be destroyed by digestive juices. The drug can have an effect on the whole body (*systemic* effect) which can be rapid, depending on the type of injection used. If the injection is made straight into the vein (*intravenously*) the body's response to the drug is almost instantaneous. This route is usually reserved for people who are severely ill. Drugs can also be injected into a muscle (*intramuscularly*), under the skin (*subcutaneously*), or into the skin (*intradermally*), but it takes longer for a drug to work by these routes.

A drug may also be injected for a local effect, for instance to deaden a nerve before dental work or to relieve an inflamed and painful arthritic joint.

● *IMPLANTS*

A tiny pellet is placed under the skin in fatty tissue from where it gradually releases the drug into the body. Some hormones are given this way when long-term treatment is needed.

● *TOPICAL ADMINISTRATION*

When a medicine is used *topically*, the drug should work only at the place where the medicine is applied. For example, when you use an ointment on the skin the drug should not get into the body. However, some absorption may occur.

Some drugs are absorbed through the skin in amounts which have a therapeutic effect in the body. This is the *transdermal* route, where absorption is intended. This route of administration, a form of sustained-release preparation, is used for only a few drugs, such as glyceryl trinitrate for preventing attacks of angina, hyoscine for preventing motion sickness and oestrogen given as hormone replacement therapy.

A drug can be put directly on the skin for a local effect to clear up a rash, infection or other skin condition. Preparations used on the skin include creams, ointment, pastes, gels, and lotions. Some medicines are used on the moist skin surfaces of the body (*mucous membranes*) for a local effect – in the mouth (oral gel), the nose (drops), vagina (pessaries or vaginal tablets) and rectum (suppositories). A drug acting on the eye has a very specific local effect, although sometimes the drug enters the body via the tear ducts or through the blood vessels.

● *INHALATION*

A medicine is breathed into the lungs where the drug can have a local effect (an aerosol for asthma) or a general effect on the body (a general anaesthetic).

Acting and leaving

● *INACTIVE INGREDIENTS*

The words 'drug' and 'medicine' are often used interchangeably, but strictly speaking medicine is the whole preparation whereas the drug is the active ingredient which is mixed with other substances to form the medicine. These other substances are called inactive ingredients or *excipients* and they help to carry the drug into the body and determine the way in which it is absorbed. Medicines designed to produce a local effect only – for example products for the skin, nose, ears and eyes – also need inactive ingredients to help deliver the drug to its site of action.

Inactive ingredients may be added to a drug to improve the taste and appearance – 'sugar-free' preparations have a sweetening agent. Liquid preparations often need a preservative to stop bacterial growth. The number of inactive ingredients in a medicine varies and depends on the form of medicine and type of drug. For example, if the amount of drug per dose is small, a tablet or capsule may need a filler or bulking agent, such as lactose or sucrose. In a tablet a drug may need an inactive ingredient to bind it together (such as gum, gelatin or sucrose) and a disintegrating agent, such as starch or sodium bicarbonate, to help it break down once the tablet is in the stomach. A tablet formulation generally contains more inactive ingredients than either a capsule or liquid.

Inactive ingredients should not produce a noticeable pharmacological effect, but some do. For example, tartrazine, the orange-yellow colourant, can cause sensitivity such as skin reactions and asthma. Although tartrazine has been removed from many products, it remains in general use both in pharmaceuticals and foods. The ointment base lanolin (wool fat) commonly causes skin problems as do some preservatives. It is often difficult to discover the inactive ingredients for yourself, but a doctor or pharmacist can help. Improved labelling of medicines in the future will enable you to see more easily exactly what you are taking.

● *REACHING THE SITE OF ACTION*

If you take a tablet, it has to reach the stomach, disintegrate and dissolve before the drug is released. How well the manufacturer mixes the drug with inactive ingredients to make the medicine has a bearing on how easily the drug reaches its site of action. This also depends on the characteristics of the drug itself, for instance the size of drug particles and how readily they dissolve. Most drugs pass across the small intestine wall into the bloodstream, a process known as *absorption*. The rate of drug absorption varies from person to person, but may also depend on whether the stomach is empty or processing food. Some medicines must be taken an hour before food or on an empty stomach because food and gastric acid reduce absorption. As the drug passes through the intestinal wall, it gets into the bloodstream and is taken to the liver and around the body through the network of blood vessels (the circulation).

● *DRUG ACTION*

Each drug has its own duration of action, which depends on the nature of the drug, how it is distributed in the body and by which route the drug is given. A drug taken by mouth takes longer to get into the bloodstream than when it is injected as a solution directly into a vein. A drug in liquid form, such as a mixture taken by mouth, is absorbed more rapidly than a drug in solid form.

Knowing how long certain drugs act in the body helps doctors and pharmacists work out how often someone has to take a medicine in one day. Drugs like penicillin or aspirin enter the bloodstream quickly, act and then leave the body rapidly. They have to be taken four times a day to be effective. On the other hand, the effects of one dose of the anti-anxiety drug diazepam linger in the body for over two days. Some drugs attach themselves to blood proteins and remain bound for prolonged periods. Other drugs are fat-soluble and are stored in the body's fat from which they will be gradually released back into the bloodstream.

Once in the bloodstream the drug reaches the body's organs and tissues where it starts to exert an effect. The strength and variety of the effects of a drug depend on the size of the dose and on how selective the drug is. Generally the desirable effects provide the benefits of the drug and the undesirable effects cause the unwanted effects, but sometimes the desirable effects can become excessive and therefore unwanted – for example, lowering blood pressure too far can cause dizziness.

● *INACTIVATION AND ELIMINATION*

The liver is the main site for dealing with foreign substances in the body. Liver *enzymes* process food and drugs, breaking them down to *metabolites* – products of the group of chemical reactions known as *metabolism*. An *inactive* metabolite has no further effect on the body, but an *active* metabolite may have a similar, but perhaps weaker, effect to the chemical from which it is derived.

The drug leaves the body mainly in urine produced in the kidneys. Blood passes through the kidneys where some of the drug and its metabolites are removed in urine. Although the kidneys are the main site for eliminating a drug from the body, it can leave in stools, sweat and other body fluids, and even on breath.

Why effects vary

How the active ingredient of a medicine works in your body depends on you and your environment as well as the medicine you take. Many factors such as your age, weight, genetics, and the state of your health are important. A drug may agree with one person whereas another cannot tolerate it. Certain medicines have more than one use: a beta blocker, for example, lowers high blood pressure but can also be used for alleviating symptoms of anxiety and nervousness, preventing migraine and for controlling the eye condition glaucoma.

● *AGE AND WEIGHT*

Children need lower doses of medicines than adults. Weight is an important factor, but so is the distribution of body fat and water, because drugs get into these fluids. The liver and kidneys of children, especially new-born babies, are not as developed as adults'. A drug may not be broken down as quickly in the liver or removed from the body by the kidneys so efficiently. The drug dosage should not be just a proportion of an adult dose based on weight, but carefully worked out to take account of age, particularly for children under one year.

As you reach middle age, your kidney and liver function start to decline. By the age of 65 there is a reduction of approximately 30 per cent in the kidney filtration rate as the blood flow to the liver and kidneys and to other parts of the body slows. In old age the total body-water decreases, but there is an increase in body-fat, particularly in men; certain parts of the body, such as the brain become more sensitive to medicines. It may be difficult to separate the effects of ageing from the effects of disease on the body or from unwanted effects of some medicines. Generally older people need less than the usual adult dose of a medicine.

The weight of a person is particularly important for certain medicines, such as antibiotics for injection during severe infection. The larger the body the higher the dose needed to achieve a specified concentration of the drug throughout the body.

● *GENETIC DIFFERENCES*

Although the same building blocks and chemicals are used to construct each human, the codes for the way the materials are put together vary. The codes are carried on genes and the differences in genetic material which account for obvious differences between people can also affect individuals' responses to different drugs. A standard dose of a medicine given to a hundred people will produce a variety of responses which may range from no response to extreme sensitivity, with most people experiencing some effect in between the two extremes. Individual variation in response to a medicine is a very important factor in drug treatment.

● *HEALTH*

The effects of a drug in your body depend on how healthy you are. Illness can alter your response to a medicine. For example, if you suffer from chronic lung disease or severe asthma you will be at risk from drugs like morphine which depress the breathing control centre in the brain. You should mention any long-term problems whenever you see a new doctor.

A reduction in liver or kidney function can affect drug treatment. As many drugs are broken down in the liver, any liver disease, such as cirrhosis or hepatitis, will alter the effectiveness of the drug. The kidneys remove most of a drug or its metabolites from the body in urine. If kidney function is reduced either through illness or old age then the body's response to drug treatment is altered. If you have liver or kidney disease, a smaller dose of drug is generally given. Some drugs must be avoided altogether.

● *ENVIRONMENT*

Response to medicines can be altered by climate and altitude. In hot places, body functions increase in activity and the body loses more water. In severe cold, there will be less blood flowing to the skin and limbs. At high altitudes less oxygen is available. These sorts of changes may modify drug effects.

Drugs and chemicals in the environment may affect some people. For instance, the general anaesthetic halothane in the air of an operating theatre has caused miscarriages in female staff who experience repeated exposure to the drug. The use of antibiotics and growth promoters in the feeds of animals which people eat is a cause for concern: antibiotic use in animals may produce drug-resistant bacteria and allow the spread of disease to humans. DDT, an insecticide now banned in Britain, accumulates in animals and in humans and modifies drug effects. DDT increases the rate at which enzymes break down some drugs so that the medicine has less time to work in the body. Smoking and alcohol have the same effect.

● *DOSAGE*

The standard dose of a drug may not produce the expected response because not all people react to a medicine in the same way. If the dose proves ineffective increasing it may well increase the intensity of the effect, but there is a limit. A bigger dose might produce a better effect on the disease or symptoms but it is more likely to cause unwanted effects. Beyond a certain level increasing the dose does not have a greater beneficial effect and unwanted effects become a nuisance, even a danger. For example, an ordinary dose of aspirin (600mg) will relieve a moderate headache, but may not be adequate for a severe one. A dose of 900mg may help, but perhaps only partially. Taking an even bigger dose will not help because the drug cannot achieve greater relief. However, the bigger dose is more likely to cause unwanted effects such as symptoms of indigestion or ringing in the ears.

The aim of drug treatment is to achieve a concentration of drug in the blood or tissue that lies somewhere between the minimum effective dose and the maximum safe dose. The difference between these two is known as the *therapeutic range* or *margin* and is unique to each drug. A drug with a narrow therapeutic range must be used with care because there is a fine line between effective treatment and risk of serious unwanted effects.

Before a medicine is marketed the manufacturer tries to find the best dose of the product. The dose of the drug that produces an effect in 90 per cent of people in the early clinical studies is usually selected. This means that some patients will find this dose too high for comfort and may experience adverse reactions. Some people may find the dose too low and the drug ineffective. Sometimes the medicine is marketed in too high a dose. This is discovered only once the drug has been in general use, sometimes for three or four years, as experience with it accumulates. The blood pressure lowering drug captopril was introduced in 1981 at a daily dose of 300mg (maximum dose 450mg), but by 1985 the dose was lowered to 50mg (maximum dose 100mg) because some patients had suffered adverse reactions to the drug.

Taking too little of a drug may also have consequences, for example taking too low a dose of an antibiotic in a serious infection. Underdosage may also occur when one drug interacts with another reducing the efficacy of the second medicine. For example, the antibiotic rifampicin reduces the effectiveness of the combined oral contraceptive pill. Similarly, relative overdosage can occur when one drug is added to another, increasing its effects: for example, the anti-arthritic drug azapropazone seriously enhances the blood-thinning effects of the anticoagulant warfarin.

Beyond the maximum safe dose overdosage and poisoning can occur, although this is not dangerous for all medicines. Taking one extra dose of a medicine is unlikely to cause problems but if you are unsure about how much you might have taken, contact your doctor or pharmacist and ask for advice. Taking more than the recommended dose or taking the medicine more often than suggested does not help you to get better more quickly.

● *BELIEF IN MEDICINE*

Believing in the healing power of the medicine you take plays an important part in the restoration of your health. The actions of the doctor giving you a prescription and of your taking a medicine or using any treatment adds to the effectiveness of the drug. This is known as the placebo response. It is particularly prominent with drugs taken to relieve pain or anxiety. Approximately one person in three responds in this way to medicine. The placebo response may be subtle, but can be surprising because you can experience unwanted effects in the same way.

Medicines in the future

Biotechnological techniques are likely to be used extensively in the development of many pharmaceuticals. Recent innovations include safer vaccines and products to replace faulty proteins. Eventually an alternative to blood may be made.

Gene therapy to correct defective genes will be the treatment of the future. There are thirty-eight inherited genetic disorders, such as *muscular dystrophy* and *cystic fibrosis*, which are serious and disabling diseases and for which there is treatment only to relieve rather than to cure. About a third of all hospital admissions of young children involve a genetic disease. As more genes are identified, the possibility of replacing any defective gene comes a step closer to reality.

THE HAZARDS OF TAKING MEDICINES

There is no such thing as a safe medicine: almost all medicines can cause unwanted effects.

Unwanted effects can generally be predicted from the drug's pharmacological activity and are usually known by the time the medicine is marketed. These effects may be inconvenient, such as slight feeling of sickness or a dry mouth, but they often fade to a 'non-worrying' level as treatment continues. Your doctor should tell you what unwanted effects to expect, so that you recognise them and are not concerned.

If unwanted effects are a nuisance and do not seem to fade with time, you need to discuss this with your doctor. A lower dose or taking the medicine less often may reduce unwanted effects, or it may be necessary to change to another preparation.

Serious unwanted effects

Serious reactions to drugs may cause a reversible illness, permanent disability or even death. Such reactions are much rarer and sometimes unpredictable. They may not have been noted during clinical trials and may not be detected until many thousands of people have used the medicine once it is on the market. An individual may interact unusually with the medicine because of the way his or her body deals with the drug, perhaps due to an inherited disorder or some extreme sensitivity, for instance, sudden collapse and shock after a dose of penicillin.

REVERSIBLE ILLNESS

Drugs can mimic disease. It can be difficult to know whether a condition is occurring naturally or whether it is caused by a drug or even worsened by it. As an example, confusion, a common problem in very old people, may fluctuate from time to time. Any variation, particularly a worsening of the condition, may be attributed to the condition rather than the medicine(s) being taken. However, pain-relievers, the heart drug digoxin, corticosteroids in high doses, anti-anxiety drugs and antidepressants can all exacerbate confusion. Other conditions aggravated by medicines that may be mistaken for the progression of natural disease include heart conditions – heart failure, abnormal rhythms angina and high blood pressure – diabetes, gout, asthma, epilepsy and depression. For example, digoxin, which is used for treating heart failure and certain types of irregular heart beats, may itself cause irregular heart rhythms. Diuretics, which reduce blood pressure by lowering the amount of water in the blood, increase uric acid levels in the blood and this can worsen gout.

Many adverse reactions are reversible once the drug has been identified as the culprit. A medicine which makes you ill should be stopped, but discuss this with your doctor.

● *PERMANENT DISABILITY*

This may occur because a medicine has been used in too high a dose and/or used for prolonged periods.

The antibiotic gentamicin is used to treat serious infections and is usually given by injection in hospital. The unwanted effects of deafness and kidney injury are dose-related; with careful control they are not generally a problem but if high doses have to be used, or if the drug is given to an elderly person or to someone with reduced kidney function, it may accumulate in the body. If deafness results it is not reversible, although kidney function is usually restored.

Chloroquine, primarily used against malaria, also affects rheumatic disease. It has to be taken for long periods and may damage the cornea (usually reversible) and the retina (generally not reversible) of the eye. Blindness can result. However, damage to the retina is rare provided the dosage is kept within recommended limits. Eye damage is more likely to occur if chloroquine treatment exceeds two years.

● *DEATH*

Death can occur as a result of overdosage or in individuals who are very susceptible to a drug.

With drugs that have a narrow therapeutic range, the difference between the desired effects and harmful ones is small. For example, barbiturates used for inducing sleep and widely prescribed until the 1970s were found to be toxic just over the maximum dose.

Susceptible individuals may without knowing take a medicine that causes very little upset in other people. Aspirin, for instance, relieves millions of peoples' headaches a year but in some people it can cause severe ulceration and bleeding in the stomach, which may be fatal. Chloramphenicol, an antibiotic frequently and safely used as drops in the eye to clear up infections such as conjunctivitis, causes toxic effects if taken into the body. It is used by mouth or injection only for very severe, life-threatening infections and only after careful consideration, because it can cause irreversible blood disorders, resulting in death.

Missed doses

It is important to take medicines in the right dose, at the right times, by the right route and in the right way whenever you can. Forty to seventy per cent of people omit some doses during long-term treatment with medicines. Even with short courses of medicine, such as a five-day supply of an antibiotic, you may miss doses or not finish the treatment.

It may not matter if you do not take every dose of your medicine, but you must find out how important it is to do so from your doctor. For certain conditions it is especially important to sustain drug levels in the body, for example anticonvulsant treatment for controlling fits. If you have high blood pressure you will need to take medicine every day to keep the pressure at a lower level. If you have a hormone imbalance, such as thyroid disease, you may need to take medicine as long as that hormone imbalance persists, perhaps for ever, and it will certainly be important to take treatment regularly. You may need treatment for a particular length of time to prevent the risk of a relapse. Find out what to do if you miss a dose of your medicine as the advice varies depending on the type of drug.

Drug interactions

A drug interaction occurs when the effects of one drug are modified by the effects of another drug. Some foods and alcohol can also interact with specific drugs. A few drug interactions are beneficial. For example, probenecid, a drug used to control gout, also delays the elimination of penicillin from the kidneys, allowing the dose of penicillin to act longer in the body. However, most significant drug interactions are adverse reactions and the more drugs you take the greater the chance of an interaction.

The absorption, distribution, metabolism and elimination of one drug may be altered by another drug. For example, rifampicin, a drug for treating tuberculosis, interferes with the metabolism of warfarin, a drug which thins the blood and affects clotting, to diminish the effect of warfarin, which could allow blood clots to form again.

Alternatively, the effects of two drugs may interact at the site of action. For example, alcohol interacts with any drug that dampens down (depresses) brain function. Alcohol should not be taken at the same time as a sleeping tablet because it enhances the effect of the medicine; the combined effects of the two lead to excessive sleepiness and even coma.

A prescribed medicine may be accompanied by a patient information leaflet or another label apart from the instructions for taking the medicine, which may warn you of a drug interaction. For instance, the antibiotic tetracycline should not be taken at the same time as milk, iron preparations or indigestion remedies because these substances reduce its absorption and therefore its effectiveness.

Some interactions may be life-threatening and if you are prescribed one of the followings groups of medicines you should be given a treatment card which lists important drug interactions, and in some cases, drug and food/alcohol interactions. You will then know which combination of medicines to avoid. Always check with your doctor or pharmacist before taking any other medicine with:

- anticoagulants
- oral corticosteroids
- monoamine oxidase inhibitor antidepressants
- lithium.

Medicines from these groups should never be stopped abruptly without consulting your doctor.

Not only do some prescription medicines interact, but those bought over the counter can also cause problems. A monoamine oxidase inhibitor antidepressant interacts with certain constituents of some cold remedies, resulting in a dangerous rise in blood pressure. If you take a prescription medicine and then want to buy a preparation over the counter always check with your doctor or pharmacist before buying. Always tell your doctor or pharmacist if you are taking any over-the-counter remedy before a prescription is written.

● *COMBINED PREPARATIONS*

Combinations of some drugs can be taken together safely and sometimes they are mixed together in one medicine. A combined preparation can be useful if one drug enhances the activity of another or moderates its unwanted effects. It is easier to take, and to remember to take, one tablet rather than several different medicines, particularly if treatment is for long periods. Furthermore, if you pay a prescription charge, you pay only one charge for a combination product but several charges for the ingredients dispensed separately.

The disadvantage of combination products is that the individual drug dosages are fixed and cannot be adjusted to suit your needs during a course of treatment. Drugs may be combined inappropriately in medicines – some combination cough and cold remedies even contain ingredients with opposing effects. Certain combination analgesic preparations, often promoted as additionally effective, are no more effective than the main ingredient, such as aspirin or paracetamol, used alone. Caffeine, for instance, adds nothing to the pain-relieving properties of aspirin and may even worsen any gastric irritation it causes.

It is difficult enough for doctors and pharmacists to remember the individual ingredients of a combination preparation, let alone for the patient, but a manufacturer's brand name masks the presence of several ingredients. Listing the components by generic name on the label of a medicine dispensed in a brown bottle is unwieldy and brand names are often preferred. The manufacturer's original pack and patient information leaflets are more informative and should give the generic name of your medicine as well as the brand name. Generic names beginning with 'co' contain two drugs in fixed proportion, for example the analgesic co-codaprin contains codeine phosphate (1 part) and aspirin (50 parts).

Polypharmacy and overprescribing

The use of several different medicines at the same time is known as polypharmacy. Certain diseases or conditions, for example chronic lung disease, congestive heart failure, high blood pressure and epilepsy, may require daily treatment with two or more medicines. The doctor balances the effects and the dosages of the medicines to provide the best treatment for the patient.

However, inappropriate or irrational use of several medicines – for example using two medicines of the same class, such as the benzodiazepines temazepam for sleep and lorazepam for its daytime tranquillising effect – can be a danger. Both drugs act in the body in a similar way and are likely to enhance each other's effects.

Polypharmacy can occur when the unwanted effects of a medicine are treated with a second medicine, which in turn produces unwanted effects requiring treatment with a third. This produces a vicious circle of unnecessary and harmful drug treatment when what is needed is a thorough assessment of all the medicines taken by the patient. Successful treatment may involve stopping all drug treatment and monitoring the patient's progress without medicines. Of course, this must only be done by your doctor.

Older people in nursing homes or on long-stay wards are particularly vulnerable to unnecessary treatment with many medicines – for example, routine doses of laxatives and sedatives may be given along with any specific treatment.

Some medicines may be used in too high a dose, particularly in older people, for example benzodiazepines and antidepressants which act on the brain and nervous system. Medicines for removing excess fluid from the body (diuretics) are sometimes used at too high a dose and for unnecessarily long periods. In older people with fluid on the legs, a few days' treatment with a diuretic may be all that is needed to remove the water, followed by gentle exercise and then resting with the legs up. Yet many people are prescribed diuretics for months.

Who is most at risk from medicine-taking?

The effects of a medicine depend on many factors. Although all people vary in their response to drugs, certain groups are more vulnerable when taking medicines than others.

● *BABIES AND CHILDREN*

Age, weight and maturity of the liver and kidneys are important factors in drug treatment of the young. Not only do babies and children need smaller doses than adults, but a medicine which may not cause any problems in an adult may adversely affect a young baby. Pseudoephedrine, a decongestant drug for drying up colds, may cause sleep disturbances and nightmares and young children seem quite sensitive to this effect. Antihistamines, also in cough and cold remedies, help the child to sleep, but they are long-acting and the effects continue the next day, interfering with muscle control, co-ordination and balance.

A baby's immune system is immature and therefore it takes time to build up resistance to every sort of infection. Immunisation against serious diseases, starting at two months, prevents major illness, but otherwise the child develops immunity to common infections as contact occurs with other children in playgroups and school. Repeated infections, such as colds, coughs, diarrhoea and skin complaints, are quite normal in childhood: a six-year-old may well have had over 30 episodes of illness by this time. Antibiotics do not cure colds: the only reason why a doctor might prescribe an antibiotic is to combat a secondary bacterial infection of the ear, throat or chest. Simple remedies, such as simple linctus for coughs or paracetamol syrup for fever and pain relief, may be all that is needed.

● *PREGNANT WOMEN*

Most women now understand that it is best to avoid taking any non-essential medicine during any stage of a pregnancy because drugs can cross the placenta and enter the baby's bloodstream. During the first three months of pregnancy some drugs can interfere with the development of the baby and cause abnormalities. They are called *teratogens*. Few drugs are proven teratogens, but no drug is beyond suspicion in early pregnancy. After the first three months of pregnancy, drugs may affect the growth and further development of the baby. It is difficult for doctors to assess whether a baby's abnormality is due to chance or to the effect of a particular drug.

The thalidomide tragedy prompted much stricter testing of drugs so that now all pharmaceutical companies must make a statement about a medicine's use in pregnancy at the time the medicine is marketed and promoted. However, it is sensible to avoid taking any medicine unless absolutely necessary before you plan to conceive or during pregnancy.

If you have a permanent condition such as diabetes or epilepsy drug treatment will be essential during your pregnancy, so you should see your doctor to discuss management of the pregnancy even before you conceive. Screening tests during pregnancy are available.

If you are planning to become pregnant or are pregnant, check with your doctor before taking any medicine, either prescribed or over-the-counter. Even vitamins which might seem beneficial during pregnancy must be treated with care. High doses of vitamin A can affect the unborn baby and cause abnormalities. Nicotine and alcohol should also be avoided as they can affect the developing baby.

● *BREAST-FEEDING WOMEN*

Some drugs can pass through the mother's milk into the baby where they may act. Some may cause toxicity, whereas others have little effect on the baby. Certain drugs can inhibit the flow of milk. Breast milk concentrates some drugs so that the baby may get a toxic dose even though the mother is taking a normal dose. Other drugs, such as antibiotics, may in theory cause an allergic reaction, even though the drug concentration may be low in the baby's blood. Tranquillisers may make the baby drowsy and less able to feed. For many drugs there is inadequate information, but these examples illustrate that it is best to avoid taking medicines while breast-feeding unless absolutely necessary. Check with your doctor or a pharmacist before taking any medicine.

● *ELDERLY PEOPLE*

Medicine use increases substantially between the ages of 65 and 80 and with it the potential for unwanted effects. On average, people over 65 take three times more prescription medicines than younger people.

As you grow older, your body and the way it works gradually change. The body's regulatory mechanisms, such as the control of temperature or blood pressure, become less efficient. This is part of the normal ageing process and is separate from the effects of diseases which become increasingly commonplace with age.

Elderly people's response to treatment with medicines and the way the body handles drugs changes. The liver and kidneys become less efficient. In particular, the decline in kidney function means that drugs are removed from the body more slowly. The brain and nervous system become more susceptible to drugs; the immune system may not protect the body reliably and drug treatment may set off an unusual response.

All these physical changes mean that drug treatment of elderly people must be approached with care. Conditions which are commonly treated include heart and blood pressure problems, nervous disorders, rheumatic diseases and digestive complaints. Older people take more medicines and for longer periods, because many diseases, such as arthritic conditions, last for a long time.

The more medicines that are taken, the greater the risk of drug interactions and other unwanted effects. The standard adult dose of some medicines may be higher than necessary; with many medicines, treatment should be started with a lower dose than that used for younger adults.

The ageing process can be mistaken for disease and inappropriate drugs may be prescribed. For example, dizziness is common in older people because of the change in the blood pressure control mechanism. Prochlorperazine has been used to treat this sort of giddiness, but the drug can cause mental confusion and symptoms of Parkinson's disease (uncontrolled movements, particularly of the face, rigidity and tremor) which may not develop until the medicine has been taken for weeks or even months. Because drugs can mimic diseases and worsen them, the patient's deterioration might not be credited to the adverse effects of the medicine, but to the condition itself. When the adverse effects of medicines are not recognised, further drug treatment might then be prescribed to deal with the patient's new symptoms. See 'Polypharmacy and overprescribing', above.

● *DRIVERS AND OTHER DECISION-MAKERS*

Any skill which requires judgement and co-ordination can be affected by a medicine which acts on the brain and nervous system. This type of medicine can affect car and train drivers, airline pilots, machine operators and many others who have to make quick decisions. Many drugs can interfere with driving skills, particularly during the first few days of treatment when the extent of unwanted effects is unknown. It is an offence to drive or be in charge of a vehicle when your ability to drive is impaired by medicines.

The following groups of prescribed medicines can affect performance of skilled tasks, mostly by causing drowsiness:

- ☐ most antihistamines
- ☐ anti-anxiety drugs
- ☐ antidepressants
- ☐ antipsychotics
- ☐ some pain-relievers
- ☐ some blood pressure lowering drugs
- ☐ some drugs for epilepsy
- ☐ some drugs to control vomiting
- ☐ some muscle relaxants.

You can become tolerant to the effects of some of these drugs, but until you are sure about your reaction to the medicine, you should avoid driving. Other medicines that affect vision (for example eye drops for glaucoma), or cause nausea or dizziness, can also impair driving ability. Ask your doctor if you can drive. Sleeping tablets can have 'hangover effects' the next day, particularly in older people, which can affect driving. You should not drive for 24 hours after a general anaesthetic. If you are a diabetic on insulin you should not drive just before a meal is due unless you take extra carbohydrate. Always carry a supply of snacks in the car to deal with symptoms of low blood sugar.

You are required to tell the Driver and Vehicle Licensing Centre (DVLC) of any disability which affects your fitness as a driver if you expect it to last longer than three months. If you suffer from epilepsy, you will need your doctor's advice about driving and operating machinery.

Over-the-counter medicines, such as preparations for hay fever, and cough and cold remedies, contain antihistamines and decongestants. These can cause drowsiness, impair judgement and affect driving skills. The effect of alcohol on driving performance is well known and even a small quantity will enhance the effects of drugs that cause drowsiness.

Putting the risks into perspective

Medicines have enormous beneficial potential: lives have been saved by antibiotics; a diabetic's daily existence depends on regular insulin injections. But the dramatic adverse effects of thalidomide, the blood pressure lowering drug practolol (brand name Eraldin) and the anti-arthritic drug benoxaprofen (Opren) have been widely publicised. All medicines, even those sold in supermarkets, carry some benefits and some risks.

It has been estimated that adverse drug reaction problems account for two to three per cent of consultations in general practice and three to five per cent of hospital admissions. Ten to twenty per cent of hospital inpatients are thought to experience adverse drug reactions. These often seriously ill patients are likely to be treated with powerful medicines which carry greater risks of adverse reactions. It is difficult to get accurate figures because the reported incidence of adverse reactions varies depending on how the information has been collected.

The most common reactions to drugs involve the skin, then the nervous system, followed by the digestive system. Non-steroidal anti-inflammatory drugs (NSAIDs) cause the most serious and life-threatening reactions, with bleeding and perforation of the intestines. There is no doubt that some medicines actually cause death and a serious amount of drug-induced (*iatrogenic*) disease and discomfort, but the overall reported risk of dying from a serious adverse drug reaction has remained at less than one in a million for most years since records began in the 1960s.

The precise number of people who die as a result of medicine-taking per year is not known. In 1987, over 16,000 adverse reactions were reported to the Committee on Safety of Medicines of which 5,000 were serious and 280 were fatal. This compares with a figure of around 5,000 deaths on British roads in the same year. In 1991 there were around 270 deaths a day in Britain from diseases caused by nicotine, tar products and carbon monoxide in cigarettes, cigars and pipe tobacco, such as cancer and heart and lung problems.

Balancing the benefits and risks of a medicine needs to be done in context of the disease being treated. Generally, more serious diseases are treated with more powerful medicines. Treatment of cancer with medicines that can make you feel very ill may be worthwhile if they prolong life. Taking aspirin for a fleeting headache is not worthwhile for people who suffer serious unwanted effects. Arthritic patients are usually prepared to put up with the unwanted effects of indigestion and tinnitus caused by NSAIDs which relieve joint pain and swelling in order to remain active and mobile. Many people are prepared to tolerate the unwanted effects of medicines so long as they understand that they will happen and know what to look out for.

Your doctor must choose the right medicine and before writing a prescription must weigh the evidence for and against the medicine. This should include an assessment of what will happen if you do not take any form of medicine. It is then up to you to use the medicine correctly.

Monitoring adverse reactions

The launch of a new medicine is often accompanied by such a fanfare and flourish in the media that the risks, even those which are well established, may not be aired. Doctors and medicine-takers ought to know the benefits and the risks of a medicine when it is marketed, but they cannot. A medicine is licensed after testing in 2,000 to 3,000 people, both healthy volunteers and people with the disease for which the medicine will be licensed. Some of the tests will be studies on what happens to a single dose of the drug in the body, while other volunteer patients may take the trial drug for a few months. The likely dose-related unwanted effects will be confirmed and others may be discovered. Yet the number of people taking part in premarketing clinical trials is not large enough to uncover the rarer, unpredictable adverse reactions. These unforeseen reactions and who will be at risk cannot be determined until larger numbers of people have taken the medicine, usually after several years.

● *CLINICAL TRIALS*

The era of modern medicines started with sulpha drugs in the 1930s and penicillin in the 1940s. At first medicines were manufactured and used without any previous clinical testing. As the therapeutic revolution progressed, there was a gradual realisation that clinical impressions of the effects of a drug in patients were not enough. Anecdotal reports of one or two cases of a medicine relieving a specific disease may be interesting, but how were doctors to tell whether the effects were due to chance, to the drug or to the placebo response?

WHAT IS A PLACEBO?

Placebo is Latin for 'I shall please'. A placebo can be a medicine which is given more to please than to benefit the patient, who believes that taking a medicine will help. The word is also used to describe a 'dummy drug', an inactive substance which has no pharmacological effect on the body and which is used in clinical trials to test the effects of a medicine. A placebo helps to sort out the true response to a medicine from the belief in medicine-taking. You can experience both beneficial and unwanted effects from a placebo, even though it does not act in a measurable way. This is particularly so when you do not know whether you are taking a placebo or the active drug in a clinical trial.

In response to this problem, Sir Austin Bradford Hill, a medical statistician, defined a *clinical trial*. It should be a carefully and ethically designed experiment with the aim of answering some precisely framed question. The drug should be tried in equivalent groups of patients treated at the same time, but in different ways. The patients should be randomly allocated to one treatment or another.

Tests of the medicine must be carried out in adequate numbers of patients to establish the true effect of a medicine. The effect must be statistically valid and not due to chance. This is particularly important because of the placebo effect.

A clinical trial aims to show:

- the value of the treatment
- whether the treatment is better than existing treatments
- the type of patient who will benefit
- in what form the drug should be taken
- the dose and how often it should be taken
- the nature of any unwanted effects and adverse reactions.

A new drug may be tried against an established treatment or it may be tested against a placebo. One group of patients may take the test drug for a particularly period while another group takes the comparison treatment or placebo. The groups then swap to treatments they have not yet had. In a *double-blind cross-over trial* neither the doctor nor the patient knows whether the trial drug or placebo is being taken until the trial has ended.

A clinical trial may take over three years to set up, to find the correct number of patients, to collate and interpret the results and to publish the findings. At every stage of a trial it is possible to introduce error and bias, even quite unintentionally. A trial costs a large amount of money to conduct. Unfortunately, some trials do not provide clear-cut answers, although the results may be presented in optimistic and glowing terms. One of the skills your doctor needs is that of interpreting the study and reading between the lines of a clinical trial. Doctors must have reliable information on the effects and hazards of treatment which they can then apply to their own practice.

Once the medicine is licensed by the Committee on Safety of Medicines, the Medicines Control Agency's adverse drug reaction section monitors reports of serious unwanted effects. Information comes from a variety of sources.

● *VOLUNTARY REPORTING BY DOCTORS*

Doctors are asked to report all cases of suspected adverse reactions to new medicines and serious or unusual reactions only with older established products. They fill in details on a special adverse reaction card (also known as a yellow card). There are four regional centres which collect adverse reaction information. The main drawback of this scheme is that the true incidence of a drug's adverse effects cannot be obtained because only 1 in 6 doctors reports adverse reactions to the Committee on Safety of Medicines. Around 20,000 adverse drug reaction reports are sent to the Medicines Control Agency each year. A new computerised monitoring system will improve the time taken to identify and analyse these reports.

● *PHARMACEUTICAL COMPANIES*

The Medicines Act requires manufacturers to report any suspected adverse reactions to their products whether in Britain or overseas.

● *WORLD HEALTH ORGANIZATION*

The Medicines Control Agency has an on-line link to the World Health Organization's database which collects information from 30 countries giving a worldwide perspective on drug safety matters.

● *POST-MARKETING SURVEILLANCE SCHEMES*

These involve independent organisations as well as the pharmaceutical industry. The Drug Safety Research Unit, an independent group, monitors prescriptions on selected medicines. Prescribers are identified and are then asked to complete a card, which names the patient and the medicine, with details of any adverse reactions.

Many general practitioners now store on computer details of

patients, records of illnesses and any medicines prescribed. Several independent companies operate a record linkage scheme where the prescriptions for the selected medicine can be linked to clinical reports and a search made for specific reactions.

Once a medicine is marketed, a pharmaceutical company may set up a post-marketing surveillance study to monitor unwanted effects. Guidelines for operating these studies are agreed by representatives from doctors' organisations, the British Medical Association and the Royal College of General Practitioners, the Committee on Safety of Medicines and the Association of the British Pharmaceutical Industry. In spite of the existence of these guidelines, some studies are thinly veiled promotional studies, encouraging the doctor to prescribe the medicine which patients may then continue to take for many years. Doctors are paid a token sum per person to enter patients into these studies. Sometimes the results remain unpublished, although the Medicines Control Agency may know them.

▼'*BLACK TRIANGLE' MEDICINES*

All new prescription medicines are marked with an inverted black triangle (▼) in the *British National Formulary* and other doctors' reference books. The triangle is an alerting device for doctors to report any adverse reaction to the new medicine to the Committee on Safety of Medicines. A medicine is marked for the first few years after it is marketed.

What if treatment goes wrong?

Doctors do not intend to harm patients with medicines, but accidents and mistakes occur. If you suffer permanent disability from the adverse effects of a medicine or you are the relative of someone who dies as result of taking a medicine, redress is difficult to obtain, expensive and time-consuming. You have to prove that the doctor was negligent and that it was this negligence which caused your present condition. It can be very difficult to prove that medical negligence caused your injuries. A court may be unable to determine whether they were a result of carelessness in the use of the medicine or a deterioration in your illness.

Yet patients who are seriously damaged by a medicine need reasonable and speedy financial compensation even if nobody is to blame. Patients should not have to take expensive legal action against the pharmaceutical industry or their doctors to prove negligence. Various 'no fault' compensation schemes have been suggested, but so far no workable arrangements have been proposed. Some of the concerns about these schemes include how they would work equitably, the expense to the taxpayer and the lack of accountability for drug manufacturers.

Consumers' Association research has shown that people want to know the risks involved in any treatment. They expected that they would feel less resentment against the doctor if they had been sensibly forewarned than if they had not been told of a serious risk which then materialised. If you have suffered avoidable harm through a prescribing error, you should expect a prompt explanation of the facts. You may be confused, angry and worried. You will want to know what went wrong and to have an assurance that all appropriate steps will be taken to prevent a repetition in other patients. It would be helpful if the doctor offered an apology, but many fear that to do so is an admission of liability. Your doctor may be able to help you, for instance by advising you to consult particular solicitors who specialise in medical negligence.

THE MEDICINES MARKET

Since the 1940s the pharmaceutical industry has been one of the successes of Britain's economy. Many multinational companies based in Britain research and develop medicines and every year around £3 billion of pharmaceuticals are consumed. How much money pharmaceutical companies make from selling medicines has always been a secret between them and the Department of Health. The government takes into account various factors, such as the amount of investment the company makes in Britain.

Most of the new products marketed are variations of established medicines, but some contain new active ingredients. In the early stages of research up to 10,000 compounds are screened for their potential as medicines, but only a small number are selected for development. Development of a new active substance may take 10 years and cost up to £150 million and even then, once commercially available, only one in five new active substances recovers the research and development costs.

The supply and use of medicines in Britain is based on the Medicines Act 1968. This means that any product for which a medicinal claim is made must be licensed by the government. Before this Act, medicines and poisons were regulated, but the tragedy of thalidomide, a sleeping tablet which caused severe abnormalities in the babies of women who took the drug during pregnancy prompted a review of how medicines reached the market. Now the Committee on Safety of Medicines, whose members are independent experts, advises ministers on the licensing of medicines. The whole system is administered by the Medicines Control Agency, a branch of the Department of Health.

The Medicines Control Agency

The Medicines Control Agency is responsible for seeing that all medicines sold or supplied for human or animal use in Britain meet certain standards. Before a medicine is marketed, as much information must be known about its quality, effectiveness and safety as possible. Assessments of quality concern the physical and chemical properties of the active ingredient and the supposedly inactive ingredients that carry the medicine into the body. Details of how the drug is to be assembled with the other ingredients, how it is to be manufactured and packed, and how long it will last once the medicine leaves the factory (its shelf-life) must be known. In assessing the safety of a drug the Medicines Control Agency has to balance the risks of medicines against their benefits in relation to the seriousness of the disease under treatment.

Laboratory and animal studies provide information on the drug's effectiveness as well as its possible harmful effects (toxicity). Then the drug must be studied in 2,000–3,000 people, both those who need treatment and healthy volunteers, who should accurately reflect the expected users of the medicine once it is licensed. Where a drug is intended for treatment of elderly people or children specific studies must be made.

At one time the very young and people over 70 were not included in these assessments, but medicine use among elderly people, in particular, is high. The Opren case highlighted the need for proper clinical assessment in the likely users of medicine. People over 70 were not included in the clinical studies of benoxaprofen (brand name Opren), which was marketed in 1980 for the treatment of arthritis; yet arthritis is a common condition of old age. Benoxaprofen stayed in the body much longer than other arthritis drugs and it lingered even longer in elderly people because the kidneys become progressively less efficient with age. Older people were therefore more likely to experience the adverse effects of benoxaprofen.

When all the tests and trials are finished, the drug company is ready to apply to the Medicines Control Agency for a licence. All the information about the medicine which has been recorded over its years of development is sent to the Medicines Control Agency for assessment. In 1988 the average size of a dossier of information on one drug was 170 volumes, each the dimensions of a telephone directory.

Medicine marketing

Every year, the industry spends around £170 million on promoting medicines; the launch campaign for a new product may cost up to £1 million in the first two years of marketing. When a company has spent so much time and money bringing a medicine to the market, it is naturally keen to sell its product. Prescription-only medicines are vigorously promoted to doctors by company representatives, by mail-shots and journal advertisements and through sponsored symposia.

Much of the promotional effort involves the company attempting to gain a larger market share than its competitors; many of the medicines promoted in Britain are 'me-too' medicines – variations of an original drug which is already available. There are, for instance, more than 18 non-steroidal anti-inflammatory drugs (NSAIDs) for the treatment of rheumatic diseases, all of which have very similar anti-inflammatory activity. It is often hard for doctors to sort out the facts – the benefits and risks of each medicine – from the material that bombards them.

About 3,500 sales reps direct their energies to promoting medicines to the country's 34,000 general practitioners. Eighty per cent of all prescriptions (for around 400 million medicines and other items per year) are written by GPs. Medical reps aim first to persuade doctors to prescribe their company's products and secondly to inform and perhaps educate. Companies also want reps to report doctors' experiences with their own and their competitors' products.

Reps are the access point for free gifts, lunches and trips to sponsored meetings which are all part of the pharmaceutical industry's advertising and promotional effort. These meetings must have a clear educational content, apart from the advertising. Entertainment and other hospitality must be secondary to the main purpose of these meetings, and should not cost more than doctors would otherwise pay for themselves. Free gifts, lunches and trips to symposia generate goodwill and many doctors see no harm in them. Yet over the years heavy promotion seems most likely to have contributed to excessive and inappropriate prescribing. Reps cannot be an impartial source of information.

Most GPs see at least one rep a week and over half of them find that reps are the source of information when deciding whether or not to prescribe a new product. It takes time and effort to read independent sources of information to judge whether a drug is useful or not; information from the rep is an easier route. Some doctors are concerned about the close relationship between prescribers and the manufacturers of medicines and do not see representatives at all. Unbiased sources of information are available and more GPs are preparing their own lists of selected or preferred medicines (*formularies*) now that the government requires them to prescribe cost-effectively. Doctors and patients need unbiased comparative information on prescription and over-the-counter medicines but this is not provided by the pharmaceutical industry.

Pharmaceutical companies have their own medical information departments staffed by doctors, pharmacists and other scientists. Part of the information department's function is to provide reps with technical data and to answer enquiries on the company's products. The company medical director is responsible for checking promotional literature and advertising copy produced by the marketing department. All promotional literature must be in line with the product licence.

DOCTORS AND REPS

Out of 229 GPs in the Greenwich and Guildford areas, 156 responded to a small survey (published in 1987) to find out what they actually thought about the quality of information given by reps. Eighty-four per cent saw reps on a regular basis, 26 per cent seeing between two and four a week and four per cent more than four per week. Sixty-three per cent felt they were 'slightly' or not at all influenced by reps, while 37 per cent felt they were swayed by reps to a moderate or large degree.

In another recent survey 79 per cent of 219 GPs felt that, during at least one visit, a rep 'made less' of the product's unwanted effects than the doctor believed was clinically justified. Furthermore, 66 per cent of 217 GPs said that a rep claimed more uses for a preparation than were justified.

Marketing regulations

Most pharmaceutical companies belong to the Association of the British Pharmaceutical Industry (ABPI) which has a voluntary Code of Practice for how products are promoted. It has been drawn up in consultation with the British Medical Association and the Department of Health and is published in the *Data Sheet Compendium*. The code is administered by an 18-member committee of whom four are independent, three are doctors and a barrister is chair. The other members are senior managers drawn from member companies.

The code regulates the standard of conduct in the marketing of prescription medicines and this includes advertising and the activities of reps. It emphasises 'the importance in the public interest of providing the medical and allied professions with accurate, fair and objective information on medical products so that rational prescribing decisions can be made. . . . Information should . . . conform not only to legal requirements but also to ethical standards and canons of good taste'. Company reps must follow the code when they talk to doctors.

An analysis of how well the code of practice was adhered to in a six-year period in the 1980s showed that there were around 300 complaints with over 370 breaches of the code, of which 270 were possible infringements of the Medicines Act. The rules of the Medicines Act forbidding misleading and unsupported information and misleading claims or comparisons were broken most often, on seven out of ten occasions. Misconduct by reps accounted for 13 breaches and there were 14 transgressions of the code on gifts, inducements and hospitality. Prescription-only medicines must not be promoted to the public, for example through press conferences, and yet there were eight breaches of this rule. Sixteen companies were found to have brought discredit on or reduced confidence in the pharmaceutical industry. Many complaints are dismissed and there are no provisions for appeal.

However, the Code of Practice Committee's hearings are held in private and companies are admonished, but rarely punished, for breaching the code. These breaches are published in professional journals, but they are rarely made public in the lay press. The Department of Health leaves regulation of the industry largely to the ABPI, and this self-regulation seems to be a service to itself rather than to the public. The committee is not publicly accountable. The majority of committee members represent the industry's interests and there are no members to represent consumers, the users of medicines. Pharmaceutical companies have been in court only seven times since the Medicines Act was passed in 1968.

Generic medicines

When a medicine is marketed, it has already been patented, so that the manufacturer has the sole right to develop and market it and the brand name is protected. Other companies may not copy this medicine or infringe the patent. In Britain, the patent life of a drug is 20 years, but many new medicines take 10–12 years to develop, because of all the tests that must be done before the medicine is licensed. Manufacturers say that selling a medicine for the remaining eight to ten years leaves too little time to recoup the huge costs of research and development and they are asking for an extension to the patent life.

Once a medicine's patent has expired, another company is free to copy the medicine. It can do so more cheaply because it does not have to fund development and initial marketing of the medicine. However, generic copies are not made for all branded medicines, even after the patent has expired. Generic copies cost the National Health Service less than brands and doctors are increasingly prescribing generics. This threatens the profits of the major pharmaceutical companies.

If you have a medical condition requiring long-term treatment, you may receive a variety of brands or the generic version of a medicine over a period of time. You may be concerned about differences between them and the relative quality of them. However, the licensing requirements for generic medicines are just as stringent as they are for branded products. The same medicine produced by separate manufacturers may differ in shape, size, colour or taste, but these differences are rarely significant; the active ingredient of the medicine is the same. A pharmacist must always dispense exactly what the doctor has indicated on the prescription. If the prescription has a particular brand name, then you will receive that brand, but if the prescription has the generic name then the pharmacist only has to dispense a medicine containing that active ingredient: you may receive a generic version or any of the branded versions.

Imported prescription medicines

Your medicine may sometimes come from another country in the European Community. the medicine and packaging may look familiar except that the wording on the pack will not be in English. The medicine will be exactly the same as the British product and the pharmacist will label the medicine with the required instructions.

The current system for buying pharmaceuticals varies throughout the European Community, which leads to discrepancies in prices. Germany, Denmark, the Netherlands and Britain have high medicine prices while those in Spain, Portugal, Italy and Greece are lower. This had led to a brisk trade in some pharmaceuticals, known as 'parallel imports'. Parallel imports are regulated by the Medicines Control Agency and each type of medicine has to have a special product licence number. Both the importer, who must hold a licence for this trade, and the pharmacist, who buys and supplies parallel imports, benefit financially. Neither the consumer nor the National Health Service gains from parallel importing. Parallel importing annoys the pharmaceutical industry considerably, because it reduces profits.

The Limited List

In 1985 the government decided to restrict some of the medicines that doctors could prescribe on the National Health Service in order to save money. The List includes all the medicines a doctor would normally require to meet the needs of all his or her patients. The Limited List has reduced duplication and the numbers of less effective medicines. Medicines are restricted in the following groups: antacids, laxatives, cough and cold remedies, analgesics for mild to moderate pain relief, vitamins and tonics and the benzodiazepine sedatives and tranquillisers. Medicines in all these categories remain available for NHS prescription (the White List) but a number of each have been blacklisted. Most blacklisted medicines can still be obtained on a private prescription and you can buy others over the counter. A doctor in the NHS cannot charge for writing a private prescription for a blacklisted medicine, but you will have to pay for the medicine and probably a dispensing fee to the pharmacist.

● *DRUG LISTS*

Of the hundreds of products available, most doctors have, in practice, prescribed from a personal list of around 200–300 medicines. Drug selection is influenced by a number of factors. These include the doctor's training at medical school, the latest medical research and current medical opinion, what the specialist recommends at the local hospital, and also the activities of the pharmaceutical industry in developing and promoting medicines.

In addition to blacklisting some medicines the government has taken measures to encourage cost-effective and rational prescribing by doctors in the new contract with GPs. Doctors are encouraged to evaluate their prescribing and set up drug lists (formularies) based on medicines which are selected for their effectiveness, safety, convenience and cost. Drug formularies allow doctors to become very familiar with a narrow range of medicines and so increase their experience in using these drugs. Generic medicines usually cost less than branded versions and are therefore likely to feature in most drug formularies. Although doctors are working within guidelines for drug costs set by Family Health Services Authorities, patients can still get the medicines they need, including the high-cost drugs.

European Community Developments

The EC is moving steadily towards a single market in pharmaceuticals. Proposals on drug licensing, distribution, pricing, advertising, labelling and patient information have been considered and some will be implemented by 1993. The Medicines Control Agency has been working with other European drug regulatory bodies in preparation for the single internal market. A single European medicines agency is planned to smooth out the present tangle created by 12 national agencies, but it will deal only with applications for products of biotechnology (genetically engineered medicines and vaccines). It will also monitor drug safety after a medicine is marketed.

Changes to the way medicines are advertised and sold in Britain are likely to be gradual. One of the problems for the single market at present is that a medicine may be available on prescription in one country, but be sold over the counter in another. A proposal for a Community-wide list of prescription-only medicines has yet to be approved. Also the way a medicine is used varies from one country to another as well as the types of symptoms treated. The single market will mean that you will get more information when you obtain a medicine, whether on prescription or over the counter.

1

DIGESTIVE SYSTEM

Indigestion Peptic ulcer
Diarrhoea Constipation
Piles and anal disorders

The digestive system (also known as the gut or *gastrointestinal* system) includes the gullet (*oesophagus*), stomach, small and large intestines, the rectum and anus. Chewed food passes from the mouth into the oesophagus, down into the stomach where digestive juices (including hydrochloric acid and the enzyme *pepsin*) break down the food into smaller particles; these pass into the small intestine, where more enzymes break them down (digest them) into molecules small enough to be absorbed through the intestinal wall into the bloodstream. These molecules go to the liver, which sorts them and breaks them down further (*metabolises* them) into nutrients for the body to use. The remnants of digestion pass to the large intestine (*colon*) where water is absorbed into the bloodstream leaving stools (or faeces), which are passed out of the body through the anus.

Indigestion

Indigestion (*dyspepsia*) is a symptom popularly attributed to difficulty with digesting food: you may experience bloating, pain under the ribs or heartburn – a burning pain in the centre of the chest which you sometimes also feel in the throat; you may have an acid taste in the mouth, burp a lot or feel sick. You may feel a burning pain after swallowing hot drinks.

Your stomach may be irritated or inflamed because you have eaten or drunk too much. Some medicines, particularly aspirin and other non-steroidal anti-inflammatory drugs (NSAIDs), can irritate the stomach and cause indigestion or even ulceration. Indigestion can be due to a condition called *hiatus hernia* – a weakness of the muscle between the gullet and the stomach which is supposed to stop food and acid leaking into the gullet. This type of indigestion (also called *oesophagitis* or *reflux oesophagitis*) is particularly noticeable after meals and when stooping or lying down, and is more likely if you are overweight.

If you have indigestion for more than a few weeks you should see your doctor. Long-term symptoms can be caused by an ulcer (see page 72), although the lining of the stomach may not be damaged as it is by a full-blown ulcer. Indigestion sometimes has other causes, such as *irritable bowel syndrome* (see page 85), but indigestion for which there is no clear explanation is called *non-ulcer dyspepsia*

HOW YOU CAN HELP YOURSELF

☐ Lose weight if you are overweight
☐ Cut down on alcohol
☐ Give up smoking or at least cut down: any form of tobacco can irritate the digestive system
☐ Sit upright when you eat your food, so that you are not pressing down on your stomach
☐ Eat at regular intervals, avoiding large meals late at night
☐ Avoid stooping forwards, especially after meals, and avoid reclining after meals; sleep with your head raised
☐ Avoid coffee, and spicy foods if you are not used to them
☐ Avoid foods and drinks you know cause you problems
☐ Eat a sensible balanced diet, with not too many fried and fatty foods – these can aggravate indigestion
☐ Avoid medicines that irritate the stomach: use paracetamol instead of aspirin, for example.

Antacids

Antacids neutralise stomach acid. They are useful once you have indigestion or if you expect symptoms. Many antacids can be bought over the counter (often for less than the cost of a prescription), but you should avoid using them for long periods without seeking advice from a doctor or pharmacist. Liquid preparations work better than tablets, although tablets are more convenient.

● *ALUMINIUM AND MAGNESIUM ANTACIDS* ●

Most antacid preparations are based on **aluminium** or **magnesium salts** or mixtures of both, sometimes with additional ingredients. Aluminium- and magnesium-containing antacids stay in the digestive system and are not much absorbed into the body. Aluminium preparations may cause constipation whereas magnesium-containing antacids tend to have a laxative effect: preparations containing both aluminium and magnesium may suit you better.

Additional ingredients

Manufacturers often add extra ingredients to aluminium and magnesium antacids. **Alginic acid** is a mucus-like substance derived from seaweed which may help to protect the lining of the stomach and oesophagus, but little evidence exists that other extras make the basic antacid work any better. Because these preparations are generally more expensive than simple antacids and have no clear advantages, many complex antacids are no longer available on prescription: your doctor only prescribes the most cost-effective.

ALUMINIUM HYDROXIDE

On prescription/over the counter
ALUMINIUM HYDROXIDE – Liquid, tablets
ALU-CAP – Capsules

Aluminium hydroxide is an antacid used to relieve indigestion which may or may not be due to an ulcer and to relieve discomfort in the oesophagus caused by excess stomach acid. Occasionally it is prescribed in large doses for removing high levels of phosphate which have formed kidney stones. Your doctor will supervise this form of treatment.

Before you use this medicine

Tell your doctor or pharmacist if you are:
☐ pregnant or breast-feeding ☐ taking any other medicines, including vitamins and those bought over the counter ☐ on a low-sodium diet – some antacids are low in sodium (Alu-Cap, for example) ☐ diabetic – some antacids are sugar-free.

Tell your doctor or pharmacist if you have or have had:
☐ severe or prolonged stomach pain ☐ blood in stools ☐ prolonged diarrhoea ☐ constipation ☐ piles ☐ metabolic bone disease – you should not take aluminium antacids ☐ kidney disease – you must not take aluminium antacids for long periods of time.

See your doctor immediately if you feel sick or vomit matter that looks like coffee grounds, suffer from stomach cramps or pain, or if you have black, tarry or speckled stools. These are signs of a bleeding ulcer.

How to use this medicine

Liquids are more effective than tablets or capsules, although these are more convenient to carry around; it is a good idea to keep a liquid at home and take tablets with you when you go out. Take four times daily about an hour after meals and at bedtime. Additional doses can be taken up to once an hour if needed. See your doctor if you take an antacid continuously for more than two weeks and feel no better.

Liquids must be shaken before use; tablets must be chewed well.

Over 65 No special requirements.

Interactions with other medicines

Antibiotics (particularly tetracyclines) and antifungals, warfarin and the heart drug digoxin Aluminium hydroxide may reduce the absorption of these and other medicines if taken at the same time.
Tablet coatings Aluminium antacids may damage enteric coatings, used to delay the release of a tablet into the gut.

Check with your doctor or pharmacist before taking an aluminium antacid with another medicine and avoid taking one within half an hour of any other medicine if possible.

Unwanted effects

Likely Constipation may develop: change to an antacid that does not contain aluminium or to one containing both aluminium and magnesium.

Lists of antacids containing both aluminium and magnesium and of those with additional ingredients appear after the profile of magnesium trisilicate on page 69.

MAGNESIUM TRISILICATE

On prescription/over the counter
MAGNESIUM TRISILICATE – Liquid, powder

Magnesium trisilicate is an antacid used to relieve indigestion which may or may not be due to an ulcer. It can also relieve discomfort caused by stomach acid in the oesophagus.

Before you use this medicine

Tell your doctor or pharmacist if you are:
☐ pregnant or breast-feeding ☐ taking any other medicines, including vitamins and those bought over the counter ☐ on a low-sodium diet – magnesium trisilicate and magnesium carbonate mixtures contain a lot of sodium ☐ diabetic – some mixtures are sugar-free.

Tell your doctor or pharmacist if you have or have had:
☐ severe or prolonged stomach pain ☐ blood in stools ☐ prolonged diarrhoea ☐ kidney disease – you must not take magnesium antacids for long periods as they stay in the body: you may feel drowsy, dizzy and weak ☐ metabolic bone disease – you should not take magnesium antacids containing aluminium.

See your doctor immediately if you feel sick or vomit matter that looks like coffee grounds, suffer from stomach cramps or pain, or if you have black, tarry or speckled stools. These are signs of a bleeding ulcer.

How to use this medicine

Liquid and powder preparations are more effective than tablets, although tablets are more convenient to carry around; it is a good idea to use liquid or powder preparations at home and take tablets with you when you go out. Take four times daily about an hour after meals and at bedtime. See your doctor if you take an antacid continuously for more than two weeks and feel no better.

Liquids must be shaken before use; tablets must be chewed well.

Over 65 No special requirements.

Interactions with other medicines

Antibiotics (particularly tetracyclines) and antifungals, the heart drug digoxin Magnesium antacids may reduce the absorption of these medicines.
Tablet coatings Magnesium antacids may damage enteric coatings, used to delay the release of a tablet into the gut.

Avoid taking a magnesium antacid at the same time as any other medicine if possible.

Unwanted effects

Likely Loose stools or diarrhoea may develop: change to an aluminium-containing antacid or to one containing both aluminium and magnesium.

Similar preparations

On prescription/over the counter
MAGNESIUM CARBONATE – Liquid

Antacids containing aluminium and magnesium

Over the counter
ALUDROX – Tablets
DIJEX – Liquid, tablets
GASTRILS – Pastilles
GELUSIL – Tablets

On prescription/over the counter
HYDROTALCITE – Liquid, tablets
MAALOX – Liquid
MAALOX TC – Liquid
MAGNESIUM TRISILICATE COMPOUND – Tablets
MAGALDRATE – Liquid
MUCOGEL – Liquid

Aluminium and magnesium with other ingredients

Over the counter
ACTONORM – Liquid
ALTACTITE PLUS – Liquid (also on prescription), tablets
ASILONE – Liquid (also on prescription), tablets
MAALOX PLUS – Liquid (also on prescription), tablets
SIMECO – Liquid, tablets
UNIGEST – Tablets

On prescription/over the counter
ALGICON – Tablets
DIOVOL – Liquid
GASTROCOTE – Liquid, tablets

Continued over

GASTRON – Tablets
GAVISCON – Liquid, powder, tablets
INFACOL – Liquid
INFANT GAVISCON – Powder
POLYCROL – Liquid, tablets (also high-dose Forte liquid, tablets)
TOPAL – Tablets

Poor choice
MUCAINE

• *SODIUM BICARBONATE* •

Taken as powder or tablets this works more quickly than either aluminium- or magnesium-containing antacids and is effective and cheap for relief of occasional indigestion. However, if taken in large doses for long periods it is absorbed into the body, where it can upset the blood chemistry. Like other carbonate-containing antacids, it releases carbon dioxide gas, which causes burping. This does not mean that the antacid is working more effectively; the gas it forms may be trapped in the stomach and add to discomfort. You should not use sodium bicarbonate if you have heart, liver or kidney problems or you are on a low-sodium diet.

• *CALCIUM AND BISMUTH* •

Some over-the-counter products contain either **calcium** or **bismuth** (see Box opposite). Short courses of a calcium-containing antacid or occasional doses are fine but high doses for long periods may rarely increase blood-calcium and upset the acid balance in the stomach. Calcium-containing antacids can also result in the stomach producing more acid after treatment although in practice this is rare.

Bismuth-containing antacids (although not **bismuth chelate**; see page 79) are best avoided, especially for prolonged use, because bismuth absorbed into the body can damage nerves. They also tend to cause constipation.

Other medicines for indigestion

• *ANTISPASMODIC MEDICINES* •

These relax the stomach and intestine's nervous control of the muscle around the stomach. They are sometimes used with other treatments for non-ulcer dyspepsia and irritable bowel syndrome.

POPULAR OVER-THE-COUNTER ANTACIDS

These antacids cost less than the prescription charge. Most contain several ingredients, such as **sodium bicarbonate + magnesium carbonate + calcium carbonate**. Here they are listed under their main ingredient.

Sodium bicarbonate-containing
BISMAG – Tablets

Calcium-containing
BISODOL – Tablets
BISODOL EXTRA – Tablets
OPAS – Tablets
RENNIE – Tablets
RENNIE GOLD – Tablets
NULACIN – Tablets
MACLEAN – Tablets
RAP-EZE – Tablets
SETLERS – Tablets, liquid
TUMS – Tablets

Also contain bismuth
MOORLAND – Tablets
BISMA-REX – Powder, tablets
JACKSON'S – Lozenges

Bismuth-containing (not recommended)
ROTER – Tablets (larger packs cost more than the prescription charge)
PEPTO-BISMOL – Liquid

They have been used for treating ulcers but the high doses needed to stop gastric acid production cause unwanted effects such as dry mouth, blurred vision, constipation and difficulty in passing urine. Older people are particularly sensitive to these effects, even at a lower dosage. If you have the eye problem *glaucoma* or a condition known as *paralytic ileus* you should not take these medicines. These medicines have been superseded by ulcer-healing drugs (see page 73) which are much more effective for treating ulcers and have fewer unwanted effects. The following over-the-counter remedies for indigestion and other stomach upsets contain small amounts of antispasmodics and are not recommended: **atropine** (brand name Actonorm), **belladonna** (Alka-Donna; Alka-Donna P; Aluhyde; Bellacarb), **homatropine** (APP Stomach Tablets and Powder) and **hyoscine** (Buscopan).

● *MOTILITY STIMULANTS* ●

Medicines that enhance or stimulate the movement of the intestine (*motility stimulants*) are used for treating non-ulcer dyspepsia and reflux oesophagitis. **Metoclopramide** and **domperidone** speed emptying of the stomach and increase the movement of the intestines thereby helping the flow of contents along the gut. They also help to enhance the narrowing of the muscle between the stomach and gullet and control acid leaking from the stomach into the gullet. Both drugs also act on the central nervous system as anti-emetics and are used for controlling nausea and vomiting (see page 227).

Metoclopramide and occasionally domperidone can cause unwanted *parkinsonian* effects (similar to the symptoms of Parkinson's disease), such as spasms of the facial muscles and abnormal movements of the eyes. Contact your doctor if these effects occur. The effects are more common in younger people (especially girls and young women) and the very old. They usually happen just after starting treatment, but will fade a day or so after stopping the drug.

Cisapride (brand names Alimix; Prepulsid) is a newer drug which is similar to metoclopramide and domperidone. It does not act on the central nervous system and is unlikely to cause parkinsonian unwanted effects.

Peptic ulcers

A peptic ulcer is a damaged section, rather like a small crater, in the lining of the stomach or intestine wall. It is caused by the irritant action of stomach acid which has broken through the layer of mucus that protects the tissue from harm. Peptic ulcers are known specifically as *gastric* or *duodenal* ulcers depending on whether they occur in the stomach or in the first part of the small intestine (*duodenum*). If an ulcer is left untreated it can burst (perforate), causing a great deal of pain, or it can bleed – sometimes severely. Most of the symptoms of indigestion can be caused by an ulcer, particularly if they go on for several weeks without relief. However, the pain from an ulcer can start suddenly and severely. A bleeding ulcer will cause you to vomit blood or matter that looks like coffee grounds or have black, tarry stools; you should see your doctor immediately if you have either of these symptoms. The

– HOW YOU CAN HELP YOURSELF –

- ☐ Give up smoking or at least cut down: any form of tobacco can irritate the digestive system
- ☐ Eat at regular intervals, avoiding large meals late at night
- ☐ Avoid alcohol
- ☐ Avoid foods and drinks you know cause you problems
- ☐ Avoid coffee, and spicy foods if you are not used to them
- ☐ Eat a sensible diet with plenty of roughage, although there is no need for a special diet
- ☐ Avoid medicines that irritate the stomach: use paracetamol instead of aspirin, for example.

causes are thought to include smoking, stress, alcohol, and some drugs, particularly aspirin and other non-steroidal anti-inflammatory drugs. Some people are prone to developing ulcers. Food, milk or antacids may relieve the pain, but you should see your doctor if you have indigestion for more than a few weeks or if it recurs regularly.

Ulcer-healing medicines

Some ulcer-healing medicines work by reducing the amount of acid in the digestive system; others form a protective layer over the ulcer. High doses of an antacid can promote ulcer-healing, but the amount of medicine that you have to take every day may be unacceptable. Sometimes several medicines are used together – for example, an antacid and an H_2-receptor antagonist – your doctor will advise you about this. You should not take these medicines for minor digestive disorders, such as occasional upset stomach, nausea or heartburn.

Before the introduction of H_2-receptor antagonists, many gastric ulcers were treated by surgical operations. Surgery can often be avoided now, but may be needed if complications develop. Your doctor may need to make sure that you have an ulcer and that there are no other underlying conditions, such as cancer, particularly if you are middle-aged or older, so you may have to attend an outpatient clinic in hospital to have a *gastroscopy* (also called *endoscopy* or OGD). This procedure involves swallowing a thin fibre-optic tube passed down the back of your throat into your stomach and duodenum, through which the ulcer can be seen. You do not need an anaesthetic for this, but you will be given a mild sedative.

● *H_2-RECEPTOR ANTAGONISTS* ●

These are *antihistamines* which block histamine receptors in the stomach to limit the flow of gastric acid (see 'Allergies and hay-fever', page 177). The H_2-receptor antagonists **cimetidine, ranitidine, famotidine** and **nizatidine** can all heal gastric and duodenal ulcers in one to two months and there is little to choose between them. They do not have many unwanted effects.

Although H_2-receptor antagonists have revolutionised the treatment of ulcers, an ulcer may recur once you finish a course of treatment. Your doctor may decide to treat you with further courses of an H_2-receptor antagonist each time this happens or put you on a lower dose for a longer period. The profile of cimetidine, over the page, is an example of how you should use any of this group of medicines.

CIMETIDINE

CIMETIDINE – Tablets
DYSPAMET – Chewable tablets, liquid
TAGAMET – Tablets, liquid, injection

Poor choice
ALGITEC – Chewable tablets, liquid
CIMETIDINE + ALGINIC ACID

Cimetidine is an H_2-receptor antagonist. It blocks the release of stomach acid and can heal ulcers in the oesophagus, stomach and duodenum.

Before you use this medicine

Tell your doctor if you if you are:
□ pregnant or breast-feeding □ taking any other medicines, including vitamins and those bought over the counter.

See your doctor immediately if you vomit blood or matter that looks like coffee grounds or if you have black, tarry stools. These are signs of a bleeding ulcer.

How to use this medicine

Your doctor will tell you for how long you must take cimetidine – it will be for at least a month, often two. Do not alter the dose without talking to your doctor. Avoid drinking alcohol or smoking. Do not stop taking this medicine before you finish the course of treatment, even if you feel much better.

Take the tablets twice a day, with breakfast and at bedtime. If you have a duodenal ulcer, you should take the whole dose at bedtime.

Over 65 You may need less than the adult dose if your kidney function is very poor.

Interactions with other medicines

Oral anticoagulants (warfarin, theophylline, phenytoin) Cimetidine increases the effects of these, so your doctor may need to adjust the dose. Other H_2-receptor antagonists, **ranitidine, famotidine** and **nizatidine**, do not interact with these medicines.

Unwanted effects

Unlikely Diarrhoea, rash, dizziness, tiredness, confusion, headache.
Rare but serious Blood disorders, muscle or joint pain, irregular heartbeat, swollen breasts. These usually occur only with high dosage and generally stop when you stop taking cimetidine.

Similar preparations

AXID – Capsules
NIZATIDINE

PEPCID PM – Tablets
FAMOTIDINE

ZANTAC – Tablets, soluble tablets, liquid, injection
RANITIDINE

● *NSAID-ASSOCIATED ULCERS* ●

Non-steroidal anti-inflammatory drugs (NSAIDs) are widely prescribed for the treatment of arthritis and other painful conditions. If you take an NSAID you may experience indigestion, which is a common unwanted effect; this does not necessarily mean that you will develop an ulcer, although it is more likely if you are over 60 or have had an ulcer previously. NSAID-induced ulcers can develop and even bleed or perforate without causing pain or any other warning symptom.

Sometimes they heal themselves despite your continuing to take an NSAID, but if you have to continue treatment you may be prescribed an H_2-receptor antagonist or one of two newer medicines – **misoprostol** (brand name Cytotec) or **omeprazole** (Losec) – to heal the ulcer. Misoprostol and the H_2-receptor antagonist ranitidine can both be prescribed to prevent this sort of ulcer in people who are at risk. Misoprostol is not very useful for treating or preventing ulcers not associated with NSAIDs and will not treat indigestion caused by an NSAID unless the person has an ulcer.

MISOPROSTOL

CYTOTEC – Tablets
NAPRATEC – **Naproxen** (an NSAID) and misoprostol tablets in a combination pack

Misoprostol works in a different way to the H_2-receptor antagonists. It is related to a substance formed in the stomach that reduces the production of stomach acid and promotes the formation of mucus and new cells. Misoprostol can be used for treating ulcers, whether or not caused by an NSAID. It can also prevent ulcers forming if taken with an NSAID, but does not relieve indigestion. If you have already had a peptic ulcer or you are elderly, and need an NSAID, your doctor may consider adding misoprostol to your prescription.

Before you use this medicine

Tell your doctor if you are:
☐ pregnant or planning to become pregnant – **misoprostol must not be taken during pregnancy**; if you still have monthly periods, you must take effective contraceptive measures to make sure that you do not become pregnant during treatment ☐ breast-feeding ☐ taking any other medicines, including vitamins and those bought over the counter.

If you have low blood pressure, heart disease, narrowing of the arteries or have had a stroke, see your doctor for regular check-ups.

How to use this medicine

The usual dose is four tablets a day: you can either take **two** tablets **twice** a day with breakfast and at bedtime or you can take **one** tablet **four** times a day with or just after meals. If you develop diarrhoea whilst on misoprostol, taking one dose four times a day after meals may help this problem. Treatment for existing ulcers usually lasts for a month or two months.

Avoid drinking alcohol or smoking. Do not stop taking this medicine until you have finished the course of treatment, even if you feel much better. If you miss a dose take it as soon as you remember, but skip it if it is almost time for your next dose. Do not take double the dose.

Over 65 No special requirements.

Interactions with other medicines

None is known, but avoid magnesium-containing antacids, especially if diarrhoea is a problem.

Unwanted effects

Misoprostol is still quite a new medicine. Tell your doctor if you experience any unwanted effects or notice any changes while taking it.

Likely Loose stools or diarrhoea – if the diarrhoea is severe, you must contact your doctor, who will decide whether you should continue treatment. Other effects include feeling or being sick, indigestion, excess wind and stomach cramps.
Unlikely Vomiting, dizziness, skin rashes.
Rare but serious There have been occasional reports of women experiencing heavier than usual monthly periods and bleeding in between periods, and of women who have stopped menstruating bleeding. See your doctor if you experience any of these effects.

OMEPRAZOLE

LOSEC – Capsules

Omeprazole blocks stomach acid production completely by binding to an enzyme which is necessary for acid manufacture. It is used for treating ulcers, including those caused by NSAIDs, oesophagitis and other rarer conditions. An ulcer will heal while you take omeprazole, but may recur after you stop treatment. Omeprazole works very specifically in the body and patients generally tolerate it well.

Before you use this medicine

Tell your doctor if you are:

☐ pregnant or breast-feeding, taking any other medicines, including vitamins and those bought over the counter.

Tell your doctor if you have or have had:
☐ kidney or liver disease.

How to use this medicine

The usual dose is one capsule daily for one month, sometimes two months, although your doctor may decide that you need two capsules a day. Take the capsule at a regular time each day. If you have reflux oesophagitis you may be given a lower dose for longer periods.

Avoid drinking alcohol or smoking. Do not stop taking this medicine until you have completed the course of treatment, even if you feel much better. If you miss a dose take it as soon as you remember, but skip it if it is almost time for your next dose. Do not take double the dose.

Over 65 No special requirements.

Interactions with other medicines

Phenytoin, warfarin Effects enhanced by omeprazole, so the doses may need reducing.
Diazepam Possible increased effects.

Unwanted effects

Omprazole is a new medicine, so its effects are being monitored. Tell your doctor if you experience any unwanted effects. Unwanted effects are rare, and those that occur seem to pass off quite quickly.
Unlikely Feeling sick, headache, diarrhoea, constipation, excess wind.
Rare Skin rashes.

• *MEDICINES THAT PROTECT THE STOMACH* •

In **bismuth chelate** (brand name De-Nol) bismuth is bound in a *complex*, unlike bismuth antacids, which means that very little is absorbed into the body. **Sucralfate** (brand name Antepsin) is an aluminium complex which must be taken four times daily, either as liquid or tablets. The tablets are large, but can be dispersed in a little water. You must not take sucralfate at the same time as other medicines, particularly antacids, phenytoin, tetracyclines, cimetidine or digoxin: allow two hours in between taking sucralfate and any other medicines. Constipation is a common unwanted effect.

BISMUTH CHELATE

DE-NOL – Liquid DE-NOLTAB – Tablets

Bismuth chelate is effective in healing gastric and duodenal ulcers. It seems to rid the stomach of a bacterium which appears to play a part in ulcer formation in some people. If this bacterium is found in your stomach, your doctor may also prescribe an antibiotic. Bismuth also seems to coat the ulcer and protect it from stomach acid.

Before you use this medicine

Tell your doctor if you are: □ pregnant or breast-feeding □ taking any other medicines, including vitamins and those bought over the counter.

Tell your doctor if you have or have had:
□ severe kidney disease.

How to use this medicine

Bismuth chelate can be taken either as liquid or tablets but always on an empty stomach, generally twice daily, half an hour before breakfast and half an hour before the evening meal. Alternatively you may take a smaller dose four times a day.

Tablets are as effective as the liquid and more pleasant to take. The liquid has a strong ammonia smell which you may find unpleasant. Each dose of tablets should be swallowed with a tumblerful of water. Each dose of liquid must be diluted with a tablespoonful of water.

You may be given one month's treatment, immediately followed by another if necessary. A further month's course may be necessary after a bismuth-free period of a month. Bismuth chelate is not given continuously as maintenance treatment.

Food interferes with bismuth chelate's action. Milk should not be drunk by itself during a course of treatment but may be taken in small amounts in tea or coffee or on cereal. Alcohol should be avoided.

Do not stop taking this medicine until you finish the full course of treatment. If you miss a dose take it as soon as you remember it, but skip it if it is almost time for your next dose. Do not take double the dose and always take the medicine on an empty stomach.

Over 65 No special requirements.

Interactions with other medicines

Antacids interfere with the action of bismuth chelate and should not be taken for half an hour before or after a dose.
Tetracyclines Effectiveness reduced by bismuth chelate.

Unwanted effects

Likely Discoloration or blackening of faeces.
Unlikely Feeling or being sick.

• *OTHER ULCER-HEALING MEDICINES* •

Pirenzepine (brand name Gastrozepin) is an *antimuscarinic* drug (see page 197) sometimes used for healing ulcers. It has fewer unwanted effects than other antimuscarinic drugs. Medicines based on **liquorice** cannot now be recommended because the H_2-receptor antagonists are more effective. **Carbenoxolone** preparations (brand names Biogastrone; Pyrogastrone) can promote ulcer-healing but their adverse effects are difficult to manage, especially for people over 65. These effects include salt and water retention, and a lowering of blood-potassium. The **liquorice derivative** Caved-S has few unwanted effects but is not very effective.

Acute diarrhoea

Diarrhoea is an increase in the frequency and looseness of your bowel movements. Water is normally absorbed from the remnants of digested food in the large intestine and the waste left over from this water recycling process becomes stools, which are then passed out of the body at regular intervals. If this absorption process is upset, less water is taken back into the body and the remainder is passed out in liquid stools. Serious loss of water is called *dehydration*; it causes thirst, dry mouth, dry skin, reduction in quantity and darkening of urine, fast breathing and fever.

Sudden (acute) diarrhoea generally lasts only a few days and may get better whether you treat it or not. However, for babies, young children, and frail or elderly people, diarrhoea can be serious and must be treated with glucose and salt solution (see page 82) to replace the body's lost water and salts if it causes dehydration or lasts for more than a few hours. Common causes include viral or bacterial infections in the digestive system (food poisoning) or a change of country and climate when your body is not yet immune to a new set of bacteria and viruses (often called 'traveller's diarrhoea').

Anxiety, alcohol, food intolerance and some medicines (for example some antibiotics, magnesium-containing antacids, the ulcer-healing drug misoprostol, stimulant laxatives, medicines for high blood pressure and those for regulating the heartbeat) can also cause acute diarrhoea.

Prolonged (chronic) diarrhoea usually has other causes and does not clear up like acute diarrhoea. Your doctor will need to diagnose and treat it; see page 85.

– HOW YOU CAN HELP YOURSELF –

• *ACUTE DIARRHOEA* •

☐ Avoid solid food for 24 hours; do not eat dairy products, spicy or fatty foods, fresh fruit and vegetables or any other food you do not tolerate well; do not drink milk, coffee or concentrated fruit juices

☐ Drink plenty of clear liquids (at least four glasses every 12 hours) – weak tea without milk, for example; children should be given extra liquids immediately – the glucose and salt solution described on page 83 is ideal

☐ Monitor your temperature

☐ Depending on the severity of the attack, you may need to stay in bed and rest

☐ If you have to remain active, you can avoid inconvenience and embarrassment by taking an antidiarrhoeal medicine

☐ Always wash your hands after you have been to the toilet to prevent the spread of infection

☐ When you begin to feel like eating again, re-introduce food gradually; start with, say, dry toast or cracker biscuits with a clear soup and leave out dairy products and fatty food until later.

Contact your doctor if:

☐ A baby or young child, a frail person (someone who is weak and ill already) or an elderly person has acute and severe diarrhoea

☐ Diarrhoea lasts for more than three days

☐ You have a fever: temperature above 38·5°C (101°F)

☐ Severe, disabling stomach pains accompany diarrhoea

☐ There is blood in your stools or they are black and tarry

☐ You have dehydration, characterised by dizziness while standing, confusion or drowsiness

☐ A medicine may be the cause of diarrhoea.

Medicines for diarrhoea

In an acute attack of mild to moderate diarrhoea, you can replace the water and salts lost from your body with a glucose and salts solution. Glucose increases the amount of water absorbed in the large intestine, which allows the salts in the solution to get into your body, too. This process is called *rehydration*. The aim of the treatment is to prevent dehydration developing, particularly in babies and the elderly, both of whom should be seen by a doctor.

The diarrhoea in these cases is the body's way of getting rid of harmful substances and it may be unhelpful to interfere with this natural response. Most people with acute but mild diarrhoea get better so quickly using oral rehydration salts and a light diet that the use of any other medicine is unnecessary. However, antidiarrhoeal medicines may sometimes be useful; they are discussed briefly after the profile of oral rehydration salts, below.

ORAL REHYDRATION SALTS

On prescription/from a pharmacy
DIOCALM JUNIOR – Soluble powder
DIORALYTE – Soluble powder, effervescent tablets
ELECTROLADE – Soluble powder
GLUCO-LYTE – Soluble powder
RAPOLYTE – Soluble powder
REHIDRAT – Soluble powder

A mixture of salts and glucose powder must be dissolved in water and made into a solution for drinking. There are several recipes for oral rehydration salts but the formula that is used most in the UK is based on sodium chloride, potassium chloride, sodium bicarbonate and glucose. You can buy sachets of ready-prepared, flavoured powders in a pharmacy.

If the diarrhoea is not too severe or you do not have a ready-prepared powder to hand, you can make your own mixture (see right). The commercial solutions should be substituted as soon as possible if the attack is prolonged, if you are more severely ill or if dehydration has already started.

Before you use this medicine

Tell your doctor or pharmacist if you are:
☐ diabetic – the glucose (sugar) content of the solution should not

cause a problem □ taking any medicines, such as laxatives or magnesium-containing antacids □ pregnant or breast-feeding.

Always contact your doctor if diarrhoea does not get better within three days or if you are suffering severe vomiting. People over 70, frail people, babies and children under three years must be seen by a doctor.

How to use this medicine

The powder in one sachet or the tablets should be dissolved in 200–250ml (7–8fl oz) of drinking water, depending on the instructions given with the particular product. Do not add extra salt, sugar or glucose: make up the solution exactly as instructed. A weaker than instructed solution will not be effective. The solution should be made just before it is needed, but can be kept in a refrigerator for up to 24 hours. If it cannot be stored in a fridge, the solution must be thrown away after one hour. For babies and children under three use freshly boiled and cooled water, but do not reboil the prepared solution.

An adult usually needs around 200–400ml (half to one pint) of prepared solution after liquid stools are passed; a child needs approximately 200ml. If you feel sick or are being sick, take sips of the solution as frequently as possible.

Over 65 No special requirements.

Unwanted effects

Likely Feeling of sickness (nausea); flavoured solutions can help to overcome the taste.

HOME-MADE SALT AND GLUCOSE SOLUTION

Use one small level teaspoon (3·5g) of salt and eight large level teaspoons (40g) of sugar – or four large level teaspoons (20g) of glucose powder – to one litre of water. A small amount of fruit juice or squash can be added to flavour the solution.

You can get a two-ended spoon, the large end for sugar and the small end for salt from Teaching Aids at Low Cost (see 'Useful addresses').

– HOW YOU CAN HELP YOURSELF –

• *TRAVELLER'S DIARRHOEA* •

☐ Avoid drinking tap water unless you are sure that it is fit to drink. Use chemical water-purifying tablets or ten drops of weak iodine solution to a litre of water in parts of the world where water supplies are suspect. In areas where amoebic dysentery is likely, boiling water for half an hour will kill the organisms and any amoebic cysts satisfactorily
☐ Avoid ice cubes in your drinks unless you are sure of the water
☐ Avoid eating unwashed salads and unpeeled fruit (even in drinks)
☐ Wash your hands before you eat, or use an antiseptic wipe
☐ Take with you a supply of salt and glucose sachets and an antidiarrhoeal medicine
☐ Do not buy or use an antibiotic to treat diarrhoea, unless under guidance from a doctor.

• *ANTIDIARRHOEAL MEDICINES* •

Treating diarrhoea with an antidiarrhoeal medicine is of less importance than rehydration and should not distract you from fluid replacement measures. For adults, it can help to overcome some of the inconvenience and embarrassment associated with an acute attack. Babies, young children, frail people and elderly people must always be rehydrated with glucose and salts solution; they should avoid antidiarrhoeal medicines.

• ***Adsorbent medicines***

These form bulk in the intestines; mixtures of chalk and kaolin are sometimes used in mild chronic diarrhoea. They are not recommended for acute diarrhoea.

• ***Antimotility medicines***

These slow down intestinal movement (*peristalsis*). Although these medicines relieve diarrhoea symptoms, they can prolong contact between harmful micro-organisms and the intestinal cells. Opioids (derivatives of the poppy plant) have long been used: these include liquid mixtures of **opium** or **morphine** (such as Kaolin and Morphine mixture BP) or tablets. Over-the-counter products include Enterosan, Diocalm, Diocare and J Collis Browne. **Codeine** (brand names Diarrest; Kaodene) and **co-phenotrope** (brand name Lomotil) are also used. These products are of limited use in controlling acute diarrhoea.

They can reduce breathing and cause constipation and even dependence after prolonged use of high doses. Lomotil was an important cause of accidental poisoning in young children before oral rehydration was introduced and symptoms of overdosage can occur after as little as one dose; children under four must not be given Lomotil.

Loperamide (brand names Imodium; Arret; Diocalm Ultra) works more specifically on the intestinal wall and does not have so many unwanted effects. It is the most useful medicine for temporarily suppressing acute diarrhoea in adults.

• *ANTIBIOTICS* •

Antibiotics were used to treat acute diarrhoea until it was realised that they seldom helped, even when a micro-organism was involved. A doctor will sometimes prescribe an antibiotic, usually after investigation of a stool sample. For example, co-trimoxazole or trimethoprim may reduce the severity and duration of traveller's diarrhoea; metronidazole is used for amoebic dysentery and *giardiasis* (see page 294).

Chronic diarrhoea

Chronic diarrhoea is a long-term condition where the stools are loose or watery, and sometimes bloody or fatty. The diarrhoea does not clear up with the usual treatment for acute diarrhoea, and can eventually result in weight loss, anaemia and various forms of malnutrition. Your doctor will need to investigate your condition carefully, because some of the causes of chronic diarrhoea are serious, and include bowel cancer.

• *Irritable bowel syndrome*

Irritable bowel syndrome (IBS) is a very common disorder of bowel movement. Its symptoms include griping, colicky pain across the lower abdomen and a disturbed bowel habit alternating between frequent, loose stools and constipation with hard, 'rabbit-pellet' stools. Diarrhoea often occurs at the onset of pain, but the pain is reduced once you have had a bowel movement. You may pass mucus and feel that you have not emptied your bowel completely. You may feel sick or have flatulence, heartburn, bloating, wind or fatigue. These symptoms can be intermittent or you may experience them all the time.

Although the cause of IBS is not clear, symptoms often start after an acute intestinal infection. Stress and some foods (although not on an allergic basis) can both trigger IBS. Women under 40 seem to suffer most from IBS and symptoms are often worse before a period. You should see your doctor if you are worried or have severe, persistent and recurrent symptoms, particularly if you are over 50 when you develop symptoms. You may need to have some tests in hospital, particularly if the first treatment has not worked.

● *Ulcerative colitis and Crohn's disease*

Ulcerative colitis and *Crohn's disease* are uncommon inflammatory bowel diseases, the causes of which are unknown. The wall of the intestine becomes inflamed, causing bouts of colicky pain and frequent diarrhoea with blood. You may feel unwell, lose your appetite and lose weight because food is not properly absorbed. Ulcerative colitis involves only the large intestine, while Crohn's disease can also affect the small intestine. *Proctitis* is a similar condition which affects only the rectum and is seldom severe.

These inflammatory bowel diseases cannot be cured, but medicines can suppress the inflammation, control the symptoms and prevent complications, such as anaemia or perforation of the intestine. Sometimes these diseases will subside, but may then recur, so prolonged 'maintenance' treatment is often needed. Surgery may be necessary to remove damaged parts of the intestine.

● *Malabsorption syndromes*

Sometimes the body cannot absorb one or more nutrients from the digestive system (*malabsorption syndrome*) and chronic diarrhoea may result. The stools are often fatty. Once the offending nutrient is known, you can avoid it, so relieving the diarrhoea, but you may need to take particular replacement products. For example, a child who is lactose-intolerant will have to avoid cow's milk as this is high in lactose, but may then need a substitute milk product which is lactose-free. *Coeliac disease* is caused by an allergy to gluten, which is found in wheat, and requires a very strict diet supplemented with special gluten-free products. Your doctor can prescribe a range of these special products.

HOW YOU CAN HELP YOURSELF

☐ Make sure you have a healthy diet with plenty of fluids, high in fibre and with foods that suit your body – a high-fibre diet is the most helpful treatment for irritable bowel syndrome
☐ Some people find that milk aggravates their system – it might be worth avoiding milk to see if it helps your condition
☐ Reduce stress in your life as far as possible, for example by taking regular exercise and using relaxation techniques – excessive stress is known to aggravate these diseases
☐ Rest in bed during acute attacks
☐ In cases of ulcerative colitis and Crohn's disease see your doctor regularly for checks – you will probably have to see a hospital doctor as well as your GP.

Medicines for chronic diarrhoeas

• *IRRITABLE BOWEL SYNDROME (IBS)* •

It may not be necessary to take a medicine to control your symptoms if they are mild and intermittent and you benefit from a high-fibre diet. An explanation of IBS by your doctor, so that you have a thorough understanding of your condition, can be very valuable. However, your doctor may decide that drug treatment can help relieve your symptoms, particularly at first while you are improving your diet. Bulk-forming preparations (see page 94) are used to improve the consistency and regularity of bowel movements because diarrhoea in the case of IBS is often related to underlying constipation. For this reason antidiarrhoeal medicines should not be used.

Antispasmodic medicines work either by slowing down intestinal movement or by exerting a direct relaxant effect on intestinal muscle; **dicyclomine** (brand name Merbentyl) appears to work both ways. They relieve stomach cramps and colicky abdominal pain. Those based on atropine have a limited use because of their unwanted effects (dry mouth, problems with vision and difficulty with passing urine). **Alverine** (brand name Spasmonal), **peppermint oil** and **mebeverine** (brand names Colofac; Colven) in particular are of some value because they act only on the digestive system. Peppermint oil is contained in capsules (brand names Colpermin; Mintec), which should be taken for two to three months. The capsules must be swallowed whole, otherwise oil released into the mouth and gullet will cause irritation. Antidepressants are used very occasionally; they may help relieve symptoms of IBS whether or not you are depressed.

MEBEVERINE HYDROCHLORIDE

COLOFAC – Liquid, tablets

COLVEN – Granules

MEBEVERINE + ISPAGHULA HUSK – see page 94

Mebeverine has a direct relaxant effect on intestinal smooth muscle. It is used for the relief of colicky abdominal pains, stomach cramps and spasm associated with irritable bowel syndrome and similar conditions. Mebeverine has few unwanted effects and does not cause the atropine-like effects of some other antispasmodics.

Before you use this medicine

Tell your doctor if you are:
□ lactose- or sucrose-intolerant – mebeverine tablets contain these sugars, but the liquid does not □ pregnant or breast-feeding □ taking any medicines, including vitamins and those bought over the counter.

Tell your doctor if you have:
□ Paralytic ileus or diverticulitis of the colon – like all antispasmodics, mebeverine should not be given to someone with these conditions
□ porphyria – mebeverine should be avoided
□ reduced kidney function – mebeverine+ispaghula granules should be avoided because of a high sodium content.

How to use this medicine

Take one tablet three times a day with a glassful of water, 20 minutes before meals. Shake the liquid suspension well before taking the dose (three 5ml spoonfuls). Your doctor will tell you how many weeks you need to take the medicine. You may be able to reduce the dose gradually once the symptoms are under control. If you miss a dose, take it as soon as you remember, but skip it if it is almost time for your next dose. Do not take double the dose.

Over 65 No special requirements.

Unwanted effects

Mebeverine can aggravate IBS if there is underlying constipation, which is commonly the case; you may be constipated even if you defaecate every day.

• *ULCERATIVE COLITIS* •

For acute attacks your doctor may prescribe a rectal *corticosteroid* enema or foam to be inserted into the rectum at bedtime or twice daily. A corticosteroid reduces inflammation of the intestinal wall and brings the symptoms under control. Administering a corticosteroid directly into the bowel avoids some of the adverse effects such as moon face, thinning of the skin and weight gain that can occur with a corticosteroid taken by mouth for long periods. Treatment is usually limited to three- or four-week courses, so the corticosteroid does not cause unwanted effects throughout the body (*systemically*). Some absorption can occur with prolonged treatment, should this prove necessary, and then you may need additional doses of a corticosteroid in times of major stress, such as surgery. Liquid and foam preparations are equally effective. Foam products are easier to use and more convenient, especially if you have difficulty retaining a liquid enema. Suppositories are prescribed for proctitis.

Sometimes it may be necessary to take the corticosteroid **prednisolone** by mouth. Your doctor should prescribe ordinary prednisolone tablets, not the red or brown *enteric-coated* type (brand name Deltacortril Enteric) as these act slowly and are less effective in diarrhoeal diseases. A corticosteroid is not taken all the time and the dose will be tapered off gradually once the disease is under control. In acute flare-ups you may need to be admitted to hospital.

Sulphasalazine (brand name Salazopyrin) or one of the newer related drugs, **mesalazine** (Asacol; Pentasa) or **olsalazine** (Dipentum) also reduce inflammation. They are widely used to prevent relapse and may also be used for treating mild ulcerative colitis. Each of these medicines has its own pattern of unwanted effects and the newer preparations often cause diarrhoea which can be confused with an exacerbation of the underlying disease.

SULPHASALAZINE

SULPHASALAZINE – Tablets
SALAZOPYRIN – Tablets, enteric-coated tablets, liquid, suppositories, retention enema

Sulphasalazine is used for reducing intestinal inflammation in ulcerative colitis and Crohn's disease. It is used for treating active ulcerative colitis and for maintenance once the disease has been controlled. Sulphasalazine splits into two chemicals in the body and unwanted effects are caused by both parts. Some unwanted effects can be diminished by a gradual increase in the daily dose to the full dosage, but in high doses unwanted effects are common. If you cannot tolerate sulphasalazine, you may be prescribed olsalazine or mesalazine; each has different unwanted effects.

Sulphasalazine is also used for treating rheumatoid arthritis (see page 374) as it has an anti-inflammatory effect and suppresses the disease process.

Before you use this medicine

Tell your doctor if you are:
☐ pregnant – sulphasalazine should be used with caution, although there is no evidence of risk to the foetus ☐ breast-feeding ☐ taking any other medicines, including vitamins and those bought over the counter.

Tell your doctor if you have or have had:
☐ severe kidney or liver disease ☐ lack of glucose-6-phosphate dehydrogenase (G6PD) ☐ a blood disorder ☐ allergy to *sulphonamides* or *salicylates* (for example, aspirin) ☐ porphyria.

How to use this medicine

Take the tablets or liquid regularly four times a day. The night-time interval between doses should be no more than eight hours. During an acute attack a corticosteroid may be prescribed alongside sulphasalazine. For ulcerative colitis treatment may be needed for several years to prevent relapse.

Suppositories may be used for treating inflammatory disease in the rectum either alone or in conjunction with tablets. They are inserted into the rectum in the morning and at bedtime after defaecation. Enemas should be given once a day towards bedtime and the liquid retained in the rectum for at least one hour.

Drink plenty of fluids while you are taking sulphasalazine. Eat plenty of green vegetables because sulphasalazine can reduce the absorption of folic acid and iron. Your doctor may check blood and liver function at the start of treatment.

Until you know how you react to sulphasalazine, do not drive or do other activities that require alertness.

Do not stop taking sulphasalazine suddenly: take the full course of treatment even if you feel better. If you miss a dose take it as soon as you remember. If your next dose is due within two hours, take the missed dose immediately and omit the next dose.

Over 65 No special dosage requirements.

Interactions with other medicines

Oral anticoagulants (such as **warfarin**), **oral antidiabetics** (such as **chlorpropamide**), **antiepileptics** (such as **phenytoin**) The sulphonamide part of sulphasalazine may increase the effects of these.

Unwanted effects

Likely Headache, feeling or being sick, loss of appetite, rash.
Unlikely Fever, temporary sterility in men – reversible on stopping treatment or changing to an alternative treatment.
Rarely Blood disorders, generalised skin eruptions, tinnitus, dizziness.

Sulphasalazine may colour the urine orange-yellow and extended-wear soft contact lenses may stain permanently. Daily-wear soft contact and gas-permeable lenses should respond to routine cleansing.

Similar preparations

ASACOL – Tablets, suppositories
MESALAZINE

DIPENTUM – Capsules
OLSALAZINE

PENTASA – Tablets, enema
MESALAZINE

Sometimes your doctor may consider trying a medicine that suppresses the immune system (*immunosuppressant*), such as **azathioprine**, if other measures have not been successful. This treatment will be closely supervised.

The symptoms of mild ulcerative colitis can be controlled with an antidiarrhoeal medicine (see page 84), such as **codeine** or **loperamide**, but not for long periods. An antidiarrhoeal should not be used alone for treating colitis because it does not reduce the inflammation and may cause constipation, which aggravates the disease. Antispasmodic medicines (see page 70) are not helpful in ulcerative colitis. Bulk-forming agents (see page 94) may be needed to adjust the consistency of stools.

• *CROHN'S DISEASE* •

If the large intestine is inflamed then treatment is similar to ulcerative colitis. Active disease of the small intestine is usually treated with a corticosteroid to damp down the inflammation. Sometimes an antibacterial may be prescribed to control bacterial overgrowth in the small intestine.

Both ulcerative colitis and Crohn's disease can cause general ill health because your body may not absorb nutrients and water properly through the intestinal wall. You may need food, mineral and vitamin supplements and rehydration treatment to prevent malnutrition. Your doctor will advise you about the supplements you need; you should not buy them over the counter without taking advice.

Constipation

Constipation is the difficult and infrequent, sometimes painful, passage of hard stools. Water and salts are absorbed into the body from the remnants of digested food in the bowel (large intestine or colon). The residue in the bowel becomes stools and as the bowel fills up, the urge to defaecate develops. If the movement of digested food through the intestines is too slow, too much water is absorbed in the bowel and the stools become hard and dry and difficult to pass.

Healthy people can have from two bowel movements a week to three movements a day. If there is a change in the frequency of your bowel movement, from every day to less than twice a week, for example, or you are having difficulty passing stools, then you are constipated. However, you do not need to treat yourself with a laxative: the commonest cause of constipation is a lack of roughage or fibre in Western diets. It is essential to include in your diet high-fibre food and plenty of liquids.

Irritable bowel syndrome often involves underlying constipation, even when loose, watery stools are being passed.

HOW YOU CAN HELP YOURSELF

☐ Eat a balanced diet high in fibre to maintain health and prevent constipation
☐ Take daily exercise to help maintain regular bowel movements
☐ Do not ignore the body's urge to pass stools
☐ Try to develop a regular time to defaecate – after a meal for instance
☐ Do not become preoccupied with your bowel function
☐ If you do become constipated, increase your daily intake of fibre and non-alcoholic liquids such as fruit juice
☐ A change in bowel habit may not necessarily be simple constipation: if you have pain, notice bleeding when you pass stools, or you are worried, see your doctor.

Laxatives

Medicines for relieving constipation are known as laxatives. They are broadly grouped as *bulk-forming medicines, stimulants, softeners* and *osmotic laxatives*, but some drugs act in more than one way. A laxative may be needed to relieve constipation or painful passage of stools when:

☐ you have an illness which causes temporary constipation (a feverish illness or one that keeps you in bed, for example)
☐ straining at stool might worsen a condition such as angina, myocardial infarction, haemorrhoids or anal fissure
☐ constipation is an unwanted effect of a medicine, such as the pain-relievers morphine, codeine and related opioids, antimuscarinics, antidepressants and aluminium antacids
☐ an elderly person develops constipation due to poor mobility.

A laxative may also be used to prepare the bowel for surgery or radiological procedures.

A laxative should only be used for a short period and once your normal bowel movement is re-established, you should maintain the routine with additional roughage in your diet. If a laxative is taken every day, your bowel will become dependent on it to function. Long-term use of regular doses of a powerful laxative will make the bowel insensitive to it. This results in constipation again. In some cases the nerves controlling the bowel muscles are destroyed and the bowel ceases to work on its own.

If a laxative is needed, bran or another bulk-forming agent is best for long-term use and is particularly suitable for people over 60. If a bulk-forming agent is ineffective or difficult to take then a stimulant laxative, such as senna, could either be added or substituted for a short time.

Children, especially young ones, should not be given laxatives, but their diet can be adjusted. If dietary changes do not make any difference, discuss your child's problem with a doctor.

BULK-FORMING MEDICINES

These retain water and increase the mass of stools and residue in the bowel, which stimulates bowel movement (*peristalsis*). They are useful for relieving constipation and in conditions where the consistency of stools needs to be improved, such as irritable bowel syndrome, and for patients with *colostomy* and *ileostomy*. Bulking agents take some days to produce an effect.

All the bulk-forming agents must be taken with plenty of water or other liquids to lubricate the bowel and to prevent them from becoming jammed in the intestine. If you have an intestinal stricture or the muscles of your bowel are damaged, you should not take a bulk-forming agent. All the products are effective and there is little to choose between them. However, there are differences in presentation and taste, so you should find a product that suits you.

Raw, unprocessed bran is slightly more effective than fine, processed bran but you may find the finer, cooked bran more palatable. You need 10–30g a day of raw bran, which can be added to any food at the table. You should increase the amount of bran you eat gradually until the passage of stools is comfortable. Do not take a whole day's dose with one meal. If you have a high requirement for calcium, iron or zinc you should take processed bran because these minerals can be removed from the intestine by coarse bran. Bran can cause excess wind and bloating, which you may find unpleasant. Do not take bran if you are gluten-sensitive or have coeliac disease.

Many cereals, breads and biscuits contain bran – you may find these as effective as raw bran and more acceptable. You can also buy medicinal bran preparations (Fybranta and Proctofibe, for example).

ISPAGHULA HUSK

On prescription/over the counter
FYBOGEL – Granules
ISOGEL – Granules
METAMUCIL – Powder
REGULAN – Powder

n.b. When buying over the counter, Isogel and Metamucil are cheaper.

Ispaghula husk is a general term for preparations containing ground seed husks of the Plantago species (plantain). The seeds swell on contact with water.

Ispaghula is a bulk-forming laxative which is used to treat constipation and other long-term conditions where stool consistency requires regulating, such as irritable bowel syndrome, ulcerative colitis, haemorrhoids and patients with colostomy or ileostomy.

While taking ispaghula you must take plenty of water or other liquids so that the bulking agent passes down the digestive tract and does not stick or cause an obstruction.

Before you use this medicine

Tell your doctor or pharmacist:
☐ whether your constipation happens often or was a sudden change.

Tell your doctor or pharmacist if you are:
☐ pregnant or breast-feeding ☐ diabetic – avoid Metamucil, which contains sugar (other preparations are sugar-free) ☐ gluten-sensitive – two preparations are gluten-free (Metamucil, Fybogel) ☐ taking any medicines, including vitamins and those bought over the counter.

Ispaghula and other bulking agents must not be used when any part of the intestine is blocked or when the stools are hard, dry and blocking the bowel (impacted). They cannot be used if the bowel's nerves and muscles are destroyed.

How to use this medicine

Take the recommended dose in half a glass of water, stir the granules or powder briskly and drink immediately. Carbonated water can be used for non-effervescent preparations or you can flavour the water with a fruit squash. Take ispaghula at meal times or just after, but not immediately before going to bed; you may need to take a dose once, twice or three times a day depending on your bowel action.

Always drink plenty of non-alcoholic drinks while you are on a course of ispaghula, so that the bulking agent passes down the digestive tract and does not stick or cause an obstruction.

Over 65 No special requirements. This is the best choice of laxative.

Unwanted effects

Likely Excess wind, flatulence, bloating.
Rarely but serious Intestinal obstruction if liquid intake is insufficient.

Similar preparations

On prescription/over the counter
CELEVAC – Tablets
METHYLCELLULOSE
FYBRANTA – Tablets (not on prescription)
BRAN
NORMACOL – Granules
STERCULIA
NORMACOL PLUS – Granules
STERCULIA+FRANGULA
PROCTOFIBE – Tablets (not on prescription)
BRAN
TRIFYBA – Powder
BRAN

• *STIMULANT LAXATIVES* •

Stimulant laxatives speed up intestinal movement (increase *motility*). Most take eight to twelve hours to work and can be taken at bedtime. When the bowel is loaded and a bulking agent is ineffective, a short course of stimulant laxative can be helpful. Stimulant laxatives must not be taken for long periods, as they can destroy the nerves to the bowel and so prevent the normal defaecation process. They must not be used if there is an intestinal obstruction and should be avoided in pregnancy.

Stimulant laxatives can cause stomach cramps and griping. If the dose is too high, diarrhoea may occur. You should start with a low dose and increase it gradually until you feel comfortable passing stools.

Senna, an established laxative since ancient times, is a good choice and is cheap to buy over the counter.

• *STOOL SOFTENERS* •

Any effective laxative softens stools, in particular bulk-forming agents, glycerol and docusate. **Liquid paraffin** has been a popular lubricant and stool softener. Once widely available, it can now be bought only from a pharmacy in small bottles because it should not be used regularly for long periods to relieve constipation. Long-term use has caused adverse effects, such as skin irritation, changes to the bowel wall due to absorption of small quantities of the paraffin, interference with the absorption of certain vitamins and a form of pneumonia. **Liquid paraffin**

STIMULANT LAXATIVES

On prescription
DANTHRON (only for constipation in patients who are very old, terminally ill or have cardiac conditions and must avoid straining to pass faeces) – available as **CO-DANTHRAMER** combined with **POLOXAMER** liquid and **CO-DANTHRUSATE** combined with **DOCUSATE** capsules.

On prescription/over the counter
BISACODYL – Tablets, suppositories
DULCO-LAX – Tablets, suppositories
BISACODYL
DIOCTYL – Liquid, tablets
DOCUSATE SODIUM
FLETCHERS' ENEMETTE – Enema
DOCUSATE SODIUM + GLYCEROL
GLYCEROL – Suppositories
MANEVAC – Granules
SENNA + ISPAGHULA HUSK
NORGALAX – Enema
DOCUSATE SODIUM
SENOKOT – Granules, liquid, tablets
SENNA
SENNA – Tablets

Not recommended
Other over-the-counter preparations containing:
☐ **CASCARA, FRANGULA, RHUBARB, SENNA** – they are unstandardised, so the laxative effect is unpredictable
☐ **ALOES** (brand names ALOPHEN; BEECHAMS PILLS; CALSALETTES), **COLOCYNTH, JALAP** – these are strong purgatives
☐ **PHENOLPHTHALEIN** (brand names BONOMINT; BROOKLAX; CORRECTOL; EX-LAX; KEST; SURE-LAX) – its laxative effect may continue for several days as it is recycled in the liver; it can cause skin rashes and colour urine pink
☐ **CASTOR OIL** – now obsolete.

emulsion (brand names Petrolagar; Agarol) should also be avoided – Agarol also contains phenolphthalein.

● *OSMOTIC LAXATIVES* ●

These work by retaining liquid, mostly water, in the bowel. They also soften stools. Commonly used osmotic laxatives include **magnesium salts** and **lactulose solution** (see over). **Sodium phosphate** or **sodium citrate** enema solutions are used for the urgent relief of constipation.

Magnesium salts

These are used to relieve constipation and when rapid bowel evacuation is needed. **Magnesium hydroxide** mixture or **liquid paraffin and magnesium hydroxide** mixture are both effective within about four hours. Repeated use of these mixtures is not recommended, although the problems associated with long-term use of liquid paraffin on its own have not been noted with the latter. **Magnesium sulphate** (Epsom salts) has a rapid effect, particularly if a dose is taken on an empty stomach before breakfast, followed by a glass of warm water. This should not be used routinely for a laxative effect.

Magnesium salts should only be used occasionally in the elderly. If you have poor kidney function, you should avoid magnesium-based laxatives. If you have poor liver function, you should avoid magnesium sulphate. Magnesium reduces iron absorption.

LACTULOSE SOLUTION B.P.

On prescription/over the counter
LACTULOSE SOLUTION B.P. – Liquid
DUPHALAC – Liquid

Lactulose is a sugar which, when broken down by bacteria in the bowel, increases stool bulk and stimulates intestinal movement. Softer stools are then passed. Lactulose solution may take up to two days to work at the start of treatment.

Before you use this medicine

Tell your doctor or pharmacist if you are:
☐ sensitive to the sugar galactose – lactulose breaks down to galactose and fructose ☐ sensitive to lactose, a similar sugar ☐ pregnant or breast-feeding ☐ taking any other medicines, including vitamins and those bought over the counter.

How to use this medicine

Take three 5ml spoonfuls twice a day to start with, but then reduce the dose to suit your needs; you can take lactulose with water or fruit juice. You should take plenty of water or other liquids whilst taking an osmotic laxative and, as with all laxatives, you should not take lactulose if you have an intestinal blockage. If you are diabetic, you can still use lactulose: a daily dose of 15ml provides 14 kcal.

Over 65 No special requirements, although some doctors think this is not an ideal laxative for older people.

Unwanted effects

Likely Flatulence, cramps and feeling sick, especially in the first few days of treatment.
Less likely Bloating and diarrhoea can occur if the dose is too high. These should ease if you reduce the dose.

Similar preparations

▼ **LACTITOL** – Powder

● *SEVERE CONSTIPATION* ●

Stools in the rectum and bowel which are very hard, dry and difficult to move are *impacted*. The intestinal tract may be temporarily blocked and you may feel uncomfortable. You may also pass loose stools which leak around the impaction and are not true diarrhoea. Faecal impaction can occur in frail, elderly people and those who are seriously ill and immobile.

Your doctor may prescribe a stimulant suppository, such as **bisacodyl** or **glycerol**, or an enema. An enema is a solution of salts – of **sodium** or **magnesium**, for example – in a disposable pack which has a nozzle for inserting into the rectum. An enema produces a speedy response and is therefore used in emergencies or to clear the bowel before an operation or childbirth.

Piles and anal disorders

Piles occur when the veins in the anus and rectum become swollen or irritated. Piles, also called haemorrhoids because the haemorrhoidal veins are involved, may be *external* (at the anus) or *internal* (within the rectum). They are purple in colour and may look like a bunch of grapes. Internal piles may not cause much trouble, but bleed, cause occasional discomfort and itch. Sometimes during defaecation, the piles are pushed down through the anus but return again spontaneously. Severe piles come down readily and need to be pushed back into the rectum.

Piles appear to occur because of prolonged local pressure on the haemorrhoidal veins. Pregnant women are prone to develop them and they are made worse by constipation and straining to pass stools. Occasionally blood clots form in the piles, which causes severe pain. Blood around the stools, or bleeding before or after defaecation are commonly caused by piles, but you should always see your doctor to confirm this, as bleeding is also a symptom of bowel cancer. Your doctor will need to examine you and may use an instrument called a *sigmoidoscope* to look into your rectum.

Sometimes surgery may be needed to relieve painful and persistent haemorrhoids. They can also be treated by *rubber band ligation*, where the haemorrhoid is tied off from the vein.

Other anal disorders include anal fissure, painful tears around the anus and anal itching (*pruritus ani*). All these are relieved by attention to cleanliness and diet.

– HOW YOU CAN HELP YOURSELF –

- ☐ Increase the amount of fibre in your diet and drink plenty of water or non-alcoholic drinks
- ☐ Use a bulk-forming laxative if necessary to soften stools
- ☐ Whenever possible, wash your anus carefully after defaecation; soap is irritant and should be avoided in conditions such as anal fissure; dry the area gently
- ☐ Always see your doctor if you have a sudden change of bowel habit or blood mixed with your stools.

Medicines for anal discomfort

Medicines used to relieve anal discomfort and irritation are soothing preparations applied locally as creams, ointments, suppositories and dusting powders. Preparations may be bland or may include a local anaesthetic. A **corticosteroid** to reduce inflammation should not be used for long periods.

• *BLAND SOOTHING PREPARATIONS* •

Some are a mixture of astringents, which cause tissue to contract; others contain astringents plus an antiseptic, or a local anaesthetic, or a vasoconstrictor (which reduces the size of blood vessels) or a lubricant. A soothing preparation is used at night and in the morning, and also after a bowel movement. An unwrapped suppository is inserted into the rectum or the cream or ointment can be used with a special applicator. You can also use the cream or ointment externally around the anus.

Bismuth subgallate, zinc oxide and **hamamelis** (witch hazel) are astringents which may relieve itching and uncomfortable piles.

A local anaesthetic (**lignocaine**, for example) can be used just before passing stools to relieve the pain associated with anal fissure. However, a local anaesthetic should only be used for a short period, no longer than two weeks, because it may cause skin sensitisation. Young children should not be treated with products containing a local anaesthetic: see your doctor about any problems your child has with defaecation.

Avoid products containing **resorcinol** because it may interfere with the thyroid gland. Other products contain a variety of ingredients which add little to their basic efficacy, such as **ephedrine** or **hexachlorophane**. **Heparinoid** is thought to relieve swelling. Always read the list of ingredients before you make a purchase.

BLAND SOOTHING PREPARATIONS

On prescription/over the counter

ANACAL – Suppositories, ointment
HEPARINOID

ANODESYN – Suppositories, ointment
LIGNOCAINE + EPHEDRINE + ALLANTOIN

ANUSOL – Suppositories, cream, ointment
BISMUTH + ZINC

BISMODYNE – Suppositories
LIGNOCAINE + BISMUTH + ZINC + HEXACHLOROPHANE

LANACANE – Cream
BENZOCAINE

LASONIL – Ointment
HYALURONIDASE + HEPARINOID

Over the counter

GERMALOIDS – Cream, ointment, suppositories
LIGNOCAINE + ZINC

HEMOCAINE – Suppositories, cream
LIGNOCAINE + BISMUTH + ZINC

PREPARATION H – Suppositories, ointment
SHARK LIVER OIL + YEAST CELL EXTRACT

Not recommended

COMPOUND BISMUTH SUBGALLATE – contain **RESORCINOL**

• *CORTICOSTEROIDS* •

Anti-inflammatory corticosteroids are combined with soothing preparations and local anaesthetics. These preparations must be prescribed by your doctor. They should only be used for short periods of about five to seven days, once infection has been excluded as a cause of the complaint. Preparations containing a corticosteroid and an antibiotic are not recommended. If infection is present, a corticosteroid should not be used because it can make the infections worse.

CORTICOSTEROID PREPARATIONS

All products contain several ingredients but we list the corticosteroid component only.

ANUGESIC-HC – Ointment, suppositories
HYDROCORTISONE

ANUSOL-HC – Ointment, suppositories
HYDROCORTISONE

BETNOVATE – Ointment
BETAMETHASONE

PROCTOFOAM HC – Aerosol foam
HYDROCORTISONE

PROCTOSEDYL – Ointment, suppositories
HYDROCORTISONE

SCHERIPROCT – Ointment, suppositories
PREDNISOLONE

ULTRAPROCT – Ointment, suppositories
FLUOCORTOLONE

XYLOPROCT – Ointment, suppositories
HYDROCORTISONE

Not recommended

UNIROID – contains an antibiotic

2

HEART AND CIRCULATION

High blood pressure Angina
Heart attack Heart failure
Irregular heartbeat Stroke
Circulatory problems Blood clots

The heart is a strong muscle which constantly pumps blood to all parts of the body, through thousands of miles of blood vessels called *arteries*. The blood fuels every cell, organ and system with oxygen and nutrients which the body needs to function. Blood from the main arteries flows into smaller and smaller vessels ending in the *capillaries*. This network of very fine blood vessels allows oxygen and nutrients to reach individual cells. The blood then takes the cells' waste products through *veins* back to the heart. The body's network of arteries, capillaries and veins is known as the circulation.

The heart has four chambers, which are really very large blood vessels. There are two on the left and two on the right. Each of the smaller top chambers is called an *atrium* while the larger, lower parts are known as the *ventricles*. The right atrium receives blood from the veins which then passes into the right ventricle. From here the blood carrying waste gas (carbon dioxide) is pumped to the lungs, where the blood cells exchange it for oxygen; blood is returned to the left side of the heart for circulation to the rest of the body. (The heart receives its own blood supply through the coronary arteries.) Inside the heart and blood vessels there are valves which ensure that the blood flows in only one direction. The heart and circulation are known collectively as the cardiovascular system.

High blood pressure

Blood pressure is the force the heart uses to pump blood around the body. During each heartbeat pressure is highest when the heart muscle contracts to push blood through the system. Blood pressure is at its lowest when the heart then relaxes before the process is repeated. The higher force is known as the *systolic* pressure, the lower as the *diastolic* pressure; both are measured when you have your blood pressure taken.

Blood pressure varies between individuals, although it generally increases with age because of changes in lifestyle: as people grow older they tend to put on weight, take less exercise and drink alcohol. An individual's blood pressure is partly hereditary, and high blood pressure tends to run in families. Blood pressure varies throughout the day and depends on what you are doing. It will rise when you take exercise because blood needs to be pumped around the body faster; when you rest, sit or lie down your blood pressure will be lower. It is only when your blood pressure is consistently higher than it should be, no matter what you are doing, that you have high blood pressure (*hypertension*). If high blood pressure is left untreated, it will reduce your life-expectancy.

MEASURING BLOOD PRESSURE

A *sphygmomanometer* is generally used to measure blood pressure. It consists of a rubber-lined cuff which is attached by rubber tubing to a small hand pump on one side and a mercury gauge on the other. The cuff is wrapped round the upper arm and inflated to stop blood flow temporarily. The doctor or nurse places a stethoscope over an artery on the arm below the cuff and listens to the heart sounds as the blood starts to flow down the artery again as air is gradually let out of the cuff. The mercury gauge shows the *systolic pressure* as a thumping noise is heard. As the pressure falls a second, more muffled sound is heard and the gauge shows the *diastolic pressure*. The readings are given in millimetres of mercury in the gauge (mmHg). You can buy do-it-yourself blood pressure measuring devices, but a *Which?* report (August 1989) found that of the seven machines tested all were unreliable compared with the sphygmomanometer. It is best, therefore to get your doctor to confirm any blood pressure measurements.

Arteries and veins are like rubber tubing with good elasticity. Blood is constantly forced through the arteries at great pressure and the artery walls gradually fur up, roughen and thicken (*arteriosclerosis*), causing narrowing of the arteries and loss of elasticity. This natural ageing process is accelerated by high blood pressure, which increases the risk of coronary heart disease. Blood clots in blood vessels are more likely to form: if this happens in an artery in the brain it may cause a stroke; a clot in the arteries to the heart is known as a *coronary thrombosis* and will cause a heart attack.

Peripheral vascular disease results from long-term reduction in blood flow to the arms and legs providing less oxygen and nutrients to feed the cells and tissues. Blood vessels may also become blocked by fatty deposits (*atherosclerosis*).

The increase in pressure puts an extra workload on the heart, making it more difficult for it to pump blood efficiently around the body, and the heart is gradually damaged. Kidney function can be reduced if high blood pressure persists and the walls of the arteries supplying blood to the kidneys thicken. A few people with high blood pressure suffer worsening eyesight because of damage to the blood vessels in the eye.

Many people with raised blood pressure have no symptoms at all. Measuring blood pressure is the only way to find out whether it is high or not. You should have your blood pressure measured on several different occasions to see if the reading is consistent; stress and anxiety (perhaps brought on by a visit to the doctor or hospital clinic) can increase blood pressure. Adults who have not had their blood pressure checked during the last five years should consider having a check-up.

Doctors generally advise patients whose diastolic blood pressure is above 110mmHg on three separate occasions or 100–109mmHg when measured over a period of four to six months that drug treatment is necessary. If your diastolic blood pressure is only mildly increased, but you have other problems, such as diabetes or high blood-fats, you are still likely to need treatment. Young men with high blood pressure appear to be at a high risk of developing heart and circulation problems and are therefore likely to need treatment. The risks are equal for older men and women. Your doctor will need to assess the benefits of treating high blood pressure against the risks of adverse effects from medicines, especially if you are over 60. If you are over 80, drug treatment is not particularly helpful.

Low blood pressure rarely requires treatment. Faintness or dizziness may sometimes be troublesome, but most people do not experience any symptoms or health problems. Very severe high blood pressure (*malignant hypertension*) needs urgent hospital treatment.

Many people have no obvious cause of high blood pressure, but a few have *secondary hypertension* caused by a disease or condition, such as kidney disease or high blood pressure during pregnancy. However, several lifestyle factors contribute to high blood pressure and these often work in combination with each other. See How you can help yourself, over the page.

HOW YOU CAN HELP YOURSELF

☐ **Lose weight** – the heart has to work much harder to pump blood around the body if you are overweight; losing weight can bring your blood pressure back to normal.

☐ **Restrict salt** – reducing your daily salt intake may be all that is required to treat mildly raised blood pressure.

☐ **Reduce alcohol** – even in moderate quantities, alcohol can increase blood pressure; try to cut down and definitely stay within the recommended weekly limit.

☐ **Stop smoking** – smokers are in a high-risk category for heart attacks and strokes.

☐ **Avoid stress and take plenty of rest** – relaxation therapy may help some people with mild to moderately raised blood pressure; you will have to persist with relaxation treatment, but it may allow your doctor to reduce or withdraw your drug treatment.

☐ **Exercise regularly** – exercise helps the circulation, improves blood flow through the muscles and helps the efficiency of the heart; regular exercise may prevent the development of high blood pressure and it can lead to a reduction in blood pressure. Avoid strenuous exercise if you are not used to it, but start gently with a brisk walk a few times a week or swimming.

Medicines for high blood pressure

Lowering blood pressure reduces the risk of stroke and cardiovascular problems. High blood pressure cannot usually be cured, but it can be kept under control. If your doctor diagnoses high blood pressure, the approach to treatment depends on how high it is. Your doctor will aim to lower blood pressure to a diastolic reading of 90mmHg, but certainly below 100mmHg. Even mildly increased blood pressure should be lowered to reduce the risk of stroke.

Most people with high blood pressure will need treatment with one or more medicines, but losing weight, controlling salt and alcohol consumption and stopping smoking may delay or limit the need for medicines. For some people with mildly raised blood pressure these measures may be all that is needed. Even if you do not have to take a medicine, your doctor will still want to see you to check your blood pressure regularly.

The various medicines used to treat high blood pressure act in different ways in the body. Your doctor may prescribe a particular type of medicine or a combination. Most of the medicines have unwanted effects and older people are especially at risk from them. Some of the unwanted effects are quite subtle, because the medicines affect the body's metabolism; other people may notice a change in you that you do not, and it is worth noting these developments on a medicines worksheet. You must tell your doctor about any unwanted effects, especially if these effects put you off taking the medicine. You may have to take a medicine for blood pressure control for the rest of your life, so it is important to find a treatment that suits you. You should work in partnership with your doctor to try to achieve a sensible blood pressure level without taking the enjoyment out of life.

Some of the medicines used to treat high blood pressure are also used to treat other heart and circulation problems, but the dosage may vary depending on the condition.

● *DIURETICS* ●

Diuretics, sometimes called 'water tablets', remove water and salts from the body. Water, mineral salts (mostly sodium and potassium) and waste products are taken out of the bloodstream as blood flows through the kidneys. Some of the water and salts are recycled back into blood (a process called reabsorption) and the rest leave the body with the waste products as urine. Diuretics interfere with the recycling process in the kidneys to increase the amounts of mineral salts and water lost from the body which reduces tension in the arteries. Diuretics also help the heart to work more efficiently and reduce extra fluid trapped in body tissues. A diuretic increases the frequency and the amount of urine you produce, particularly at the start of treatment.

There are several types of diuretic. The main classes are *thiazides, loop diuretics* and *potassium-sparing diuretics*. They work at slightly different places in the kidney, but all block sodium and water reabsorption. Loop diuretics (except **piretanide**; brand name Arelix) are not generally used to lower high blood pressure, but they are used to remove excess water from the body, especially in heart failure (see page 139).

The unwanted effects of diuretics are sometimes troublesome, although lower doses may lessen them. Not only is there the inconvenience of more frequent and larger volumes of urine, but diuretics may also upset the balance of the body's chemistry. Older people are particularly sensitive to these effects; they need lower doses and should not take diuretics for long periods without their doctor reviewing the need for treatment.

Potassium is lost from the body when you take a diuretic other than the potassium-sparing type. The body needs potassium for the proper functioning of muscle, especially heart muscle. The rhythm of the heart may be upset by low potassium levels, which can be dangerous. If blood levels of potassium fall, you may feel weak, dizzy, sick and even vomit. You must see a doctor if you get these symptoms.

Thiazide diuretics

Thiazide diuretics are very effective in low doses for controlling high blood pressure. All the thiazides are similar in action although they may vary in how long they work. **Bendrofluazide** and **hydrochlorothiazide** are the most commonly prescribed.

BENDROFLUAZIDE

BENDROFLUAZIDE – Tablets
APRINOX – Tablets
BERKOZIDE – Tablets
CENTYL – Tablets
NEO-NACLEX – Tablets

Poor choice: bendrofluazide with potassium
CENTYL K
NEO-NACLEX K

Bendrofluazide is a thiazide diuretic widely used in low doses to reduce high blood pressure. It is used on its own in mild cases and with other medicines when high blood pressure is more severe. Bendrofluazide is also used to remove excess fluid (oedema) from the body, for example in mild to moderate heart failure. It starts to act within one or two hours of taking it by mouth and is effective for 6–12 hours.

Bendrofluazide can upset the body's chemistry and metabolism particularly if taken for long periods, although low doses may avoid this. Older people are particularly sensitive to these metabolic effects. A number of preparations combine potassium and bendrofluazide in the same tablet as a sustained-release product. These products may not contain enough potassium for people who need supplementation. Many people taking a low dose of thiazide only need to take in potassium as part of their diet.

Before you use this medicine

Tell your doctor if you are:
☐ pregnant ☐ breast-feeding – large doses may stop milk production ☐ restricting salt or sugar in your diet – bendrofluazide affects salt and sugar levels ☐ taking any other medicines, including vitamins and those bought over the counter.

Tell your doctor if you have or have had:
☐ diabetes ☐ pancreatitis ☐ gout ☐ kidney disease ☐ liver disease ☐ sensitivity to any thiazide diuretic or a sulphonamide ☐ high blood-calcium levels ☐ the hormone disorder Addison's disease ☐ porphyria ☐ the arthritis-like condition systemic lupus erythematosus.

If you have to take bendrofluazide for long periods or in high doses, you should ask your doctor about potassium supplementation. Bendrofluazide removes potassium from the body as well as sodium and water (see 'Keeping potassium in balance', page 111).

How to use this medicine

Take the tablet in the morning with breakfast, so that night-time sleep is not interfered with by additional visits to the toilet: during the first few days of treatment, you will produce a larger volume of urine and need to go to the toilet more often than usual. If you are away from home, make sure you know where the toilet facilities are for emergencies.

Because a diuretic helps you to lose water, you may lose too much and become dehydrated. You may feel thirsty and your skin may look and feel dry. Check with your doctor to see that your daily fluid intake is appropriate. You will lose potassium from your body; make sure that you eat foods rich in potassium every day. If you reduce salt intake your body will lose less potassium, but discuss salt restriction with your doctor. Your doctor should check your blood potassium levels after about a month of treatment; if potassium is low discuss whether you can adjust this by dietary intake.

You may feel dizzy or faint when you get up from sitting or lying down, especially during the first few days of treatment. Get up slowly and stay beside the chair or bed until you are sure you are not dizzy.

Alcohol intake should be kept low: loss of body fluids increases the effects of alcohol.

Over 65 You need as small a dose as possible. You may be able to take bendrofluazide every other day; check with your doctor. Bendrofluazide should be used very cautiously if you have poor kidney function. Your doctor should take a blood sample to check your kidney function and potassium levels periodically.

Interactions with other medicines

Thiazide diuretics interact with a number of medicines, but only the important interactions are given here. Do not take any other medicines, such as those bought over the counter, without checking with your doctor or pharmacist.

Lithium Bendrofluazide stops lithium from leaving the body; the amount of lithium in the blood may increase to toxic levels.

Heart drugs If bendrofluazide causes low potassium levels in the body, the adverse effects of certain heart drugs increase. These include digoxin, amiodarone, disopyramide, flecainide and quinidine.

Other blood pressure lowering drugs can be given with bendrofluazide but this will enhance its unwanted effects, such as the dizziness and faintness.

Unwanted effects

Likely Muscle cramps, weakness.

Unlikely Dizziness, feeling or being sick, loss of appetite, diarrhoea, impotence, skin rashes. Contact your doctor if you develop a rash. Problems of impotence should always be discussed.

Bendrofluazide may aggravate diabetes and increase blood-sugar levels. Symptoms may appear if you are on the threshold of developing diabetes. The blood-sugar lowering effect of antidiabetic medicines is opposed by bendrofluazide and this may upset the control of diabetes. Blood levels of uric acid may be increased, causing or aggravating gout. Bendrofluazide may cause or aggravate high blood-fat levels (*hyperlipidaemia*).

Similar preparations

BAYCARON – Tablets
MEFRUSIDE

DIUREXAN – Tablets
XIPAMIDE

ENDURON – Tablets
METHYCLOTHIAZIDE

ESIDREX – Tablets
HYDROCHLOROTHIAZIDE

HYDRENOX –Tablets
HYDROFLUMETHIAZIDE

HYDROSALURIC – Tablets
HYDROCHLOROTHIAZIDE

HYGROTON – Tablets
CHLORTHALIDONE

METENIX 5 – Tablets
METOLAZONE

NATRILIX – Tablets
INDAPAMIDE

NAVIDREX – Tablets
CYCLOPENTHIAZIDE

NEPHRIL – Tablets
POLYTHIAZIDE

SALURIC – Tablets
CHLOROTHIAZIDE

XURET – Low-dose tablets
METOLAZONE

Keeping potassium in balance

Potassium is an essential mineral for keeping the body healthy. Too little or too much potassium can trigger irregular heart rhythms. The mild loss of potassium that occurs with diuretic treatment usually has no symptoms, although elderly people may experience muscle weakness and confusion. However, you may need to change your diet if it is low in potassium.

POTASSIUM-RICH FOODS		
almonds	coconut	peas
apricots (dried)	dates and figs (dried)	pork
avocados	fish (fresh)	potatoes
bananas	ham	prunes (dried)
beans	lentils	raisins
beef	liver	shellfish
bran	melon	spinach
broccoli	milk	tomato juice
Brussels sprouts	oranges and lemons	turkey
carrots (raw)	peaches	veal
chicken	peanut butter	

For example, six halves of dried apricots, a glass of fresh orange juice and a medium size banana per day should provide enough potassium to prevent low blood levels, but taking potassium in your daily diet may not be sufficient if your potassium loss is moderate to severe. Your doctor will need to assess blood-potassium levels and replacement treatment may be needed:

☐ for older people with a poor diet
☐ if you take high doses of a diuretic or the heart drug digoxin or an anti-arrhythmic drug
☐ if the body's potassium control is disrupted – by severe liver disease, for example
☐ if you lose potassium in faeces through an illness such as chronic diarrhoea, or experience vomiting or diarrhoea while taking a diuretic.

Some drugs taken for long periods (anti-inflammatory corticosteroids, for example) produce further potassium loss, so replacement must be given.

Restricting your salt intake helps to maintain potassium levels while lowering body sodium. A salt substitute, such as Losalt or Ruthmol contain large amounts of potassium chloride and may be used as an additional source of potassium. However, you should not use a salt substitute if you have poor kidney function or you are already taking a potassium supplement or potassium-sparing diuretic.

Potassium replacement is usually given as potassium chloride in liquid form to minimise harmful effects on the lining of the stomach and intestines. Tablets or granules should be dissolved in a tumblerful of water before swallowing the solution. Potassium chloride solution can be taken with or after food to lessen the effect on the stomach. Slow-release potassium chloride tablets have caused ulceration of the gullet and intestines and are not recommended. Some diuretics are combined with potassium, which is unnecessary in most cases and often too little to be useful when replacement is needed. It is better to take the diuretic and the potassium separately.

POTASSIUM CHLORIDE PREPARATIONS

On prescription/from a pharmacy
KAY-CEE-L – Syrup (sugar-free)
KLOREF – Effervescent tablets
KLOREF-S – Effervescent granules (sugar-free)
SANDO-K – Effervescent tablets

Not recommended
Modified-relase preparations:
LEO-K; SLOW-K; NU-K

Potassium chloride can make you feel sick or be sick and you should tell your doctor if this happens. Your doctor may recommend a potassium-sparing diuretic as an alternative to a potassium supplement to overcome this problem.

● *Potassium-sparing diuretics*

Amiloride and **triamterene** are weak diuretics on their own and are therefore used in combination with thiazide or loop diuretics. They conserve the body's potassium supplies and must not be taken with potassium supplements as the body would then retain too much potassium. **Spironolactone** is used to remove excess fluid in severe heart failure and also in liver disease.

AMILORIDE

AMILORIDE – Liquid, tablets
MIDAMOR – Tablets

Amiloride is a weak diuretic with a potassium-conserving action. It may be used alone to remove excess fluid in heart failure or liver disease. However, it is used more often in combination with a thiazide or loop diuretic to retain potassium in the body which would otherwise be lost. Amiloride starts to work within two hours and its effect may last for 12–24 hours.

Before you use this medicine

Tell your doctor if you are:
☐ pregnant – not usually prescribed ☐ breast-feeding – amiloride passes into breast milk ☐ taking any other medicine, including vitamins and those bought over the counter, or a salt substitute.

Tell your doctor if you have or have had:
☐ long-term kidney problems ☐ diabetes mellitus ☐ gout.

How to use this medicine

Take the tablet in the morning, usually as a single dose. Sometimes your doctor may prescribe a twice-daily dose. Take the second dose of the day no later than mid-afternoon because night-time sleep may be disrupted by additional visits to the toilet. Amiloride can be taken at the same time as another diuretic.

Until you know how you react to amiloride, do not drive or do other activities that require alertness. Alcohol should not cause problems with amiloride.

Do not stop taking this medicine without discussing this with your doctor. If you miss a dose take it as soon as you remember, but no later than mid-afternoon. Otherwise skip this dose and take the next one as usual.

Over 65 Amiloride is likely to conserve more potassium in the body because the kidneys work less efficiently. Your kidney function and potassium levels should be checked before you start treatment. You may need less than the usual adult dose.

Interactions with other medicines

ACE inhibitors increase blood pressure lowering effect and blood potassium levels.
Lithium Amiloride increases the amount of lithium in the blood, so there is a risk of toxic levels building up.

Unwanted effects

Unlikely Feeling sick, dry mouth, dizziness or faintness, loss of appetite, stomach upsets, confusion, rashes, high blood levels of potassium (particularly if kidney function is reduced).

See your doctor if you develop a rash, muscle weakness or confusion. Too much potassium in the body causes irregular heartbeats, muscle weakness or heaviness and numbness or tingling in the hands and feet.

Similar preparations

ALDACTONE – Tablets
SPIRONOLACTONE

DYTAC – Capsules
TRIAMTERENE

SPIROCTAN – Tablets, capsules
SPIRONOLACTONE

SPIROCTAN-M – Injection
POTASSIUM CANRENOATE

SPIRONOLACTONE – Tablets, liquid

Combined preparations

Many products combine a potassium-sparing diuretic with a thiazide, a loop diuretic such as frusemide or a beta blocker in a fixed dose. Amiloride is combined in one tablet with the thiazide diuretic hydrochlorothiazide and this combination now has the generic name of **co-amilozide**. There are two tablet strengths of co-amilozide, but they do not allow for treatment with, say, a low dose of hydrochlorothiazide and a standard dose of amiloride.

Fixed-dose preparations seem an attractive way to improve reliability in medicine-taking by reducing the number of medicines a patient has to take. Yet these combinations encourage the use of a potassium-sparing diuretic when a thiazide with a potassium-rich diet might be appropriate. Unwanted effects are more troublesome with combination preparations; they do not control blood levels of potassium reliably and doctors have reported both high and low levels. Low levels of blood-sodium are more frequent in older people given co-amilozide than in those treated with a thiazide alone. Low sodium also occurs when these combinations are given with the antidiabetic drug chlorpropamide.

Some preparations contain three drugs – a potassium-sparing diuretic, a thiazide and a beta blocker. This combination should only be used when blood pressure has not been controlled by dietary measures and a thiazide *or* a beta blocker alone (see **atenolol**, page 117).

Older people for whom dietary measures have failed to control high blood pressure may find a low dose of a thiazide diuretic adequate. If the thiazide diuretic does not control blood pressure, changing to a different type of blood pressure lowering drug (a beta blocker or a calcium channel blocker, for example) might be more appropriate than adding a further diuretic. Ask your doctor if it is possible to take just one drug for high blood pressure. If it is not, your doctor should at first prescribe the second drug separately, so that the dose of each drug can be adjusted to meet your needs.

CO-AMILOZIDE

CO-AMILOZIDE – Tablets
MODURET 25 – Tablets
MODURETIC – Tablets, liquid

● *SIMILAR PREPARATIONS* ●

ALDACTIDE – Tablets
SPIRONOLACTONE + HYDROFLUMETHIAZIDE
DYAZIDE – Tablets
TRIAMTERENE + HYDROCHLOROTHIAZIDE
DYTIDE – Capsules
TRIAMTERENE + BENZTHIAZIDE
KALSPARE – Tablets
TRIAMTERENE + CHLORTHALIDONE
NAVISPARE – Tablets
AMILORIDE + CYCLOPENTHIAZIDE

● *BETA BLOCKERS* ●

Beta blockers or *beta adrenergic* blocking drugs block receptors to dampen the effects of *noradrenaline*, a *neurotransmitter* – one of the body's chemicals produced in the adrenal glands – which plays a part in controlling the heart, blood vessels, lungs and muscles. Together with adrenaline it prepares the body for 'fight and flight', when the heart beats faster and more strongly, and other parts of the body are prepared for action. Beta blockers oppose this stimulating effect by slowing the heart rate and decreasing the force of the heartbeat.

All beta blocker preparations act in much the same way. They vary in their effects on the receptors and how long they work in the body, and different beta blockers suit different conditions and patients. **Oxprenolol, acebutolol** and **pindolol** stimulate beta receptors as well as block them; this lessens some of the unwanted effects, such as coldness in the hands and feet, but the heart is not slowed as much as with other preparations. **Propranolol, metoprolol** and **pindolol** are lipid-soluble (they dissolve in body fat); others are water-soluble. Solubility affects a drug's distribution throughout the body systems and how it leaves the body. The most water-soluble beta blockers, **atenolol, nadolol** and **sotalol**, cause less sleep disturbance because they are less likely to enter the brain than lipid-soluble preparations. However, they stay in the body longer if kidney function is poor and the dosage must be reduced.

● *Some cautions with beta blockers*

Beta blockers must not be used if you have asthma, chronic bronchitis, emphysema or any other breathing difficulties (respiratory disease) or have a history of obstructive airways disease: a beta blocker may narrow the airways in the lungs. Even the beta blockers that do not have such a marked effect on the lung beta receptors should not be used. However, there may be a rare occasion when your doctor feels that a beta blocker is the only treatment for you, in which case special precautions (such as additional use of your inhaler) must be taken.

Beta blockers make the heart pump blood through the body at a slower rate and less oxygen is required to do the work. This may worsen the effects of heart failure or heart block. A beta blocker will also worsen poor circulation to the hands and feet or Raynaud's phenomenon (see page 121) because it constricts the blood vessels, preventing blood flow to your extremities.

If you take a beta blocker for a long time – for angina for example – you must not stop taking it suddenly, as this has been known to worsen symptoms and even cause a heart attack. Your doctor will supervise a gradual withdrawal of the beta blocker if treatment needs to be stopped.

● *Combined preparations*

Preparations of a beta blocker with a potassium-sparing diuretic and a thiazide diuretic may make it easier to take a number of drugs if your doctor prescribes them after high blood pressure has not been controlled by dietary measures and a thiazide diuretic or a beta blocker alone. A combination of a beta blocker with a calcium channel blocker (**atenolol** and **nifedipine**) is also used only if one or the other has not controlled blood pressure. Combined preparations increase the likelihood of unwanted effects and do not allow the dose of an individual drug to be varied.

ATENOLOL

ATENOLOL –Tablets
TENORMIN – Tablets, liquid, injection

Combined with a calcium channel antagonist
BETA-ADALAT – Capsules
ATENOLOL + NIFEDIPINE
TENIF – Capsules
ATENOLOL + NIFEDIPINE

Combined with a diuretic
CO-TENIDONE – Tablets
ATENOLOL + CHLORTHALIDONE
KALTEN – Capsules
ATENOLOL + CO-AMILOZIDE
TENORETIC– Tablets
CO-TENIDONE
TENORET 50 – Tablets
CO-TENIDONE

Atenolol is a beta blocker used to treat high blood pressure, angina, and irregular heartbeats (*arrhythmias*). It prevents the heart from beating too quickly and is also used to prevent further damage to the heart after a heart attack (*myocardial infarction*). Beta blockers are also used for thyroid disorders, for preventing migraine and for relieving some of the symptoms of anxiety such as tremor and palpitations. A beta blocker is also used in the eye in the management of glaucoma.

Atenolol starts to act within two to four hours of taking it by mouth and is effective for longer than a day (20–30 hours). It stays in the body longer if kidney function is reduced.

Before you use this medicine

Tell your doctor if you are:
☐ pregnant – atenolol would only be used under close medical supervision ☐ breast-feeding – atenolol passes into the milk, but is unlikely to cause problems at normal doses ☐ taking any other medicines, especially medicines for controlling appetite and over-the-counter remedies for colds, coughs, hay fever and sinus problems.

Do not use if you have:
☐ asthma ☐ chronic bronchitis, emphysema or other breathing problems ☐ congestive heart failure

Tell your doctor if you have or have had:
☐ poor blood circulation ☐ Raynaud's phenomenon ☐ poor kidney function ☐ diabetes – atenolol may interfere with the body's response to low blood-sugar.

How to use this medicine

The tablets are usually taken once a day, but twice a day for angina. It may take one or two weeks of treatment before the full effect of atenolol is felt. A modest intake of alcohol will not cause problems.

If you miss a dose take it as soon as you remember. Skip the dose if your next dose is due within eight hours and take that as usual. Do not take double the dose. Do not stop taking this medicine suddenly: to prevent a worsening of your condition your doctor will give you a schedule to decrease the dose of atenolol gradually if you are on long-term treatment. Make sure you do not run out of tablets.

Over 65 You may need a lower dose of atenolol, especially if your kidney function is reduced.

Interactions with other medicines

Anaesthetics enhance the blood pressure lowering effect of atenolol and other beta blockers. Tell your doctor or dentist that you take atenolol before you have surgery.
Heart drugs such as those for controlling the heart rhythm (**amiodarone** and **disopyramide**, for example) increase the risk of reducing and slowing heart activity.
Calcium channel blockers: **diltiazem** affects heart activity; **nifedipine** may induce severe low blood pressure and heart failure; **verapamil** should not be used with a beta blocker.
Other blood pressure lowering drugs enhance the effect of atenolol.
Appetite suppressants and cough and cold remedies containing **phenylpropanolamine**, **phenylephrine** or **pseudoephedrine** taken with a beta blocker can cause a severe rise in blood pressure. They must not be taken together.

Unwanted effects

Likely Cold hands and feet, muscle ache.
Unlikely Sleep disturbances, skin rashes and/or dry eyes, depression and confusion, dizziness, slow pulse, breathing problems.

You should contact your doctor if you have severe breathing difficulties, a skin rash, or dizziness or confusion.

Similar preparations

BETA-CARDONE – Tablets
SOTALOL
BETALOC – Tablets, modified-release tablets
METOPROLOL
BETIM – Tablets
TIMOLOL
BLOCADREN – Tablets
TIMOLOL
CARTROL – Tablets
CARTEOLOL
▼CELECTOL – Tablets
CELIPROLOL
CORGARD – Tablets
NADOLOL
EMCOR – Tablets
BISOPROLOL
INDERAL – Tablets, modified-release capsules
PROPANOLOL
KERLONE – Tablets
BETAXOLOL
LABETALOL – Tablets
LASIPRESSIN – Tablets
PENBUTOLOL
LOPRESOR – Tablets, modified-release tablets
METOPROLOL
METOPROLOL – Tablets
MONOCOR – Tablets
BISOPROLOL
OXPRENOLOL – Tablets
PROPANOLOL – Tablets
SECTRAL – Tablets
ACEBUTOLOL
SOTACOR – Tablets, injection
SOTALOL
TRANDATE – Tablets, injection
LABETALOL
TRASICOR – Tablets, modified-release tablets
OXPRENOLOL
VISKEN – Tablets
PINDOLOL

Combined with a diuretic

CO-BETALOC – Tablets, modified-release tablets
METOPROLOL + HYDROCHLOROTHIAZIDE
CORGARETIC – Tablets
NADOLOL + BENDROFLUAZIDE
INDERETIC/INDEREX – Capsules
PROPANOLOL + BENDROFLUAZIDE
LOPRESORETIC – Tablets
METOPROLOL + CHLORTHALIDONE
MODUCREN – Tablets
TIMOLOL + CO-AMILOZIDE
PRESTIM – Tablets
TIMOLOL + BENDROFLUAZIDE
SECADREX – Tablets
ACEBUTOLOL + HYDROCHLOROTHIAZIDE
SOTAZIDE – Tablets
SOTALOL + HYDROCHLOROTHIAZIDE

Continued over

TOLERZIDE – Tablets
SOTALOL + HYDROCHLOROTHIAZIDE

TRASIDREX – Tablets
OXPRENOLOL + CYCLOPENTHIAZIDE

VISKALDIX –Tablets
PINDOLOL + CLOPAMIDE

• *CALCIUM CHANNEL BLOCKERS* •

Calcium is an important mineral which the body needs for the proper functioning of muscles. Calcium channel blockers interfere with the flow of calcium through special channels in the cells of the heart and the smooth muscle of blood vessels to relax them. **Verapamil** (see page 147) and **diltiazem** have more of an effect on the heart than the *peripheral* arteries (those furthest from the heart); they also maintain the rhythm and pace of the heart. **Nifedipine** and related medicines, which do not act on the heart's rhythm, are used for treating angina, high blood pressure and Raynaud's phenomenon.

NIFEDIPINE

NIFEDIPINE – Capsules
ADALAT – Capsules, modified-release tablets
CORACTEN – Modified-release capsules
NIFENSAR XL – Modified release tablets
NIFEDIPINE + BETA BLOCKER – See **ATENOLOL**, page 117.

Nifedipine is a calcium channel blocker which relaxes arterial smooth muscle of the heart and peripheral blood vessels. It is used for the control of high blood pressure, for the prevention and treatment of chest pain (angina) and Raynaud's phenomenon. Nifedipine is used mainly to prevent and treat anginal attacks, but is also useful when either a thiazide diuretic or beta blocker has not controlled raised blood pressure. Unlike beta blockers, nifedipine is suitable for treating asthmatics with high blood pressure.

Nifedipine starts to work in about half to one hour and its effects last up to about 12 hours. Minor unwanted effects are quite common and are more likely in older people.

Before you use this medicine

Tell your doctor if you are:
☐ pregnant – not usually prescribed ☐ breast-feeding – nifedipine passes into the milk but amounts are too small to be harmful ☐ taking any other medicines, including vitamins and those bought over the counter.

Tell your doctor if you have or have had:
☐ heart failure ☐ low blood pressure ☐ diabetes ☐ poor liver or kidney function.

How to use this medicine

For high blood pressure or to prevent angina Tablets are usually used, taken twice daily with or after food.
For relief of angina and Raynaud's phenomenon Capsules are taken three times daily with or after food. For immediate relief of angina, bite into the capsule and swallow the liquid.

You may feel dizzy or faint when you get up from sitting or lying down, especially during the first few days of treatment. Get up slowly and stay beside the chair or bed until you are sure you are not dizzy. Avoid alcohol which may lower blood pressure further. Until you know how you react to nifedipine, do not drive or do other activities that require alertness.

If you miss a dose, take it as soon as you remember. Skip the dose, if it is almost time for your next dose and take that as usual. Do not take double the dose. Do not stop taking this medicine suddenly; your doctor will give you a schedule to decrease the dose gradually.

Over 65 You may need a lower dose, particularly if unwanted effects are troublesome. If you have poor liver function, you may need a lower dose and your doctor will need to follow your progress.

Interactions with other medicines

Beta blockers Occasionally severe low blood pressure and heart failure.
The heart drug digoxin Blood levels of digoxin may rise, increasing its unwanted effects.

Unwanted effects

Likely Headache, a feeling of warmth, flushing, dizziness.
Less likely Feeling sick, rashes, lethargy, swollen ankles, increased desire to urinate.

Contact your doctor if nifedipine makes you feel dizzy and this does not fade after the first few days of treatment, or if your chest pains (angina) get worse when you start taking nifedipine.

Similar preparations

CARDENE – Capsules
NICARDIPINE

ISTIN – Tablets
AMLODIPINE

NIMOTOP – Tablets, injection
NIMODIPINE

PLENDIL – Tablets
FELODIPINE

PRESCAL – Tablets
ISRADIPINE

• *ACE INHIBITORS* •

Angiotensin converting enzyme (ACE) inhibitors dilate blood vessels by blocking an enzyme that helps produce a body chemical that normally narrows (constricts) the blood vessels together and so increases tension. When the chemical (angiotensin II) is prevented from working, the blood vessels widen (dilate), reducing resistance to the flow of blood around the body, and blood pressure falls. Generally, ACE inhibitors are used for lowering blood pressure only if a thiazide diuretic or beta blocker has not worked, is not tolerated or cannot be used.

All the ACE inhibitors can be used for lowering blood pressure and a few are also used for treating heart failure. Treatment of heart failure is generally started in hospital under a doctor's close supervision. All the ACE inhibitors can cause a sudden drop in blood pressure, particularly with the first dose – this should be taken at bedtime or when you can lie down for a few hours afterwards. ACE inhibitors can sometimes damage kidney function, an effect which is more likely in older people and anyone who already has poor kidney function or kidney disease.

ACE inhibitors can be used with some diuretics, but not generally with a potassium-sparing diuretic because the ACE inhibitors keep potassium in the body as well. Two ACE inhibitors, **enalapril** and **captopril** are combined with a thiazide diuretic (hydrochlorothiazide) for treatment as a single daily dose.

However, it is better to take the individual drugs separately so that the dosages can be tailored to your needs. For example, captopril is normally given as a twice-daily dose and hydrochlorothiazide as a daily dose and it is uncertain whether the single dose of captopril in the combined preparation is adequate.

There are few differences between the ACE inhibitors and all act in a similar way in the body.

ENALAPRIL

INNOVACE – Tablets

Combined with a diuretic
INNOZIDE – Tablets
ENALAPRIL + HYDROCHLOROTHIAZIDE

Enalapril is an ACE inhibitor used for lowering high blood pressure when other methods such as dietary control, diuretics or beta blockers have not worked or cannot be used. In the treatment of congestive heart failure enapril is used with digoxin and/or diuretics. Enalapril starts to work within an hour and its effect lasts about 24 hours. Like other ACE inhibitors, enalapril can produce a rapid drop in blood pressure (*hypotension*) in some people at the first dose, causing dizziness and fainting. Older people and those with poor kidney function should take a lower dose or avoid enalapril altogether.

Before you use this medicine

Tell your doctor if you are:
☐ pregnant – enalapril and other ACE inhibitors should not be used ☐ breast-feeding ☐ on a low-salt diet ☐ taking potassium supplements ☐ taking any other medicines, particularly diuretics, and including vitamins and those bought over the counter.

Tell your doctor if you have or have had:
☐ severe kidney disease or poor kidney function ☐ allergy or hypersensitivity to an ACE inhibitor ☐ porphyria.

Before you start an ACE inhibitor, your blood levels of sodium and potassium and your kidney function should be assessed.

How to use this medicine

Take the tablets once a day, with a glass of water; the first dose should be taken at bedtime or when you can lie down for a few hours afterwards. You may feel dizzy or faint when you get up from sitting or lying down, especially during the first few days of treatment. Get up slowly and stay beside the chair or bed until you are sure you are not dizzy. Alcohol and other medicines for lowering blood pressure enhance this effect.

If you are on a low-salt diet or dehydrated before taking enalapril, it may cause a sudden drop in blood pressure. If enalapril is added to treatment with a diuretic, this should be stopped for a few days before the ACE inhibitor is introduced. If you have poor kidney function, you should start treatment with a low dose. Until you know how you react to enalapril, do not drive or do other activities that require alertness.

Do not stop taking this medicine suddenly; your doctor will give you a schedule to decrease the dose gradually. If you miss a dose, take it as soon as you remember, but skip it if your next dose is due within eight hours. Do not take double the dose.

Over 65 You should start treatment with a low dose.

Interactions with other medicines

Anaesthetics enhance the blood pressure lowering effect of enalapril. Tell your doctor or dentist that you take an ACE inhibitor before you have surgery.
Diuretics enhance the blood pressure lowering effect. ACE inhibitors keep potassium in the body, so if enalapril is taken with a potassium-sparing diuretic, blood-potassium levels may rise and cause unwanted effects.
Lithium blood levels increase because ACE inhibitors prevent its removal from the body and it may reach toxic levels.
Potassium salts, including low-sodium salt substitutes, and enalapril together increase the blood levels of potassium.

Unwanted effects

Likely Dry cough, headache, dizziness.
Unlikely Feeling sick, diarrhoea, muscle cramps, skin rash, loss of taste, cough, chest pain, fast or irregular heartbeat, swelling of the face, lips and mouth.

Contact your doctor if these effects are severe or they do not fade as treatment continues. Contact your doctor immediately if you experience dizziness or faintness, indicating a severe fall in blood pressure, particularly at the start of treatment; swelling of the face, lips and mouth (*angioneurotic oedema*).

Similar preparations

ACCUPRO – Tablets
QUINAPRIL

CAPOTEN – Tablets
CAPTOPRIL

CARACE – Tablets
LISINOPRIL

COVERSYL – Tablets
PERINDOPRIL

▼STARIL – Tablets
FOSINOPRIL

▼TRITACE – Capsules
RAMIPRIL

▼VASCACE – Tablets
CILAZAPRIL

ZESTRIL – Tablets
LISINOPRIL

Combined with diuretic

CAPOZIDE – Tablets
CAPTOPRIL + HYDROCHLOROTHIAZIDE

CARACE PLUS – Tablets
LISINOPRIL + HYDROCHLOROTHIAZIDE

ZESTORETIC
LISINOPRIL + HYDROCHLOROTHIAZIDE

● *OTHER VASODILATORS* ●

Calcium channel blockers and ACE inhibitors are both *vasodilators* – that is, they open up the blood vessels. This leads to an improvement in blood-flow around the body and better oxygen supply. A calcium channel blocker acts directly on the muscle surrounding the blood vessel while an ACE inhibitor blocks an enzyme in the blood. Some other vasodilators have a direct effect on the muscles around the blood vessels (**hydralazine**, for example); others affect the nerves which control blood vessel muscles. They were all in use before beta blockers, calcium channel blockers and ACE inhibitors were developed.

Clonidine and **rauwolfia** are not used much nowadays. **Methyldopa** can be given to asthmatics and to control high blood pressure during pregnancy. **Guanethidine, bethanidine** and **debrisoquine** all cause too sudden a drop in blood pressure and are used only with other treatments when blood pressure has not been controlled by other means. Alpha blockers (**doxazosin, indoramin, prazosin** and **terazosin**, for example) are sometimes used on their own, but are more usually given with a thiazide diuretic or a beta blocker. The older alpha blockers (**phenoxybenzamine** and **indoramin**) are only used in the management of high blood pressure crises.

HYDRALAZINE

HYDRALAZINE – Tablets
APRESOLINE – Tablets, injection

Hydralazine is a vasodilator which relaxes the muscle surrounding small arteries, allowing them to widen and so improving blood flow. Hydralazine tablets are used to treat moderate to severe high blood pressure, usually with a beta blocker or a thiazide diuretic. In emergency situations when blood pressure suddenly increases, for example during pregnancy (*eclampsia*), hydralazine can be given by injection.

Unwanted effects can be minimised if low doses are given. Sometimes during long-term treatment an auto-immune, arthritis-like syndrome, *systemic lupus erythematosus*, develops, although this usually disappears when hydralazine is stopped.

Before you use this medicine

Tell your doctor if you are:
☐ pregnant or breast-feeding ☐ taking any other medicines, including vitamins and those bought over the counter.

Tell your doctor if you have or have had:
☐ heart disease ☐ stroke ☐ congestive heart failure ☐ poor liver or kidney function ☐ severe kidney disease ☐ systemic lupus erythematosus ☐ porphyria.

How to use this medicine

Take the tablets twice daily with water at mealtimes. You may feel dizzy or faint when you get up from sitting or lying down, especially during the first few days of treatment. Get up slowly and stay beside the chair or bed until you are sure you are not dizzy. Alcohol and other medicines for lowering blood pressure enhance this effect: avoid alcohol. Until you know how you react to hydralazine do not drive or do other activities that require alertness.

If you are on long-term treatment, you may need occasional blood tests.

Do not stop taking this medicine suddenly; your doctor will give you a schedule to decrease the dose gradually. If you miss a dose, take it as soon as you remember, but skip it if it is almost time for your next dose. Do not take double the dose.

Over 65 You may need a lower dose if you have poor kidney or liver function.

Interactions with other medicines

Anaesthetics enhance the blood pressure lowering effect of hydralazine. Tell your doctor or dentist that you take hydralazine before you have surgery.

Unwanted effects

Likely Dizziness, headache, rapid or irregular heartbeat.
Unlikely Feeling or being sick, loss of appetite, diarrhoea or constipation, stuffy nose, skin rashes, fluid retention, joint pains, fever and sore throat, numbness and tingling of the hands and feet.

Headache and dizziness may occur at the start of treatment, but then fade. Contact your doctor if you experience any of the unlikely effects.

PRAZOSIN

HYPOVASE – Tablets

Prazosin is a vasodilator alpha blocker which blocks the nerve stimulus that tightens the muscles around blood vessels. As the muscles relax, the blood vessels widen, blood flow improves and blood pressure is reduced. Prazosin can be used on its own or with another blood pressure lowering medicine. It is also used to treat congestive heart failure, Raynaud's disease and in low doses to ease the symptoms caused by an enlarged prostate gland. Prazosin can cause a marked fall in blood pressure (*hypotension*) on starting treatment, resulting in dizziness and fainting.

Before you use this medicine

Tell you doctor if you are:
☐ pregnant or breast-feeding ☐ on a low-salt diet ☐ taking any other medicines, including vitamins and those bought over the counter.

Tell your doctor if you have or have had:
☐ heart disease ☐ poor kidney or liver function.

How to use this medicine

Treatment is started with a low dose two or three times a day. The dose is gradually increased over a period of a week depending on the response to treatment. If you have liver disease or poor kidney function you may need a reduced dose.

The first dose should be taken at bedtime to avoid fainting and collapse. Take the tablets with a glass of water with food. If you have congestive heart failure, your doctor may ask you to take the tablets up to four times a day.

You may feel dizzy or faint when you get up from sitting or lying down, even after the first dose and especially during the first few days of treatment. Get up slowly and stay beside the bed or chair until you are sure you are not dizzy.

Alcohol and other medicines for lowering blood pressure enhance this effect: avoid alcohol.

Over 65 Older people are more susceptible to dizziness and fainting which may continue beyond the first dose. You should always start treatment with the lowest possible dose.

Interactions with other medicines

Beta blockers and diuretics increase the risk of dizziness or faintness with the first dose.

Unwanted effects

Likely Dizziness, headache, drowsiness, weakness, lack of energy, feeling sick, palpitations.
Unlikely Skin rash, dry mouth, stuffy nose, numbness and tingling of the hands and feet, inability to control urination.

Dizziness and headache should fade as treatment continues. Contact your doctor if these effects are severe and they do not fade or if you develop a rash.

Similar preparations

HYTRIN – Tablets
TERAZOSIN

CARDURA – Tablets
DOXAZOSIN

Angina

Chest pain or angina occurs when the supply of oxygen to heart muscle is restricted by a narrowing of the heart's own blood vessels, the coronary arteries. Angina usually strikes when you exert yourself – running for a bus, for example – or in times of emotional stress, when the heart has to beat faster. If you have angina, the narrowed arteries cannot supply sufficient blood and oxygen during periods of exercise or stress. When you rest, the heartbeat slows, less oxygen is needed and the pain disappears.

During an angina attack, you may experience a tightening or choking feeling which lasts about five to ten minutes and then fades as you rest. You may feel pain in the middle of the chest, or it may spread to your jaws and down your arms; you may get breathless, become pale and perspire. Angina may warn of an approaching heart attack, which can occur if a narrowed artery becomes completely blocked. You must therefore see a doctor at the first sign of any symptoms. If angina comes on suddenly and intensely or occurs when you are not exerting yourself, you must seek help immediately; this may be a sign of an imminent heart attack.

The coronary arteries tend to fur up with fatty deposits of cholesterol as you grow older – this is part of the normal ageing process, but the way we live, what we eat and drink and how much exercise we take all affect how quickly this happens. Ways to avoid or reduce some of the risk factors that encourage heart and circulatory diseases are given in 'How you can help yourself' page 106. The most important risk is smoking, which is a major cause of coronary artery narrowing.

Medicines for angina

Medicines are used to relieve the discomfort of an attack of angina (**glyceryl trinitrate**, for example) or to prevent an attack (a beta blocker or calcium channel blocker, for example). Your doctor may recommend surgery for very severe angina. Although angina is not cured by taking a medicine, most people manage the condition successfully with a nitrate, a beta blocker or a calcium channel blocker.

● *NITRATES* ●

Nitrates are vasodilators with a direct effect on blood vessels and have been in use for well over a hundred years. They are still an important group of medicines for preventing angina before exertion and for relieving chest pain when angina occurs at rest. A nitrate compound, such as glyceryl trinitrate may be used with other medicines or it can sometimes be used on its own, especially for older people with occasional symptoms. Glyceryl trinitrate works for a short time in the body but if a longer action is needed your doctor may prescribe modified-release tablets or a related compound, **isosorbide dinitrate** or **isosorbide mononitrate** tablets.

Glyceryl trinitrate (also known as GTN, nitroglycerin, trinitroglycerin or trinitrin) can be taken by a variety of routes – a common way is under the tongue or between the teeth and cheeks. These methods provide almost immediate relief of symptoms and the effect lasts up to 30 minutes. Modified-release tablets have a longer effect, to prevent an attack. Skin preparations may be helpful if you have angina at rest, for example at night. However, ointment is messy to use and transdermal plasters or patches may have to be removed for part of the day or night because tolerance can develop, reducing the drug's effectiveness.

All the nitrates can cause tolerance, but this tends to happen more with longer-acting nitrates (isosorbide dinitrate and mononitrate), modified-release products and skin preparations. The solution is to allow the body nitrate levels to fall between doses by not taking the tablets as often during the day or by taking the plaster off for several hours each day. Your doctor will guide you on any dosage changes.

GLYCERYL TRINITRATE

On prescription/from a pharmacy
GLYCERYL TRINITRATE – Short-acting tablets
CORO-NITRO SPRAY – Spray
DEPONIT – Plasters
GLYTRIN SPRAY – Spray
GTN 300mcg – Short-acting tablets
NITROCONTIN CONTINUS – Modified-release tablets
NITRO-DUR – Plasters
NITROLINGUAL SPRAY – Spray
PERCUTOL – Ointment
SUSCARD – Modified-release tablets
SUSTAC – Modified-release tablets
TRANSIDERM-NITRO – Plasters

Prescription only
GLYCERYL TRINITRATE – Injection
NITROCINE – Injection
NITRONAL – Injection
TRIDIL – Injection

Glyceryl trinitrate is a vasodilator which relieves an attack of angina or prevents one developing. It is also used to treat heart failure. When the tablets are dissolved in the mouth or the spray used, glyceryl trinitrate starts to work almost at once and acts for about half an hour. Modified-release tablets are used for a longer action, and one of these preparations (Suscard) can be dissolved in the mouth for immediate as well as longer-term relief.

Before you use this medicine

Tell your doctor if you are:
☐ pregnant or breast-feeding ☐ taking any other medicines, including vitamins and those bought over the counter.

Tell your doctor if you have or have had:
☐ severe anaemia ☐ head injuries or internal bleeding ☐ glaucoma.

How to use this medicine

To relieve an angina attack Dissolve a tablet slowly under the tongue. Do not chew, crush or swallow the tablet. You should feel the effects of glyceryl trinitrate in about five minutes. You can spit out the remains of the tablet as soon as the pain is relieved. If the pain does not go away in five minutes, take a second tablet. Alternatively, use the spray, applying one or two doses under the tongue and closing the mouth after each dose. Do not take more than three doses of the spray at one time. **If you still have pain after 10 to 15 minutes, contact your doctor.**
To prevent angina Take the modified-release tablets two or three times a day. Detailed instructions on how to apply skin preparations are supplied with the manufacturers' packs. Avoid putting the plaster on the same part of the skin every time. The ointment must be carefully measured, put on the body without rubbing in and dressed with a clean dressing.

You may feel dizzy or faint during the first few days of treatment. Try to sit down to take the dose of medicine. If you feel dizzy, lie down or put your head between your knees, breathe deeply and move your arms and legs about. Alcohol and other medicines for lowering blood pressure may make you feel more dizzy: avoid alcohol. Until you know how you react to glyceryl trinitrate do not drive or do other activities that require alertness. Do not stop taking this medicine suddenly; your doctor will give you a schedule to decrease the dose gradually without chest pains recurring.

Storage Glyceryl trinitrate tablets lose their strength once the bottle is opened to the air. The tablets must not be put into any other container and the bottle must always be kept tightly closed. Eight weeks after opening, replace any unused tablets with another supply. The spray preparation can be kept for up to three years and might be better if you only need glyceryl trinitrate occasionally. However, the spray products are flammable and must not be used near a naked flame.

Over 65 You may be more susceptible to dizziness or fainting, especially if glyceryl trinitrate is given with a beta blocker. You may need a lower dose.

Interactions with other medicines

Anaesthetics enhance the blood pressure lowering effects of glyceryl trinitrate. Tell your doctor or dentist that you take glyceryl trinitrate before you have surgery.
Blood pressure lowering medicines enhance the effect of glyceryl trinitrate.
Dry mouth Some medicines make your mouth dry (antidepressants, for example): glyceryl trinitrate may not dissolve so easily and may be less effective.

Unwanted effects

Likely Dizziness, lightheadedness, flushing of the face and neck, throbbing headache, palpitations.

Unwanted effects are quite common during the first few days of treatment, but usually fade with time. If any of the effects continue to trouble you, contact your doctor.

Similar preparations

On prescription/from a pharmacy
ISOSORBIDE DINITRATE
Brand names (short-acting tablets):
CEDOCARD; ISORDIL; SORBICHEW; SORBITRATE; VASCARDIN
(modified-release tablets and capsules):
CEDOCARD RETARD; ISOKET RETARD; ISORDIL TEMBIDS; SONI-SLO; SORBID SA

ISOSORBIDE MONONITRATE
Brand names (short-acting tablets):
ELANTAN; ISMO; ISOTRATE; MONIT; MONO-CEDOCARD

(modified-release tablets and capsules):
ELANTAN LA; IMDUR (prescription only); ISMO RETARD; MCR-50; MONIT SR
PENTAERYTHRITOL TETRANITRATE
Brand names CARDIACAP; MYCARDOL

Heart attack

Heart attack occurs when the blood supply to the heart is cut off because the coronary artery becomes blocked. In arteries that have already narrowed, a sudden blood clot can stop the blood flow (*coronary thrombosis*). Part of the heart muscle that has been starved of blood and oxygen then becomes permanently damaged (*myocardial infarction*). If you have angina, narrowing of the arteries restricts blood supply, but does not stop it completely and this leaves the heart undamaged.

Although angina may warn of a heart attack, it is possible to have chest pains for years without suffering an attack. Many people show no direct signs of an impending heart attack; some have a heart attack without realising – only tests show that the heart has been damaged. It is important to recognise the signs of a heart attack, to know what is happening to you or to someone who is with you: there may be crushing pain in the middle of the chest which extends to the jaw and down the left arm; you may look pale, feel faint and unwell and you may be breathless and perspire.

After an attack there is a high risk of complications and treatment will be needed urgently. Once the heart is damaged, its cells often generate erratic electrical impulses, disrupting the heart's beat and rhythm. These *arrhythmias*, particularly *ventricular fibrillation*, prevent the heart from working properly. At this stage the heart may stop suddenly (*cardiac arrest*), causing death (see 'Could you save a life?', page 134).

When medical help arrives, the doctor will usually give you an *analgesic*, a pain-relieving injection of morphine or diamorphine before you have further treatment, usually in hospital. Sometimes you may feel sick and vomit, which may be treated with an anti-sickness medicine (*anti-emetic*). In hospital you may be given a diuretic (frusemide, for example) to reduce the body's fluid and the load on the heart. An *anti-arrhythmic* drug may be given to counter irregular heartbeats. *Fibrinolytic* drugs, also called *thrombolytics*, break up blood clots (*thrombi*) in the coronary artery and

COULD YOU SAVE A LIFE?

Many people die in the first minutes after a heart attack. Once the heart is damaged, the regular rhythm and pace may be disrupted and the heart may suddenly stop beating. Without proper blood flow the organs, particularly the brain, are damaged by lack of oxygen. Heart–lung massage (*cardiopulmonary resuscitation*) given before the doctor or ambulance crew arrives could save the person's life. Delays in reviving and treating people who have had a heart attack results in 20,000 deaths a year. The 'Save a Life' campaign was launched in 1986 to encourage members of the public to train in the technique. To find out how you could help in an emergency, contact the British Heart Foundation for information. Courses in resuscitation techniques are run by The British Red Cross Society, St John's Ambulance, The Royal Life Saving Society and St Andrew's Ambulance Association in Scotland. The Resuscitation Council produces a booklet. See 'Useful addresses'.

minimise long-term damage to the heart muscle; they are used as early as possible after a heart attack. You may be given a *beta blocker* to help to stabilise the heart, first by injection and later by mouth. Some people may have to take a beta blocker for at least a year or possibly longer to control high blood pressure, or angina or irregular heartbeats. Aspirin is also a valuable treatment, but your doctor will guide you about how and when to take it.

A heart attack is serious, but on recovery you should be able to lead an active life. You may need to change your lifestyle – eating a balanced diet, taking regular exercise and giving up smoking.

Reducing the risk of heart attack

Britain has one of the highest rates of coronary heart disease in Europe: one in three men die of it and one in four women. Under the age of 50, men are more likely to die of a heart attack than women, but after the menopause the women's rate begins to increase. Some people are at risk because there is a strong family history of heart disease or they have a medical condition, such as diabetes or gout, which speeds up the process of arterial narrowing. Some women who take the contraceptive pill are at risk, particularly if they are overweight and smoke. Other people are at risk because they smoke, or have high blood pressure or an inappropriate diet. A combination of these factors puts you in the very high risk group for a heart attack.

● *Stop smoking*

Each cigarette contains over 3,000 chemicals of which nicotine and carbon monoxide are the most significant causes of cardiovascular disease. Nicotine increases the heart rate, raises the blood pressure and slowly tightens the blood vessels, so reducing blood flow around the body, especially to the hands and feet. Carbon monoxide gas binds tightly to *haemoglobin* (a constituent of blood) to form *carboxyhaemoglobin*. This decreases the amount of oxygen circulating in the blood and all parts of the body, including the heart, are deprived of oxygen. Carboxyhaemoglobin and nicotine significantly increase the risk of angina and heart attacks. Circulatory problems lead to peripheral vascular disease which may result in gangrene and ultimately limb amputation.

The best thing you can do for your heart is to stop smoking. Although lung cancer is a well known adverse effect of smoking, you are just as likely to suffer cardiovascular disease. Smokers are twice as likely to have a heart attack as non-smokers and if you are under 50, you are ten times more likely to die from a heart attack than a non-smoker of the same age. If you have high blood pressure or raised blood-cholesterol levels, smoking adds to the risk of a heart attack. It is never too late to give up smoking: the heart and blood vessels start to recover immediately and the risk of heart disease diminishes.

● *Reduce high blood pressure*

The risks of high blood pressure have already been discussed; see 'How you can help yourself', page 106.

● *Reduce blood cholesterol*

Inappropriate diet and in particular high blood levels of cholesterol (a type of fat) are important risk factors for heart disease. Lowering high levels of cholesterol appears to reduce the risk of developing coronary heart disease and can slow its progress. Eating too much fat, especially saturated fat, stimulates the liver to produce more cholesterol than the body needs. This additional cholesterol is carried around in the blood and eventually deposited in the arteries as *atheroma*. As this process (*atherosclerosis*) continues over a long period, the arteries narrow and the blood flow becomes restricted and slows. When blood flows less freely and has to be squeezed through narrow vessels it is more likely to form abnormal clots. It is these abberrant clots that can trigger a heart attack or stroke if the blood vessel becomes blocked completely.

Cholesterol is transported in the blood by two kinds of carriers. *Low-density lipoproteins* (LDL) take cholesterol from the liver to the arteries and deposit it along the walls of the blood vessels. *High-density lipoproteins* (HDL) carry cholesterol from the arteries to the liver where it is broken down. High levels of HDL are therefore associated with a lower risk of heart disease, whereas high levels of LDL increase the risk.

Cutting down on fatty foods and replacing saturated fats with unsaturated fats can help to reduce blood levels of cholesterol. Do not cut fat out of your diet altogether: a small amount is necessary for a healthy diet. Saturated fat is found in butter, hard margarine, milk, hard full-fat cheeses, lard, cream, palm oil, sausages, pies and red meat. Unsaturated fat is found in polyunsaturated margarines, in corn, sunflower and safflower oils, and in oily fish, such as tuna, herring and mackerel. Some evidence exists that eating oily fish such as mackerel or herring, which contain particular unsaturated fatty acids (*omega-3 marine triglycerides*), may help to prevent heart disease. Replacing saturated fats with monosaturated fats, such as olive oil and rapeseed oil can also reduce LDL levels.

• *LIPID-LOWERING MEDICINES* •

People who have high blood-fat levels in spite of dieting, stopping smoking, and reducing high blood pressure may need treatment with a fat- (lipid-) lowering medicine. They may have a condition that puts them at risk, such as diabetes or an inherited disorder of fat metabolism. A family history of coronary heart disease, especially if someone had a heart attack before the age of 50, puts young men at risk. Illness can disturb the body's handling of fat: your blood-fat levels may be altered for up to 3 months after a heart attack and during acute pancreatitis. People on long-term kidney dialysis may also have high blood-fats.

Treatment begins after blood tests to determine your blood-fat levels and which type of fat is raised. A lipid-lowering medicine will not affect existing cholesterol deposits, but may stop new ones forming. You may have to take the medicine for a long time: blood-fats usually return to a high level once you stop treatment.

Cholestyramine and **colestipol** bind with cholesterol-containing bile acids which help with the digestion of fat in the intestine. As the drug plus cholesterol and bile acids are removed from the body, the liver converts more cholesterol into bile acids to replace the lost amount. These drugs increase the amount of LDL-cholesterol broken down in the liver resulting in lower blood-cholesterol levels. Fibric acid drugs (**clofibrate**, **bezafibrate**, **fenofibrate** and **gemfibrozil**) and the nicotinic acid group (**nicotinic acid**, **acipimox** and **nicofuranose**) interfere with the conversion of fatty acids to different types of lipids in the liver. A newer group, the statins (**pravastatin** and **simvastatin**), block an enzyme in the cholesterol production process, mostly in the liver. The statins lower LDL-cholesterol better than the cholestyramine group, but are not so effective in raising HDL-cholesterol and reducing triglycerides as the fibric acid drugs.

BEZAFIBRATE

BEZALIP – Tablets
BEZALIP–MONO – Modified-release tablets

Bezafibrate affects the blood cholesterol levels by reducing LDL-cholesterol levels and increasing HDL-cholesterol. Its main action is to decrease blood levels of another type of fat, triglyceride. Bezafibrate should only be used if dietary measures have failed, for example in people who have inherited disorders of fat metabolism, and where high levels of blood fats are a risk.

Before you use this medicine

Tell your doctor if you are:
☐ pregnant – bezafibrate is not recommended ☐ breast-feeding ☐ taking any other medicines, including vitamins and those bought over the counter.

Tell your doctor if you have or have had:
☐ gallstones ☐ gallbladder disease ☐ kidney or liver disease – bezafibrate is not recommended in severe cases.

How to use this medicine

Take the tablets three times daily with or after meals. Bezalip-Mono must be swallowed whole, not chewed, and can be taken once a day with an evening meal. You will need to continue on a low-fat diet.

If you have mild to moderate impairment of kidney function, you may need a lower dose of bezafibrate. You may need periodic blood tests to assess blood-fat levels and liver function.

Over 65 No special requirements.

Interactions with other medicines

Anticoagulants (for example **warfarin**) Their effect is enhanced by bezafibrate and the dose of the anticoagulant will need to be reduced.

Unwanted effects

Likely Feeling sick, abdominal pains, bloating or discomfort.
Unlikely Aching or muscle cramps, impotence, skin rashes, hypersensitivity.

The incidence of unwanted effects is low. Bezafibrate is related to an older drug, clofibrate, which can encourage gallstone formation, but bezafibrate does not appear to do this.

Similar preparations

ATROMID-S – Capsules
CLOFIBRATE

LIPANTIL – Capsules
FENOFIBRATE

LOPID – Capsules
GEMFIBROZIL

SIMVASTATIN

ZOCOR – Tablets

Simvastatin is a new lipid-lowering drug. It lowers blood levels of cholesterol and LDL-cholesterol by suppressing a liver enzyme needed for their production. Simvastatin may help people with very high blood levels of cholesterol who have not responded to diet or other treatments. Unwanted effects of simvastatin are mild and may disappear as treatment continues. Muscle pain may be a problem and you should tell your doctor about this.

Before you use this medicine

Tell your doctor if you are:
☐ pregnant or planning to become pregnant – do not take

simvastatin; women of child-bearing age must use reliable contraception other than an oral contraceptive ☐ breast-feeding ☐ taking any other medicines, including vitamins and those bought over the counter.

Tell your doctor if you have or have had:
☐ liver disease ☐ porphyria.

How to use this medicine

Simvastatin treatment is started at a low dose, which is increased depending on blood-fat levels. The tablets are taken once a day with the evening meal. You will need to continue on a low-fat diet and avoid alcohol. You should have periodic blood tests to assess blood-fat levels and liver function.

Over 65 No special requirements.

Interactions with other medicines

Anticoagulants (**warfarin** and **nicoumalone**, for example). Simvastatin may enhance their effect and their dosage may need altering.

Unwanted effects

Likely Digestive disorders such as flatulence, indigestion, stomach pain, constipation, diarrhoea and feeling sick.
Unlikely Headache, insomnia, skin rash, muscle pains or weakness.

Tell your doctor if you have any muscle pains or weakness.

Similar preparations

▼LIPOSTAT – Tablets
PRAVASTATIN

Heart failure

Chronic heart failure is a gradual process which develops when the heart cannot pump blood efficiently. The left side of the heart pumps blood from the lungs to the rest of the body; if it cannot do this effectively, the lungs become congested, causing breathlessness. In addition, the rest of the body does not receive all the oxygen it needs, which leads to tiredness and causes excess fluid (*oedema*) to accumulate, mainly in the ankles. Acute heart failure can be sudden and severe and must be treated quickly. The main effect is excess fluid on the lungs. High blood pressure, narrowing of the coronary arteries or damage to the heart valves may cause the heart to fail.

HOW YOU CAN HELP YOURSELF

☐ **Lose weight** if you are overweight, to reduce the load on the heart

☐ **Restrict salt**, but discuss this with your doctor

☐ **Avoid alcohol**

☐ **Stop smoking**

☐ **Exercise** within your capabilities – take gentle walks, for example.

Medicines for heart failure

DIURETICS

First of all you may be given a diuretic to remove excess fluid from the body. This will reduce the pressure in the heart, ease congestion in the lungs and remove accumulated fluid from the ankles. A loop diuretic, such as **frusemide** is generally used in both acute and chronic heart failure. For longer term treatment, your doctor may give you a thiazide diuretic or a potassium-sparing diuretic (see pages 107–115). A vasodilator may be added to treatment with a diuretic (see 'Calcium channel blockers', 'ACE inhibitors' and 'Other vasodilators', pages 120–128, and 'Nitrates', pages 129–133).

FRUSEMIDE

FRUSEMIDE – Liquid, tablets, injection
LASIX – Liquid, tablets, injection

Combined with potassium-sparing diuretic
FRUMIL – Tablets
FRUSEMIDE + AMILORIDE

FRUSENE – Tablets
FRUSEMIDE + TRIAMTERENE
LASILACTONE– Capsules
FRUSEMIDE + SPIRONOLACTONE
LASORIDE – Tablets
FRUSEMIDE + AMILORIDE

Poor choice – frusemide with potassium
DIUMIDE-K CONTINUS
LASIKAL
LASIX+K

Frusemide is a loop diuretic, so called because it acts on the looped part of the kidney tubule. It stops sodium, potassium and water being taken back into the body, so they are lost as urine. Frusemide is a powerful diuretic used to remove extra fluid from the heart, lungs, liver, kidneys and the periphery of the body (the ankles, for example). The tablet acts within an hour and continues working for about four hours; the injection is used for emergencies when prompt and effective diuresis is needed. The body's salt and water balance may be upset, particularly with long-term treatment. You may need to take extra potassium (see page 111), but not combined with frusemide in one tablet.

Before you use this medicine

Tell your doctor if you are:
☐ pregnant or breast-feeding ☐ on a low-salt or low-sugar diet ☐ taking any other medicines, including vitamins and those bought over the counter.

Tell your doctor if you have or have had:
☐ diabetes ☐ gout ☐ kidney or liver disease (especially liver disease caused by alcohol) ☐ prostate trouble ☐ hearing loss ☐ porphyria ☐ hypersensitivity to frusemide or an antibacterial sulphonamide.

How to use this medicine

Take the tablet once a day in the morning. If you have to take another dose, try to take it by mid-afternoon, so that night-time sleep is not disturbed by extra visits to the toilet; during the first few days of treatment, you will produce a larger volume of urine and may need to go to the toilet more often than usual.

You will lose potassium while taking frusemide so eat plenty of potassium-rich foods (see page 111). Your doctor may prescribe a potassium supplement. Because a diuretic helps you to lose water, you may lose too much and become dehydrated – you will feel thirsty and your skin may look and feel dry. Make sure that your daily fluid intake is adequate. Dehydration is likely to make you more susceptible to alcohol: drink only small quantities.

You may feel dizzy when you get up from sitting or lying

down, especially during the first few days of treatment. Get up slowly and stay beside the chair or bed until you are sure you are not dizzy. Do not drive or do other activities that require alertness until you know how you react to frusemide.

Over 65 You may need a lower dose. Older people are more susceptible to the unwanted effects, such as dizziness and mental confusion.

Interactions with other medicines

Digoxin becomes more toxic if frusemide causes low blood-potassium levels. Potassium supplements must always be taken if digoxin and frusemide are used together.
Anti-arrhythmic drugs Their action is upset if frusemide causes low blood-potassium levels.
ACE inhibitors Their blood pressure lowering effect is enhanced by frusemide, which should be stopped for at least three days before you take an ACE inhibitor.
Lithium stays in the body longer and may reach toxic levels.
Some hospital antibiotics (**gentamicin** and **amikacin**, for example) Frusemide or bumetanide, a similar loop diuretic, increase the risk of hearing loss.

Unwanted effects

Likely Dizziness, upset in body's salts – loss of sodium, potassium and calcium.
Unlikely Feeling sick, digestive disorders, confusion, headache, muscle cramps, unusual tiredness or weakness.
If any of the unwanted effects are troublesome, discuss them with your doctor. If skin rash occurs, stop taking frusemide.

Similar preparations

ARELIX – Capsules
PIRETANIDE

BURINEX – Tablets, liquid, injection
BUMETANIDE

EDECRIN – Tablets, injection
ETHACRYNIC ACID

Combined with a thiazide diuretic

BURINEX A – Tablets
BUMETANIDE + AMILORIDE

• *DIGOXIN* •

Digoxin has been widely used to treat heart failure, but it is no longer so popular. It is not generally used on its own to treat heart failure, but may be prescribed with a diuretic. Digoxin is an age-old remedy from a species of the foxglove family and is also used to control heart rhythm disorders. It makes the heart beat more forcefully and simultaneously reduces the flow of electrical impulses which stimulate the heart to beat. When the heart rhythm is disrupted (in *atrial fibrillation*, for example) digoxin is very useful for controlling it, especially if heart failure is involved. Once heart failure is under control, your doctor will generally stop digoxin, because the margin between a harmful and a helpful dose is small. Unwanted effects limit digoxin's usefulness for treating heart failure, especially for older people.

DIGOXIN

DIGOXIN – Tablets, injection
LANOXIN – Tablets, injection
LANOXIN-PG – Liquid, tablets (for children and elderly people)

Digoxin makes the heart muscle contract more forcefully and improves the pumping of blood through the heart. Digoxin slows the heart rate by affecting the nervous and electrical control of the heart. It can relieve heart failure and control certain types of irregular heart rhythm (*atrial fibrillation*, for example).

Digoxin must be used carefully because the margin between its helpful effects and harmful ones is small. Older people are especially susceptible to the toxic effects of digoxin.

Before you use this medicine

Tell your doctor if you are:
☐ pregnant or breast-feeding ☐ taking any other medicines, including vitamins and those bought over the counter.

Tell your doctor if you have or have had:
☐ Wolff-Parkinson-White syndrome (a particular type of heart rhythm irregularity) ☐ toxic effects from digoxin or other *digitalis* preparations ☐ a recent heart attack ☐ thyroid problems ☐ poor kidney or liver function.

How to use this medicine

The dose and the timing of each dose varies at the start of treatment depending on the heart's requirements. Take the tablets or liquid on an empty stomach. If digoxin makes you feel sick, then you can take it with food. Eat plenty of potassium-rich foods (see page 111); your doctor may prescribe a potassium supplement, especially if you are taking a diuretic as well.

Do not drive or do other activities that require alertness until you know how you react to digoxin. Do not stop taking this medicine suddenly as symptoms may recur; your doctor will give you a schedule to decrease the dose gradually. If you miss a dose, take it as soon as you remember, but skip it if it is almost time for your next dose – do not take double the dose.

If you have kidney disease or poor kidney function, you will need less than the adult dose. You may need periodic blood tests to monitor digoxin and potassium blood levels.

Over 65 You are more likely to experience unwanted effects and adverse reactions with digoxin, so should have a reduced dose. Check with your doctor that you really need to take digoxin.

Interactions with other medicines

Digoxin interacts with many other medicines. Do not take other medicines without checking with your doctor or pharmacist. The following are the most important.

Anti-arrhythmics, **calcium channel blockers**, **quinine** (and possibly **chloroquine**) increase the blood levels of digoxin and therefore the toxic effects. The dose of digoxin must be reduced.

Unwanted effects

Likely Loss of appetite, feeling or being sick, diarrhoea, irregular heartbeats.

Unlikely Slow pulse, weakness, blurred vision or coloured 'haloes', confusion, headache, bad dreams, hallucinations.

Unwanted effects may be due to an increase in the level of digoxin in the blood; contact your doctor to discuss them. Irregular heartbeats need emergency action.

Similar preparations

DIGITOXIN – Tablets

Irregular heartbeat

The pumping action of the *atria* and *ventricles* is co-ordinated by electrical impulses generated by the nerves to the heart. Specialised heart cells act as pacemakers to control the flow of electrical impulses across the heart muscle cells. Irregular heart rhythms (*arrhythmias*) occur if the co-ordination of the heart's pumping action is upset or interrupted in any way. The heart may beat too slowly (*bradycardia*), too quickly (*tachycardia*) or irregularly. 'Missed beat', 'jumped beat' or palpitations which you can feel are not serious; the occasional missed beat rarely needs treatment. Rhythm disturbances which you cannot feel, but which cause the heart to pump blood around the body less efficiently usually do need medical treatment. Abnormal rhythms should be diagnosed accurately with an electrocardiograph (ECG) – a machine which measures the heart's electrical activity.

Some babies are born with irregular heart rhythms, but for many people, abnormal rhythms develop when the heart is damaged or diseased. Other causes include caffeine in tea and coffee, alcohol, smoking and thyroid disease. Arrhythmias can occur at any age and may not always need drug treatment.

Irregular heart rhythms are named after the part of heart they affect and the type of beat abnormality: *supraventricular* or *atrial* arrhythmias occur in the atria, *ventricular* in the ventricles; *tachycardia* is fast co-ordinated beating; *fibrillation* or flutter is rapid unco-ordinated beating. *Bradycardia* is slow beating – below 60 beats per minute. Heart block (*atrioventricular block*) occurs when electrical impulses are not passed from the atria to the ventricles. The ventricles beat at a slower rate. An artificial pacemaker may be fitted.

Anti-arrhythmic medicines

Anti-arrhythmic medicines are grouped either according to their effects on the electrical activity of heart cells (four classes) or, more usually, the arrhythmias they control. Anti-arrhythmics

NORMAL HEART RHYTHM

An adult heart beats at the rate of 70–80 beats per minute, whereas a child's heart rate may be 90 beats per minute. The rate of the heartbeat varies with activity. During exercise, stress or anxiety the rate increases and while you are asleep or resting it decreases.

Count the number of beats your pulse makes per minute at the wrist to find your heart rate. If the rate is more than 120 beats per minute or less than 60, get medical advice.

may be given to treat a single episode of heart rhythm irregularities or, if these become established, to prevent them happening. Low levels of blood-potassium increase the anti-arrhythmic effects of many of these medicines: a daily diet with some potassium-containing foods is advisable, but discuss this with your doctor. Most or all anti-arrhythmics are also capable of provoking arrhythmias in certain circumstances.

• *Supraventricular arrhythmias*

Atrial fibrillation occurs when the atria beat rapidly and are not co-ordinated with the ventricles. **Digoxin** is usually used to control electrical activity, sometimes with **quinidine**. *Supraventricular tachycardia* happens when extra electrical impulses arise in the heart's pacemaker region to stimulate the ventricles. The calcium channel blocker **verapamil** is often used. A beta blocker slows the heart and dampens increased nervous activity to the heart.

• *Ventricular arrhythmias*

Ventricular tachycardias range from minor to life-threatening problems. Various drugs, such as **lignocaine** are given by injection in hospital to control abnormal rhythms. The underlying heart disorders that contribute to rhythm irregularities are treated, for example with **amiodarone**.

• *Supraventricular and ventricular arrhythmias*

A variety of medicines is used when these two types of arrhythmia occur simultaneously – **amiodarone**, a beta blocker, **disopyramide**, and less commonly **flecainide**, **procainamide** and **quinidine**.

VERAPAMIL

VERAPAMIL – Tablets
BERKATENS – Tablets
CORDILOX – Tablets, injection
SECURON – Tablets, injection
For high blood pressure and angina
SECURON SR – Modified-release tablets
UNIVER – Modified-release capsules

Verapamil is a calcium channel blocker which affects the flow of calcium across the cells of blood vessels and heart muscle. It can be used to lower high blood pressure and to treat and prevent angina or supraventricular arrhythmias. Verapamil can be used by asthmatics.

Before you use this medicine

Tell your doctor if you are:
☐ pregnant or breast-feeding ☐ taking any other medicines, including vitamins and those bought over the counter.

Tell your doctor if you have or have had:
☐ kidney or liver disease.

Do not take it if you have or have had:
☐ heart failure ☐ very slow heart rate (*bradycardia*) ☐ low blood pressure ☐ Wolff-Parkinson-White syndrome or heart block ☐ sick sinus syndrome ☐ porphyria.

How to use this medicine

Take the tablets two or three times daily. You may be given the injection in hospital to control arrhythmias and then change to tablets. You may feel dizzy or faint when you get up from sitting or lying down, especially during the first few days of treatment. Get up slowly and stay beside the chair or bed until you are sure you are not dizzy.

Do not drive or do other activities that require alertness until you know how you react to verapamil. Alcohol and other blood pressure lowering medicines increase verapamil's effect: avoid alcohol.

Do not stop taking this medicine suddenly as this may change the heart rhythm. Your doctor will give you a schedule to decrease the dose of verapamil gradually. If you miss a dose, take it as soon as you remember. If your next dose is due within three hours take the missed dose and skip the next one.

If you have poor liver function, you will need a reduced dose.

Over 65 Take the same as the adult dose, unless your liver or kidney function is reduced.

Interactions with other medicines

General anaesthetics Verapamil enhances the blood pressure lowering effects; tell your doctor or dentist that you take verapamil before you have surgery.
Anti-arrhythmics, such as **quinidine** increases the blood levels of verapamil; a severe drop in blood pressure may occur.
Beta blockers used with verapamil may cause irregular heartbeats, a severe drop in blood pressure and heart failure.
Digoxin Blood levels increase, with a risk of toxicity.
Theophylline (used for asthma) Blood levels increase, with a risk of toxicity.

Unwanted effects

Likely Constipation.
Unlikely Headache, feeling or being sick, dizziness, tiredness or weakness, ankle swelling.
Rare but serious Allergic reactions, reversible impairment of liver function. Long-term treatment can cause reversible breast-swelling in elderly men and overgrowth of the gums.

Contact your doctor if you feel dizzy whilst taking verapamil. Discuss troublesome unwanted effects with your doctor.

AMIODARONE

CORDARONE X – Tablets, injection

Amiodarone is used for the treatment of irregular heart rhythms, especially the Wolff-Parkinson-White syndrome, where extra electrical impulses travel from the atria to the ventricles and upset the rhythm. Amiodarone can be used to control supraventricular and ventricular tachycardias, atrial fibrillation and recurrent ventricular fibrillation. It is generally used when other medicines cannot be used or have proved ineffective. When taken by mouth amiodarone's effects are felt gradually, but it may stay in the body for up to three months after treatment is stopped. Intravenous amiodarone acts quite rapidly. Because amiodarone can cause a number of adverse effects, such as thyroid problems and eye, liver and lung damage, treatment is usually started by a specialist.

Before you use this medicine

Tell your doctor if you are:
☐ pregnant or breast-feeding – you should not use amiodarone ☐ taking any other medicines, including vitamins and those bought over the counter.

Tell your doctor if you have or have had:
☐ liver disease ☐ heart failure ☐ reduced kidney function ☐ eye problems ☐ lung conditions, such as asthma ☐ thyroid problems ☐ heart block ☐ extremely low heart rate ☐ porphyria.

How to use this medicine

The tablets are taken on a long-term basis to prevent attacks. To begin with they are taken three times a day, then the dosage is reduced to twice a day and finally once a day or every other day. You should have the lowest possible dose to control arrhythmias and to minimise unwanted effects. If you miss a dose and the next dose is due within 12 hours, do not take it. Do not take double doses: take your next scheduled dose as usual.

If you have poor liver function, you may need a lower dose. You should have periodic tests to assess liver function. Your doctor will also monitor thyroid function. Amiodarone can cause both high and low thyroid levels in the body. It also interferes with some of the tests for thyroid function and so you should be alert for changes in how you feel while you take amiodarone.

Over 65 You may need less than the adult dose. You are most likely to experience unwanted reactions. There may be another anti-arrhythmic drug that is more suitable to take than amiodarone.

Interactions with other medicines

Anticoagulants (**warfarin** and **nicoumalone**) Effects increased by amiodarone.
Phenytoin Effect increased by amiodarone.
Heart drugs (**digoxin, beta blockers** and **calcium channel blockers**) Amiodarone increases the risk of very low heart rate and heart block.

Unwanted effects

Likely Sensitivity to light – you should protect your skin from sunlight with a reliable sunscreen preparation. During long-term treatment tiny spots appear on the cornea; they rarely interfere with sight, although occasionally may cause 'haloes'. Drivers may be dazzled by headlights at night. These spots fade when amiodarone is stopped. Routine eye examinations are advisable.
Unlikely Slate-grey or bluish discoloration of the skin, skin rashes, numbness and tingling in the limbs, shortness of breath, thyroid problems, feeling or being sick, headache, metallic taste, nightmares, dizziness, tiredness.

While you are taking amiodarone you will need to see your doctor for routine checks. Low doses minimise unwanted effects which usually disappear once you stop taking amiodarone. You should contact your doctor if you develop any of the unlikely effects.

DISOPYRAMIDE

DISOPYRAMIDE – Capsules, modified-release capsules
RYTHMODAN – Capsules, modified-release tablets
DIRYTHMIN SA – Modified-release capsules

Disopyramide is used for the treatment of irregular heart rhythms, including ventricular arrhythmias – especially after a heart attack – and supraventricular arrythmias. When given by injection, disopyramide can worsen heart failure and low blood pressure.

Before you use this medicine

Tell your doctor if you are:
☐ pregnant or breast-feeding ☐ taking any other medicines, including vitamins and those bought over the counter.

Tell your doctor if you have or had:
☐ heart failure ☐ low blood pressure ☐ prostate trouble (an enlarged prostate, for example) ☐ urinary retention ☐ glaucoma ☐ poor kidney function ☐ poor liver function ☐ high or low blood-potassium ☐ sick sinus syndrome.

How to use this medicine

Take the capsules three or four times a day depending on your response to treatment. Sustained-release preparations are taken twice a day, every 12 hours. They must be swallowed whole, not crushed or chewed. If you miss a dose take it as soon as you remember. Skip it, if it is less than four hours (eight hours for sustained-release preparations) until your next scheduled dose. Do not take double the dose.

You may feel dizzy or faint when you get up from sitting or lying down, especially during the first few days of treatment. Get up slowly and stay beside the chair or bed until you are sure you are not dizzy. Avoid alcohol, as it enhances the effect of disopyramide.

Do not drive or do other activities that require alertness until you know how you react to disopyramide. Do not stop taking disopyramide suddenly: your doctor will give you a schedule to decrease the dose gradually. If you have poor kidney function, you will need a reduced dose.

Over 65 You are likely to need less than the standard adult dose. Unwanted effects may be more troublesome.

Interactions with other medicines

Diuretics If low blood levels of potassium develop, the toxicity of disopyramide increases.
Antibacterials: rifampicin reduces blood levels of disopyramide making it less effective; **erythromycin** increases blood levels of disopyramide and therefore increases the risk of toxic effects.

Unwanted effects

Likely Dry mouth, blurred vision, constipation, difficulty passing urine, dizziness, faintness.
Unlikely Mental effects, confusion, low blood-sugar, irregular heart rhythms.

Similar preparations

KINIDIN DURULES – Modified-release tablets
QUINIDINE

KIDITARD – Modified-release capsules
QUINIDINE

QUINIDINE SULPHATE – Tablets

PROCAINAMIDE DURULES – Modified-release tablets
PROCAINAMIDE

PRONESTYL – Tablets, injection
PROCAINAMIDE

Stroke

Stroke or a *cerebrovascular accident* is damage to the brain caused by bleeding or a blocked blood vessel in the brain. If the blood supply to a part of the brain is interrupted for longer than 24 hours, a stroke has occurred. If the blood supply is cut off for a shorter time, this is known as a *transient ischaemic attack*. Most people who have a transient ischaemic attack begin to improve within minutes and have often recovered by the time they see a doctor; there is no lasting damage to the body. If you suffer a stroke, you may not recover completely.

The right side of the brain controls the functions of the left side of the body and vice versa. The part of the body controlled by the damaged area of the brain will be affected. Weakness or paralysis of one side of the body is common, although other faculties may be lost – for example, control of mental and emotional processes or the ability to speak or understand language. Sight, sound, smell, taste and touch may be affected. If brain cells die, then other areas of the brain try to compensate and take over their role. Recovery depends on how well the brain can do this and it may take several months before you know what parts of the body have been affected permanently.

Stroke rarely happens to young people: it is a condition of old age. Twenty per cent of stroke victims die within a month and about 40 per cent recover almost completely. The remaining 40 per cent (around 200,000 people at any one time) become disabled in some way.

When fatty deposits build up inside blood vessels and cause them to narrow, a blood clot (*thrombus*) may block a vessel. Other parts of the brain may not be able to compensate for the lost brain cells because the remaining arteries are also likely to be diseased.

Recovery from stroke caused by thrombosis is therefore difficult.

Haemorrhage occurs when a blood vessel ruptures and blood leaks out into the brain. The blood starts to clot and pressure from the clot also damages the brain. Unlike thrombosis, which may develop over some hours or days, a brain haemorrhage usually happens suddenly.

Part of a blood clot or collection of blood cells may break off from a blood vessel and travel round the bloodstream until it gets stuck in a smaller artery. If the collection of cells (*embolus*) is very small, it may disperse, letting the blood flow return to normal. This happens in a transient ischaemic attack.

HOW YOU CAN HELP YOURSELF

● *PREVENTING STROKE* ●

☐ Reduce high blood pressure
☐ Lose weight – reduce fat and salt intake
☐ Stop smoking
☐ Take regular exercise
☐ A daily dose of aspirin may prevent a recurrence of stroke; discuss this with your doctor.

Treatment for stroke

Medicines cannot cure a stroke once it has happened. Many drugs have been tried, but none has been shown to improve the final outcome. Drug treatment has only a small role to play in the management of a person after a stroke – for example in maintaining regular bowel movement or in managing muscle spasms.

The success of rehabilitation depends on the patient's physical and mental condition and social circumstances, and not on the type of stroke. Good nursing and co-ordinated remedial therapy help early recovery and can prevent disablement. Morale is important in achieving the best recovery and planning for a worthwhile future is important. A hopeful, but realistic approach from nurses, therapists and doctors towards the patient can prevent depression. Treatment with an antidepressant medicine may help but the patient must have a chance to vent anger, frustration or misery and to ask questions.

For the relatives of stroke victims, the aftermath of stroke is a difficult and worrying time. The Chest, Heart and Stroke Association has information which will help patients and their relatives to understand the illness better. The Association also runs the Volunteer Stroke Service which helps people with speech difficulties.

There are also pilot schemes running which aim to ease the change from hospital to home, from professional to family care and to improve support for the families of stroke victims.

Circulatory problems

• PERIPHERAL VASCULAR DISEASE •

As people grow older, the arteries narrow, harden and lose their elasticity (*arteriosclerosis*) or the artery walls may suddenly contract (go into spasm). Either process causes reduced blood flow to many parts of the body, but most noticeably the arms and legs. The arteries may 'silt up' with fatty deposits (*atherosclerosis*) leading to sluggish blood flow. A blood clot or part of one may block the artery and prevent blood flow. If this happens suddenly the arm or leg becomes pale, painful and pulseless. More usually, the restriction of blood supply happens gradually, to produce a long-term (chronic) condition. This can range from muscle pain when walking which is relieved by rest (*intermittent claudication*), to pain even when the limb is at rest, to non-healing ulcers on the legs. A completely obstructed blood flow may cause gangrene.

Untreated high blood pressure is an important cause, but the most significant contributor to peripheral vascular disease is smoking. See the sections on 'High blood pressure' and 'Heart attacks'. Treatment of a condition such as intermittent claudication is not helped by medicines. There are a number of drugs which increase the blood flow, particularly when the limb is at rest, but rarely help pain. They do not improve walking distance or help the blood flow to the muscles during exercise and cannot be recommended. These peripheral vasodilators are **cinnarizine** (brand names Stugeron; Stugeron Forte) **nicotinic acid** preparations (Bradilan; Hexopal; Ronicol), **oxpentifylline** (Trental) and **thymoxamine** (Opilon). Stopping smoking and keeping active are the best treatments for peripheral vascular disease.

• RAYNAUD'S PHENOMENON AND RAYNAUD'S DISEASE •

These are conditions of the hands and sometimes the feet in which the small blood vessels (*arterioles*) constrict or squeeze together and restrict blood flow. The fingers become pale, then blue and finally red as the attack passes. It is sometimes painful and you may have pins and needles, numbness and a burning sensation. Cold or emotion are the most common triggers for an attack. **Raynaud's phenomenon** is associated with many other disorders, such as rheumatoid arthritis or atherosclerosis. People in certain occupations are prone to develop the condition, for example chainsaw or pneumatic drill operators and pianists. Excessive vibration may be the cause in these cases. **Raynaud's disease** occurs mostly in young women and more commonly affects the hands. There is no underlying disease associated with the condition. The cause is unknown.

Severe symptoms may be helped by a vasodilator, for example, **nifedipine** (see page 120), **prazosin** (see page 127) or **thymoxamine**. You should not take a beta blocker as this will worsen the condition. **Cyclandelate** (brand name Cyclobral), **naftidrofuryl** (brand name Praxiline), **oxpentifylline** and **nicotinic acid** preparations have all been tried, but have not proved to be helpful.

HOW YOU CAN HELP YOURSELF

- ☐ Avoid exposure to cold
- ☐ Wear warm clothing including gloves
- ☐ Avoid working with vibrating machinery
- ☐ Stop smoking.

Blood clots

When you cut yourself, the blood flow stops eventually because the blood clots. Special blood cells called *platelets* act as a plug to stem the initial blood flow; they activate clotting factors to form *fibrin* which meshes in with red blood cells to form a clot. Sometimes a blood clot forms inside a blood vessel where it is not wanted, for example deep in a leg vein, and part of the leg below the clot swells as fluid is retained. The blood clot (*thrombus*) is a danger not only because it affects the flow of blood, but also because a piece of the blood clot (*embolus*) may break off and travel to other parts of the body, such as the brain, heart or lungs. This process is called *embolism* and causes damage if the embolus blocks the blood supply to an organ.

Clots deep in a leg vein (*deep vein thrombosis*) or the abdomen can occur after an operation, injury, childbirth or after long periods of inactivity when the blood flow to the legs has slowed. There is also a small risk of blood clots developing in women taking the combined oral contraceptive pill.

Anticoagulants

Blood moves more slowly back to the heart through the veins than it does when pumped through the arteries. A clot in the veins consists of a fibrin web with platelets and red cells. Anticlotting medicines (*anticoagulants*) are used to prevent blood clots forming, for example during surgery, or from getting bigger in the veins, but they cannot dissolve blood clots once formed.

Deep vein thrombosis in the legs is sometimes a serious complication of surgery, but it can be prevented by an anticoagulant. Patients suffering from major trauma, a heart attack, stroke or cancer and people who are overweight, aged over 40 or have had deep vein thrombosis before are particularly at risk. Lengthy operations, including those on the pelvis, hips or knees are especially likely to lead to deep vein thrombosis. Ask the surgeon whether you need anticoagulant cover before you have an operation. Other measures, such as anti-embolism stockings, can also be used.

Heparin is used to start anticoagulation treatment. It acts rapidly in the body to prevent clots from forming, but it is effective for only a short time and has to be given by injection. Heparin treatment is generally given in hospital and has to be carefully supervised: too much causes bleeding, such as nose bleeds, blood in the urine and bruising. These effects are soon reversed by stopping the drug or by giving a specific antidote – **protamine sulphate**. At the same time as heparin is started, an anticoagulant is given by mouth. Heparin is used for an immediate effect because oral anticoagulants take time to work in the body (36–48 hours).

Vitamin K is absorbed from the digestive system in fats and is essential for the formation of certain clotting factors. Oral anticoagulants appear to interfere with certain stages of the clotting factor formation in the liver. **Warfarin** and **nicoumalone** are commonly used; **phenindione** is less used because it may cause hypersensitivity reactions, such as skin rashes, fever, diarrhoea and liver and kidney damage.

An oral anticoagulant such as warfarin is often life-saving, but its use has to be monitored carefully. At the start of treatment this involves frequent blood tests to measure its effect on clotting time; the dosage is adjusted during this phase. Bleeding is the main adverse effect of oral anticoagulants and will usually require hospital treatment. Your doctor should give you an emergency plan of what to do in the event of bleeding. You may need to stop the drug for a day or two and possibly have a vitamin K injection or a transfusion of fresh frozen plasma in hospital.

Many drugs either enhance or reduce the effect of anticoagulants. Illness, such as diarrhoea may reduce the body's intake of vitamin K, which in turn affects the clotting factors. Liver or kidney damage alter the body's response to warfarin. If you are on long-term oral anticoagulation treatment it is essential to carry an anticoagulation treatment card – this gives advice about the treatment and will be given to you by your doctor or your pharmacist.

In the arteries blood flow is faster and clots that form are made up of clumps of platelets with little fibrin. *Antiplatelet* drugs, such as **aspirin** may stop clot formation in arteries by lessening platelet stickiness. **Dipyridamole** (brand name Persantin) is used with an anticoagulant to stop clots forming on artificial heart valves.

Fibrinolytic drugs, or 'clot-busters', dissolve blood clots once they have formed. The drugs **streptokinase** (brand names Kabikinase; Streptase), **alteplase** (Actilyse) and **anistreplase** (Eminase) have to be injected into the vein and are therefore used mainly in hospital. They are useful for dissolving blood clots after a heart attack.

WARFARIN

WARFARIN WBP – Tablets
MAREVAN – Tablets

Warfarin is an oral anticoagulant used for treating or preventing the development of blood clots deep in the leg veins and fragments of clot in the lungs. Warfarin is used to prevent blood clots forming in people with rheumatic heart disease, atrial fibrillation and after operations to insert artificial heart valves.

Warfarin takes 36–48 hours to work in the body, but continues to act for 48 hours after it is stopped. The dosage must be carefully adjusted for each person. You should see your doctor regularly to monitor progress and to have blood tests.

Before you use this medicine

Tell your doctor if you are:
☐ pregnant – you should not take warfarin in the first three months nor during the last few weeks of pregnancy ☐ breast-feeding ☐ taking any other medicines, including vitamins and those bought over the counter.

Tell your doctor if you have or have had:
☐ poor liver or kidney function ☐ recent surgery ☐ peptic ulcer ☐ severe high blood pressure ☐ infection of the heart (*bacterial endocarditis*) ☐ blood disorders.

How to use this medicine

Take the tablets exactly as directed. The dosage may be adjusted from time to time. Eat a well-balanced diet. Do not change your diet or take nutritional supplements or vitamins without checking with your doctor or pharmacist. Avoid alcohol – the anticlotting activity may be increased. Be careful doing activities that may cause bruising or bleeding.

Carry an anticoagulation card stating that you take warfarin. A medical identification bracelet may also be helpful. If you have to have an operation, tell your doctor or dentist that you take warfarin.

Do not stop taking this medicine suddenly as this may cause a worsening of your condition. See your doctor regularly for blood tests. If you miss a dose take it as soon as you remember.

Over 65 You may need less than the adult dose, especially if your liver or kidney function is impaired.

Interactions with other medicines

Warfarin interacts with many medicines. Do not take any other medicines, including over-the-counter remedies, such as aspirin, cold remedies, antacids, laxatives. Do not change the dose of any medicine you are taking. Always check with your doctor or pharmacist.

Warfarin's anticlotting effect is enhanced by:

☐ **Anabolic steroids**

☐ **Analgesics and antirheumatics**, especially aspirin, azapropazone and phenylbutazone; possibly diflunisal, flurbiprofen, mefenamic acid, piroxicam, sulindac and some other NSAIDs

☐ **Anti-arrhythmics**, such as amiodarone

☐ **Lipid-lowering medicines**: clofibrate and simvastatin; cholestyramine may both enhance or reduce anticoagulant effect

☐ **Antibacterials**, such as ciprofloxacin, co-trimoxazole, erythromycin, metronidazole, sulphonamides, trimethoprim

☐ **Antidepressants**: fluvoxamine and paroxetine

☐ **Antifungals**, such as fluconazole, itraconazole, miconazole

☐ **Hormone blockers**: danazol, flutamide, tamoxifen

☐ **Ulcer-healing drugs**: cimetidine, omeprazole

☐ **Alcohol dependence treatment**: disulfiram

☐ **Thyroid supplement**: thyroxine

☐ **Gout treatment**: sulphinpyrazone and possibly allopurinol

Warfarin's anticlotting effect is reduced by:

☐ **Antibacterial**: rifampicin

☐ **Antiepileptics**, such as carbamazepine, phenobarbitone, primidone; phenytoin both enhances and reduces effects

☐ **Antifungal**: griseofulvin

☐ **Barbiturates**

☐ **Hormone blocker**: aminoglutethimide

☐ **Oral contraceptives**
☐ **Ulcer-healing drug**: sucralfate
☐ **Vitamin K**

Unwanted effects

Likely Loss of appetite.
Unlikely Skin rashes, hair loss, diarrhoea, abdominal pain, feeling or being sick. You should see your doctor if any of these develop.

Contact your doctor immediately if you have signs of bleeding – for example bleeding gums, nosebleeds, heavy bleeding from cuts or wounds, abdominal pain, sudden lightheadedness, weakness, blood in urine, swelling of the ankles, feet or legs, purple toes.

Similar preparations

SINTHROME – Tablets
NICOUMALONE

DINDEVAN – Tablets
PHENINDIONE

3

BREATHING PROBLEMS

Asthma
Allergies and hay fever
Coughs, bronchitis and emphysema
Colds

The lungs are the body's breathing machine. As you breathe air in through your nose or mouth, it passes down the back of the throat (*pharynx*), past the vocal cords (*larynx*) into the windpipe (*trachea*) and down into the lungs. Two lungs hang in the chest cavity above the heart. The windpipe branches into each lung through an airway called a *bronchus*. The bronchus divides into smaller and smaller air passages, the *bronchioles*, which in turn branch into air sacs (*alveoli*). The lungs resemble sponges made up of thousands and thousands of air sacs.

Each air sac is surrounded by a network of blood vessels. As air reaches the air sacs oxygen passes into red blood cells flowing through the blood vessels; carbon dioxide, waste gas that the body no longer needs, leaves the bloodstream and goes into the air sacs. As you breathe out carbon dioxide is squeezed out of the lungs back into the surrounding air.

Asthma

Asthma is a long-term disturbance of the airways in the lungs. The cells of the airways become swollen. Plugs of phlegm or mucus are produced which sometimes block the air passages preventing the exchange of oxygen and carbon dioxide. The muscles of the bronchioles tighten, narrowing the airways. The inflamed airways become hyper-reactive: they are irritable and twitchy and narrow easily if they come into contact with any one of a number of trigger factors (see opposite).

The main symptoms of asthma are wheezing, chest tightness, shortness of breath and coughing. Any one of these symptoms may indicate asthma, but your doctor will need to find out from you how and when chest problems occur and how long they last. Other conditions, such as bronchitis, have similar symptoms and must be distinguished from asthma. Symptoms are usually worst at night and first thing in the morning: they vary in severity and can even be life-threatening. Attacks may happen occasionally or you may live with regular symptoms. The bronchial airways usually recover from an attack and the narrowing reverses. If you have chronic asthma, the airways may stay inflamed, even if you have no symptoms or only mild ones occasionally and usually feel perfectly well. All grades of asthma need treatment.

● *WHAT CAUSES ASTHMA?* ●

Even though asthma is a common condition, its cause is not completely understood. Asthma does run in families, often with other allergic conditions, such as hay fever and eczema, but it can affect people who have no family history of the condition or other allergic problems. Many factors can trigger an attack of asthma – you may find that any one of them or a combination sets off an attack or that none of them does. Try to find out what makes you feel worse and tell your doctor. If you know that certain situations, such as a smoke-filled room, trigger an asthmatic attack, then you should obviously try to avoid them.

● *Allergies*

Common triggers include house dust which carries microscopic house dust mites, animals such as cats, dogs and birds, and pollen and fungal spores. When a susceptible person breathes in air full of house dust mites, for example, this may start an asthmatic attack. Occasionally, some foods and drinks, such as fruits, milk, cheese, fizzy drinks, peanuts and alcohol, may trigger asthma. Airborne triggers are by far the most common cause.

FOOD ADDITIVES

Tartrazine – a dye that is often used to colour food, soft drinks and medicines – can trigger asthma. It can be identified on the label of packaged foods as E102, but it is not always obvious which medicines contain tartrazine. If you know you react to the dye, and you are not sure whether a medicine contains it, check with the pharmacist. Other similar dyes are E104 and E110. *Sodium metabisulphite* and its related compounds (E220–227) are preservatives commonly used in wines and beer and can also trigger asthma. The *benzoate* preservatives (E210–219) may also cause problems.

• *Illness*

Colds, flu and viral infections can trigger an asthma attack due to allergy to the virus, particularly in young children. Wheeziness and persistent coughing at night are common signs. About one in ten children has wheeziness that needs medical treatment at some time. Yet many wheezy babies with mild symptoms grow out of them as resistance to colds and coughs builds up by about the age of seven. In one study eight out of ten children who wheezed in their first year, no longer had asthma by the age of ten. *Atopic* children (those who have a tendency to develop other allergies) are more likely to have asthmatic symptoms when they are older.

• *Occupation*

A number of manufacturing processes can involve breathing in the fumes or dusts of particular substances which can trigger asthma. When you leave work for a weekend or holiday, your symptoms improve, but on return your condition worsens. People working in industries such as plastics, electronics and pharmaceutical manufacturing are likely to meet these *sensitising agents*. If you develop wheeziness or chest tightness during the week (the symptoms may be worse at night) see your doctor. You may be able to get compensation if you are working with a recognised sensitising agent and your symptoms are clearly caused by it. Your asthma may clear up completely if you avoid working with a particular sensitising agent.

• *Smoke*

Most asthmatics are made worse by smoke, especially cigarette smoke. Children are particularly affected by smoke-filled rooms. You should avoid smoke and smoking.

• *Medicines*

Beta blockers must not be taken by asthmatics because they can cause narrowing of the airways and provoke an asthma attack. Beta blocker eye drops for treating glaucoma (see page 392) should also be avoided. Aspirin and related medicines for rheumatic problems (non-steroidal anti-inflammatory drugs) can worsen asthma. If you are sensitive to aspirin, you may also react to ibuprofen, an over-the-counter NSAID for rheumatic and muscular pains. Paracetamol is the best choice of pain-reliever for asthmatics.

Other causes

Emotion and stress can both start an asthmatic attack in someone who already suffers from asthma, but cannot cause asthma. Going out suddenly into cold air can trigger asthma, as can a change in the weather or the different seasons. Many forms of exercise can provoke an attack.

HOW YOU CAN HELP YOURSELF

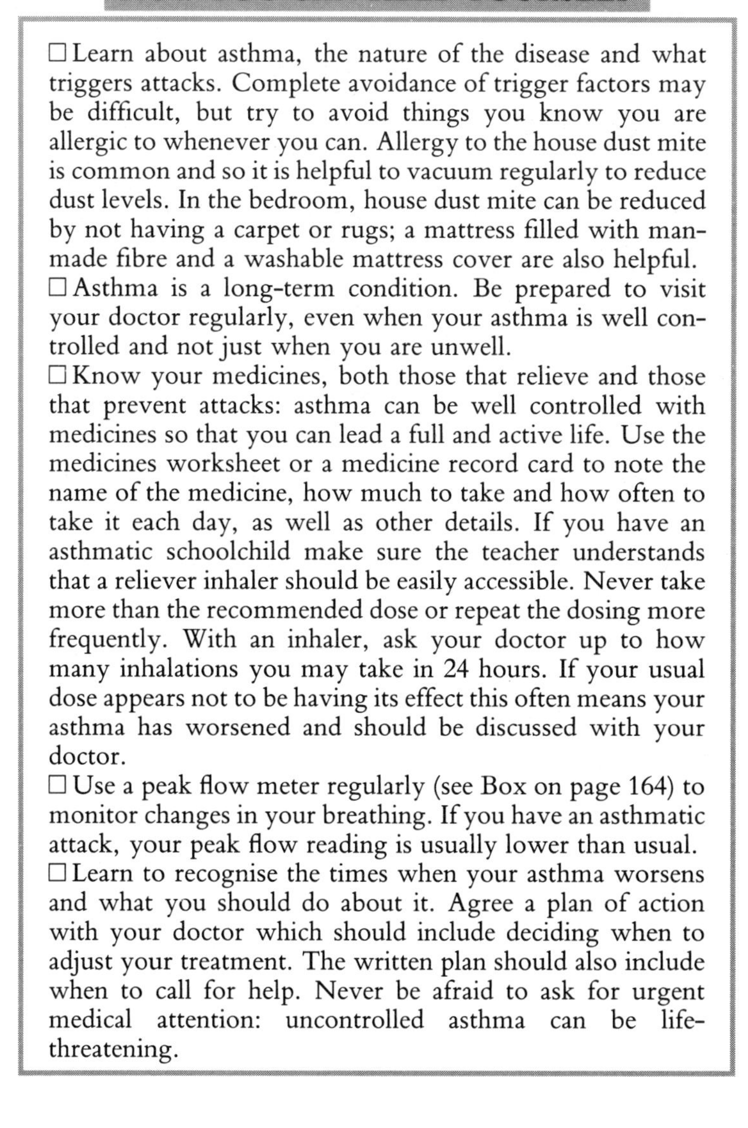

☐ Learn about asthma, the nature of the disease and what triggers attacks. Complete avoidance of trigger factors may be difficult, but try to avoid things you know you are allergic to whenever you can. Allergy to the house dust mite is common and so it is helpful to vacuum regularly to reduce dust levels. In the bedroom, house dust mite can be reduced by not having a carpet or rugs; a mattress filled with man-made fibre and a washable mattress cover are also helpful.

☐ Asthma is a long-term condition. Be prepared to visit your doctor regularly, even when your asthma is well controlled and not just when you are unwell.

☐ Know your medicines, both those that relieve and those that prevent attacks: asthma can be well controlled with medicines so that you can lead a full and active life. Use the medicines worksheet or a medicine record card to note the name of the medicine, how much to take and how often to take it each day, as well as other details. If you have an asthmatic schoolchild make sure the teacher understands that a reliever inhaler should be easily accessible. Never take more than the recommended dose or repeat the dosing more frequently. With an inhaler, ask your doctor up to how many inhalations you may take in 24 hours. If your usual dose appears not to be having its effect this often means your asthma has worsened and should be discussed with your doctor.

☐ Use a peak flow meter regularly (see Box on page 164) to monitor changes in your breathing. If you have an asthmatic attack, your peak flow reading is usually lower than usual.

☐ Learn to recognise the times when your asthma worsens and what you should do about it. Agree a plan of action with your doctor which should include deciding when to adjust your treatment. The written plan should also include when to call for help. Never be afraid to ask for urgent medical attention: uncontrolled asthma can be life-threatening.

HOW TO USE A PEAK FLOW METER

Peak expiratory flow rate or 'peak flow' is a measure of how quickly you can blow air out of your lungs. Your lung function depends on your age, height and sex and varies a great deal between people, even in those who have good lung function. If you have asthma, peak flow varies between morning and night as well as from day to day. Peak flow readings can help confirm the diagnosis of asthma, show you how good your lung function is, and help your doctor to assess both the severity of your asthma and the success of treatment.

If you have asthma the airways are narrowed and it is more difficult to blow air out. Your doctor may assess your peak flow at the surgery but you may also be asked to measure peak flow yourself for a couple of weeks at home and to keep a diary of measurements. Your doctor can prescribe a peak flow meter; with careful use it can last about three years.

To measure peak flow:

☐ stand or sit upright
☐ fit the mouthpiece (cardboard or plastic collar) around the neck of the meter
☐ make sure the marker or indicator is at the bottom of the scale
☐ check that your fingers are not over the scale
☐ take a good breath in and place your lips firmly around the mouthpiece
☐ blow out with a short, sharp blast (but not a cough)
☐ remove the meter from your mouth and take the reading
☐ note the reading, repeat the procedure twice more and record the best of the three readings.

Medicines for asthma

Asthma can be treated by using medicines regularly. Some relieve asthmatic symptoms (cough, chest tightness, wheezing and breathlessness) and the others prevent symptoms developing. Although there is no cure for asthma, symptoms can be controlled so well with medicines that you should not have any constraints on your life. With the help of your doctor you should aim to be free from the symptoms of asthma night and day, have no restrictions on the way you live, have no emergency treatments or trips to hospital and maintain your best possible peak flow rate.

Asthma treatments work on the inflamed cells of the air passages. When inhaled, small doses of medicine are very effective; much larger doses have to be used when medicine is given by mouth, because the drug reaches the lungs only after it has been absorbed into the body and distributed by the bloodstream. Getting the drug directly to where it is needed means not only that a smaller dose can be used but that unwanted effects are lessened. Medicines used simply to relieve symptoms – bronchodilators – also act more quickly when inhaled than when taken as tablets. There are various types of inhaler systems, so you should be able to find one that suits you and that you can manage easily. If you have mild symptoms, using a reliever inhaler well may reduce the need for other treatment.

● *'STEPWISE' APPROACH TO TREATMENT* ●

Guidance to doctors on how to help people with long-term asthma suggests a 'stepwise' approach to treatment. Each step represents recommended treatment according to the severity of the asthma symptoms. Your doctor will tailor treatment to your symptoms depending on how troublesome they are. Asthma is a variable condition and so you may go up and down treatment steps. The aim is to keep you feeling well using as few medicines as possible at the lowest doses possible.

Step 1 For mild symptoms or occasional bouts of coughing, wheezing and breathlessness, you may need only a 'reliever' inhaler, such as one containing **terbutaline** or **salbutamol**. You should always keep an inhaler on hand so that any developing symptoms can be relieved speedily.

Step 2 If you find that you need to use your reliever inhaler more than once a day or have night-time symptoms, tell your doctor. At this stage you may start regular treatment with an inhaled 'preventer' medicine, such as **sodium cromoglycate** or a corticosteroid. The daily dose of corticosteroid may vary depending on your symptoms and your peak flow meter readings.

Step 3 If symptoms do not improve or control is inadequate, you may need to increase the dose of the inhaled corticosteroid. A spacer may help to get the drug into the lungs and will reduce the risk of throat infections and absorption of corticosteroid into the body.

Step 4 If your asthma needs further control, your doctor may consider adding another bronchodilator, such as inhaled **ipratropium** or a beta$_2$-adrenoceptor stimulant by mouth. **Salmeterol** (brand name Serevent) is a newer type of bronchodilator with some anti-inflammatory effect on the airways. It works in the body much longer than salbutamol but it cannot replace an inhaled corticosteroid, and is sometimes added to one. If night-time symptoms are still troublesome, your doctor might try a modified-release **theophylline** preparation. Higher doses of a bronchodilator reliever may be used, sometimes by nebuliser, but only after careful consideration by your doctor. A high-dose corticosteroid inhaler may be tried. Short courses of corticosteroid tablets may be necessary from time to time, but would be considered for longer periods only if other treatments proved inadequate.

Your doctor will want to review your treatment from time to time. You may be able to step down treatment gradually if your symptoms are well controlled. Measuring your peak flow rate will be especially important during these periods and you should have a clear understanding of the signs that show your asthma is worsening:

☐ **Night-time symptoms** – waking up with shortness of breath
☐ **Morning symptoms lasting longer than usual**
☐ **Increased need for your reliever inhaler** and symptoms not as well as relieved
☐ **Fall in peak flow** and an increasing variation between morning and evening readings.

● *Aerosol inhalers*

A pressurised aerosol inhaler (or metered-dose inhaler) delivers a measured quantity of a drug carried by the aerosol propellant. Each time the canister is pressed, a dose is released. You need careful instruction on how to use an aerosol inhaler (see Box) and your technique should be checked regularly. Inhaler systems are now supplied with good instructions. Even with correct use only about ten per cent of the dose reaches the lungs; much of the drug catches on the back of the mouth and throat and is then swallowed. To use an aerosol inhaler you have to press the canister and breathe in at the same time. Children, older people and those with arthritic hands may find this a problem. A breath-controlled device, such as an Autohaler, fires a dose as you breathe in and this may be helpful for those who find inhalers hard to use.

Spacers are helpful if you find it difficult to co-ordinate your breathing in at the same time as firing a dose. A spacer extends the gap between the aerosol and the mouth and slows the speed at which the propellant and drug travel to the back of the mouth. There is also more time for the propellant to start evaporating, leaving a higher proportion of the drug in the dose you inhale. Some people find the propellant causes irritation or that the cold blast inhibits breathing in as fully as possible. A spacer may be useful for people who have to use high doses of inhaled corticosteroids because it reduces the chances of thrush in the mouth and throat. A spacer must be washed regularly in warm water.

HOW TO USE AN AEROSOL INHALER

☐ Sit upright or stand so that you are comfortable with your chin slightly raised
☐ Shake the inhaler well before each dose
☐ Hold the canister upright with the thumb at the base below the mouthpiece and the forefinger on top of the canister
☐ Breathe out as much as is comfortable
☐ Put the mouthpiece in your mouth between your teeth, but do not bite it; close your lips firmly around the mouthpiece
☐ Start breathing in through your mouth and press down on the top of the inhaler to release the dose while you continue breathing in slowly
☐ Hold your breath for as long as is comfortable, but up to 10 seconds if possible.

If you have to take a second puff, keep the inhaler upright and wait 30 seconds before repeating the procedure. This interval is necessary as a measured dose takes this time to be loaded automatically within the inhaler.

● *Dry powder systems*

With these systems you breathe in dry powder and do not need to rely on co-ordinating the dose with your breathing. Coughing may be a problem with these inhalers.

The Spincaps and Rotacaps systems have a small device which breaks open a capsule containing the powdered drug in a sugar (lactose) carrier. You will need to be shown how to load the capsule and to manage breathing in the dose. You can get a whistle attachment for the Spincaps system that sounds to let you know the dose has been taken properly.

After each dose, a fresh capsule has to be loaded, which can be inconvenient, and the Rotacaps may absorb moisture in humid climates. To overcome these disadvantages, several doses of dry powder are packed on a disk for use with the Diskhaler system.

The Turbohaler inhaler delivers the drug from a canister without a propellant or carriers and without the need to co-ordinate breathing in and pressing the canister.

● *Nebulisers*

Air or oxygen is forced through a drug solution and delivered through a mask. Breathing does not need to be co-ordinated, so a nebuliser may be very useful for emergency treatment in an acute attack of asthma, particularly for some people with chronic asthma or for young children who may be unable to manage other inhaler systems easily. A nebuliser should be used only after taking guidance from your doctor.

• *MEDICINES WHICH RELIEVE ASTHMA* •

Medicines that do not reduce inflammation of the airways but relax and open up the narrowed air passages (*bronchi*) are called *bronchodilators*. They relieve asthmatic symptoms of coughing, wheezing and breathlessness. If you have mild asthma a bronchodilator may be all you need. It may also be added to other treatments and is used to treat an acute attack. There are three types of bronchodilator medicines – the adrenaline-like *beta-adrenoceptor stimulants* (or $beta_2$-agonists), *antimuscarinics* and *theophylline* preparations.

• *Beta-adrenoceptor stimulants*

The body's chemicals act on *receptor* sites at the ends of nerves. Adrenaline and noradrenaline act on the $beta_1$- and $beta_2$-receptors to prepare you for activity ('flight or fight'). Among other effects, the airways open up, your heart beats faster and blood vessels dilate to allow blood to flow more easily around the body. Early bronchodilator treatments, such as **isoprenaline** and **ephedrine**, mimicked adrenaline by working at both types of beta-receptor site. These *sympathomimetic* drugs relieve airway narrowing, but also affect the heart, sometimes adversely by disrupting its rate and rhythm. They should be avoided if possible. Drugs that stimulate mainly the $beta_2$-receptors to relax the bronchioles, such as **salbutamol** and **terbutaline**, have much less of an effect on the heart. They may occasionally cause palpitations and fine tremor, usually of the hands, but when they are inhaled directly into the lungs they give fast relief and unwanted effects are rarely troublesome.

SALBUTAMOL

SALBUTAMOL – Inhaler, tablets, liquid, injection
AEROLIN – Inhaler and breath-controlled Autohaler
SALBULIN – Inhaler, tablets

SALBUVENT – Inhaler, tablets, liquid, nebuliser solution, injection
VENTODISKS – Dry powder inhaler (Diskhaler)
VENTOLIN – Inhaler, dry powder inhaler (Rotacaps), tablets, liquid, nebuliser solution, injection
VOLMAX – Sustained-release tablets

Useful devices
Haleraid – For use with aerosol inhalers if your hands are too weak to press the canister
Rondo – Spacer device for Salbuvent inhaler
Volumatic – Spacer device for use with Ventolin inhaler

Poor choice
VENTIDE – Contains a corticosteroid (better used separately)
SALBUTAMOL + BECLOMETHASONE

Salbutamol is a beta$_2$-adrenergic stimulant (also called beta$_2$-agonist) which opens up the airways in the lungs by relaxing the muscles around the bronchioles. It is used to relieve symptoms of asthma such as shortness of breath and wheezing. Salbutamol may also be used to treat chronic bronchitis and emphysema. It is also useful for preventing exercise-induced asthma if taken about 20 minutes before exercise. Salbutamol is very effective when given by inhaler with few unwanted effects, although fine tremor of the hands may be noticeable.

Before you use this medicine

Tell your doctor if you are:
☐ pregnant – asthma must be well controlled. Inhalation of salbutamol means that very small doses can relieve asthma symptoms without high blood levels of the drug reaching the developing baby. Salbutamol is sometimes used by injection in an attempt to prevent premature labour ☐ breast-feeding ☐ taking any other medicines, including vitamins and those bought over the counter.

Tell your doctor if you have or have had:
☐ high blood pressure ☐ an overactive thyroid ☐ diabetes ☐ heart problems ☐ an allergy to salbutamol or to other adrenaline-like drugs, such as the decongestants **pseudoephedrine** or **phenylpropanolamine**.

How to use this medicine

Use one or two puffs of the inhaler as directed (see 'How to use an aerosol inhaler' page 167). If you use a corticosteroid inhaler and a reliever bronchodilator inhaler, use the bronchodilator first. Allow about 15 minutes between inhaling the two medicines. If you need to use your inhaler more than once a day to relieve symptoms, see your doctor. Do not use more often or in a higher dose than that prescribed by your doctor. Contact your doctor if you do not feel better after taking your usual dose or your asthma worsens. Do not drive or do any other activities which require concentration until you know how you react to salbutamol.

Low blood levels of potassium may result from treatment with high doses of beta$_2$-stimulants. If you take a beta$_2$-stimulant with high doses of a corticosteroid, **theophylline** or a diuretic, blood levels of potassium may be further reduced; your doctor should monitor your blood levels of potassium.

Over 65 If unwanted effects are troublesome you may need less than the adult dose.

Interactions with other medicines

Other adrenaline-like drugs enhance the effects of salbutamol, increasing the risk of unwanted effects.

Unwanted effects

Likely Fine tremor of the hands, headache, restlessness, anxiety.
Unlikely Palpitations.

Contact your doctor if any of the likely symptoms are severe or if you have palpitations.

Similar preparations

BEROTEC – Inhaler, nebuliser solution
FENOTEROL

▼BRELOMAX – Tablets
TULOBUTEROL

BRICANYL – Inhaler, dry powder inhaler (Turbohaler), tablets, liquid, injection, nebuliser solution
TERBUTALINE

BRONCHODIL – Inhaler, tablets
REPROTEROL

EXIREL – Inhaler, capsules
PIRBUTEROL

MONOVENT – Tablets, liquid
TERBUTALINE

PULMADIL – Inhaler, breath-controlled inhaler
RIMITEROL

▼SEREVENT – Inhaler, dry powder inhaler (Diskhaler)
SALMETEROL

Poor choice
Preparations of the following are less safe and more likely to cause unwanted effects:
ADRENALINE; EPHEDRINE; ISOETHARINE; ISOPRENALINE; ORCIPRENALINE

● *Antimuscarinic bronchodilators*

These block the nerve chemicals that control muscle contraction, which allows the air passages to open up. **Ipratropium** (brand name Atrovent) and **oxitropium** (Oxivent) are antimuscarinic drugs used to relieve blocked airways, and are sometimes helpful for chronic bronchitis. They may be added to other treatments for asthma.

IPRATROPIUM

ATROVENT – Inhaler, high-dose inhaler, nebuliser solution
RINATEC – Nasal spray

Ipratropium relieves tightened air passages and is added to other asthma treatments. It is also used to treat chronic bronchitis where airway obstruction is reversible. Ipratropium acts more slowly than salbutamol or terbutaline but it continues to work for four to six hours. It is therefore used for long-term rather than rapid relief. Ipratropium nasal spray can help to dry a runny nose caused by perennial non-allergic rhinitis.

Before you use this medicine

Tell your doctor if you are:
☐ pregnant or breast-feeding ☐ taking any other medicines, including vitamins and those bought over the counter.

Tell your doctor if you have or have had:
☐ glaucoma ☐ prostate disorders ☐ sensitivity to atropine.

How to use this medicine

Inhaler Use one or two puffs three or four times a day as directed (see 'How to use an aerosol inhaler' page 167). Your doctor will usually suggest a trial period of inhaled ipratropium with peak flow measurements before prescribing a long-term course.
Nasal spray Use one or two puffs in the affected nostril up to four times a day. You may use a lower dose once symptoms are controlled.

For both preparations do not use more often or in a higher dose than that prescribed by your doctor. If you miss a dose, take it as soon as you remember, but skip it if it is almost time for next dose. Do not take double the dose. Do not stop taking this medicine suddenly without discussing treatment with your doctor.

Over 65 You may be more sensitive to ipratropium than younger people.

Unwanted effects

Likely with inhaler Dry mouth; **with nasal spray** Dry nose.
Unlikely with inhaler Difficulty passing urine, constipation; **with nasal spray** Stuffiness, irritation, burning sensation, bleeding.

If any unwanted effects are severe, discuss them with your doctor.

Similar preparations

▼OXIVENT – Inhaler
OXITROPIUM

Theophylline preparations

Theophylline and related medicines have a direct relaxing effect on the muscles surrounding the air passages. They relieve the symptoms of asthma and are sometimes used in the evening to control night-time symptoms and early-morning wheezing. The longer-acting or modified-release preparations can be useful.

Theophylline has a narrow therapeutic range: the margin between helpful and harmful effects is small and blood tests may be needed to monitor levels in your body. There is also considerable variation between people's responses to the drug, particularly smokers and those with impaired liver function or heart failure.

Furthermore, theophylline interacts with a number of other drugs, so medicines containing it need to be used with your doctor's or pharmacist's guidance. It may be added to small doses of a beta$_2$-agonist, but the risk of unwanted effects, including feeling sick, digestive disorders, effects on the heart rhythm, headache and sleeplessness, may increase.

Aminophylline, a more soluble form of theophylline, is sometimes used by injection to treat severe attacks of asthma.

THEOPHYLLINE

On prescription/from a pharmacy
BIOPHYLLINE – Liquid, modified-release tablets
LABOPHYLLINE – Injection (prescription only)
LASMA – Modified-release tablets
NUELIN – Liquid, tablets, modified-release tablets
PRO-VENT – Modified-release capsules
SLO-PHYLLIN – Modified-release capsules
THEO-DUR – Modified-release tablets
UNIPHYLLIN CONTINUS – Modified-release tablets

Over the counter
DO-DO – Tablets
ANESTAN – Tablets, capsules

Theophylline is related to caffeine in tea and coffee and theobromine in chocolate. It relaxes the air passages in the lungs and stimulates breathing and the heart rate, but cannot be used for immediate relief of asthmatic symptoms. It is added to other asthma treatments only when further control of chronic symptoms is needed. A related preparation, aminophylline, may be used by injection to treat acute severe asthma. The margin between helpful and harmful effects is narrow. Blood tests are usually needed to monitor theophylline levels.

Before you use this medicine

Tell your doctor if you are:
☐ a regular smoker ☐ pregnant or breast-feeding ☐ taking any other medicines, including vitamins and those bought over the counter.

Tell your doctor if you have or have had:
☐ liver disease ☐ irregular heartbeat ☐ peptic ulcer ☐ heart disease

☐ thyroid disease ☐ prolonged fever ☐ epilepsy ☐ porphyria ☐ an allergy to caffeine or theobromine.

How to use this medicine

Tablets or liquid Take three or four times daily, after meals.
Modified-release preparations Take once or twice a day; swallow whole with plenty of water and do not chew or crush. Do not change brands or dosage forms without checking with your doctor or pharmacist. If you leave hospital after your condition is stabilised with a particular brand, make sure you know the name of the theophylline preparation. Use a medicines worksheet to note details.

Do not use more often or in a higher dose than that prescribed by your doctor. Do not take several theophylline preparations together and always check with your doctor before using any theophylline-containing medicine, such as an over-the-counter product. Keep off charcoal-broiled foods and drinks containing caffeine, such as coffee, tea, chocolate, cocoa and colas. Alcohol and smoking may increase the need for theophylline, so discuss the dose with your doctor.

Do not stop taking this medicine suddenly without discussing treatment with your doctor. If you miss a dose, take it as soon as you remember, but skip it if it is almost time for your next dose. Do not take double the dose.

Over 65 You may need less than the normal adult dose.

Interactions with other medicines

Theophylline interacts with many medicines. Check with your doctor and pharmacist. Low blood levels of potassium may result from treatment combined with high doses of **beta$_2$-stimulants**. If you take theophylline with a beta$_2$-stimulant such as **salbutamol** or **terbutaline** in high doses, your doctor should monitor your blood levels of potassium and theophylline.
Theophylline's effects are enhanced by:
Antibacterials – ciprofloxacin, enoxacin, norfloxacin, erythromycin
Anthelmintic – thiabendazole
Calcium channel blockers – diltiazem, verapamil
Disulfiram (used to treat alcoholism)
Oral contraceptives
Ulcer-healing drug – cimetidine.
Theophylline's effects are reduced by:
Antituberculosis medicine – rifampicin

Antiepileptics – carbamazepine, phenobarbitone, phenytoin, primidone
Aminoglutethamide (used to treat breast cancer)
Sulphinpyrazone (used to treat gout).

Unwanted effects

Likely Feeling or being sick, headache, digestive disorders.
Unlikely Palpitations, irregular heartbeat, sleeplessness, diarrhoea.

Contact your doctor if you feel unwell when taking a theophylline preparation. The margin between helpful and harmful effects is narrow and your doctor should monitor blood or saliva theophylline levels.

Similar preparations

On prescription/from a pharmacy

AMINOPHYLLINE – Tablets, injection (prescription-only)

CHOLEDYL – Tablets, liquid
CHOLINE THEOPHYLLINATE

PECRAM – Modified-release tablets
AMINOPHYLLINE

PHYLLOCONTIN CONTINUS – Modified-release tablets
AMINOPHYLLINE

SABIDAL SR 270 – Modified-release tablets
CHOLINE THEOPHYLLINATE

● *Compound preparations*

Compound bronchodilator medicines are poor choices. These include Bronchilator, Duovent, Franol and Franol Plus. Although some of the drugs may be effective, the dose of the individual ingredients cannot be adjusted to suit different people.

● *MEDICINES WHICH PREVENT ASTHMA* ●

There are two main types of medicines which help to prevent asthmatic symptoms – *corticosteroids* and *cromoglycate* preparations.

● *Corticosteroids*

Corticosteroids, sometimes called 'steroids', reduce both inflammation of the air passages and the production of extra fluid and mucus. They have been used to treat asthma for many years. You may be concerned about having to take a corticosteroid because of the adverse effects of this group of medicines. However, inhaling a corticosteroid directly into the lungs is effective in very small doses and the drug has a local effect (like smoothing a cream directly on to a skin complaint), so that very little of it is absorbed into the body. Unwanted effects are rarely a problem, particularly at low doses. The corticosteroids used are **beclomethasone** and **budesonide**, which are similar in effect.

An inhaled corticosteroid is a very important treatment if you need to use an inhaled bronchodilator more than once a day or have night-time symptoms. The inhaled corticosteroid must be used regularly because it takes time to work and will not relieve sudden wheeziness or breathlessness. Some corticosteroid inhalers are available in high doses for those people who might otherwise have to take corticosteroid tablets. Occasionally, short courses of high-dose corticosteroid tablets may be necessary if symptoms increase and are not controlled by your usual medicines. High doses, in tablets, by injection or both, may be needed during a severe acute attack of asthma, which should be treated in hospital. Short courses rarely cause adverse effects.

BECLOMETHASONE

AEROBEC – Inhaler, high-dose inhaler
BECLOFORTE – High-dose inhaler
BECODISKS – Dry powder inhaler (Diskhaler)
BECONASE (*for allergic symptoms*) – Nasal spray
BECOTIDE – Inhaler, dry powder inhaler (Rotacaps), nebuliser solution
PROPADERM (*for skin disorders*) – Cream, ointment, ointment with antibacterial

Poor choice
VENTIDE
BECLOMETHASONE + SALBUTAMOL

Useful devices
ROTAHALER (*for Rotacaps*)
VOLUMATIC – spacer

Beclomethasone is a corticosteroid used for the prevention of asthma when a bronchodilator reliever does not fully control symptoms. In the lungs, it reduces inflammation of the air passages, as well as production of fluid and phlegm. On the skin it is used for severe inflammatory conditions such as eczema. Beclomethasone nasal spray helps the symptoms of an itchy, blocked nose in the hay fever season or due to perennial rhinitis. For maximum benefit beclomethasone must be used regularly. Relief of symptoms may not begin for three to seven days after the start of treatment and may take four weeks to reach full effect. The drug is used locally in very small doses and there are few local unwanted effects. Budesonide is similar.

Before you use this medicine

Tell your doctor if you are:
☐ pregnant or breast-feeding ☐ taking any other medicines, including vitamins and those bought over the counter.

Tell your doctor if you have or have had:
☐ tuberculosis of the lung ☐ viral, bacterial or fungal infections ☐ nasal disorders or surgery.

How to use this medicine

Inhaler Use regularly twice a day, in the morning and evening as directed (see 'How to use an aerosol inhaler', page 167). If your asthma symptoms are not controlled by lower-dose corticosteroid inhalers, using a high-dose inhaler may avoid the need to take a corticosteroid by mouth for long periods. If you are taking a regular dose of over 1500 micrograms a day, some suppression of the body's adrenal function can occur (see page 326). You should therefore carry a 'steroid card' and may need extra corticosteroid (a short course of tablets) during periods of stress, such as an operation or an episode of infection. You may need to have a reserve supply of tablets.
Nasal spray Apply two puffs into each nostril in the morning and evening. When symptoms are controlled you may be able to reduce the dose to one puff twice a day.
Cream/ointment Apply thinly to the affected area twice daily. Beclomethasone is a potent corticosteroid (for further information on the use of corticosteroid skin preparations see page 420).

Do not stop taking this medicine suddenly without discussing treatment with your doctor. It may be possible to step down treatment but only with guidance from your doctor (see 'Stepwise approach to treatment', page 165). Do not use more often or in a higher dose than that prescribed by your doctor. If you miss a dose, take it as soon as you remember, but skip it if it is almost time for your next dose. Do not take double the dose.

Over 65 No special requirements.

Unwanted effects

Likely with inhaler Hoarseness or huskiness of the voice – if this persists you should tell your doctor.

An inhaled corticosteroid sometimes causes a sore throat due to a fungal infection (thrush) which can be treated with an antifungal drug. Rinsing your mouth out with water after inhalation can be helpful. Using a spacer with an aerosol inhaler helps the corticosteroid to reach the lungs and lessens fungal infections. If you use an aerosol inhaler and your daily corticosteroid dose is 1000 micrograms or more, you should use a spacer. This reduces unwanted absorption of corticosteroid into the body.

Likely with nasal spray Sometimes sneezing attacks immediately after using the aerosol, drying and crusting inside the nose and sometimes bleeding. This can be reduced by pointing the spray away from the nasal septum. You should ask the doctor or pharmacist to show you how to operate the nasal aerosol.

Similar preparations

BETNESOL – Drops
BETAMETHASONE

▼FLIXONASE – Nasal spray
FLUTICASONE

PREFERID (for skin disorders) – Cream, ointment
BUDESONIDE

PULMICORT – Inhaler, dry powder inhaler (Turbohaler)
BUDESONIDE

RHINOCORT – Nasal aerosol
BUDESONIDE

SYNTARIS – Nasal spray
FLUNISOLIDE

VISTA-METHASONE – Drops
BETAMETHASONE

● *Cromoglycate preparations*

Sodium cromoglycate (brand name Intal) inhibits the release of body chemicals involved in allergic reactions. It also helps to prevent narrowing of the airways. It may be useful if asthma has an allergic basis, but does not help everyone. Children seem to respond to sodium cromoglycate better than adults. Sodium cromoglycate can only prevent an asthma attack and is no use for relieving symptoms; it is also used to prevent allergic nose and eye symptoms associated with hay fever (see page 179). **Nedocromil** is similar to sodium cromoglycate.

● *OTHER TREATMENTS* ●

Antihistamines such as **ketotifen** (brand name Zaditen) ought in theory to be helpful in treating asthma because of their anti-allergic action. In practice, antihistamines are disappointing in the treatment of asthma; they are poor choices and are not much used. Some people with asthma claim to benefit from the use of ionisers, acupuncture, homoeopathy and other forms of complementary treatment. The evidence is anecdotal and clinical trials have so far been disappointing. If you decide to try any of these treatments, you must continue to take any medicines prescribed by your doctor.

Allergies and hay fever

Allergy or *hypersensitivity* means that the body's immune system reacts excessively to an **allergen** – a harmless substance, usually a protein, which the immune system mistakes for an invading organism, such as a bacterium or a virus. When one of these foreign substances first gets into the body, white cells (*lymphocytes*) in the blood produce *antibodies*, which attach themselves to 'mast' cells, another type of white blood cell. When the same foreign substance enters the body for a second time it binds to the antibodies made on the first visit. This process causes the mast cells to release chemicals including histamine into the bloodstream. These chemicals help to destroy invading organisms and are an important defence mechanism in protecting the body from infection.

When the body responds to an allergen, the reaction is caused mainly by the effects of excess histamine, which acts at many places in the body on two types of cell receptor: H_1 and H_2. H_1-receptors are found in the skin, nose, blood vessels and airways; H_2-receptors are in the stomach lining, salivary and tear glands. *Antihistamines* block H_1-receptors to prevent the symptoms of allergic disorders. (H_2-receptor antagonists are used for healing peptic ulcers – see page 73). **Sodium cromoglycate** inhibits the release of chemicals from the mast cells. *Corticosteroids* reduce inflammation both internally and externally.

There are four common types of allergic disorder, although many substances can cause more than one type of response in any one person. Except for *anaphylaxis*, the severity of an allergy can vary from person to person. Some people have mild symptoms occasionally while others may be severely affected.

● *Hay fever*

Typical symptoms of hay fever are runny nose and eyes, blocked nose, sneezing, itchy eyes, nose and palate and a tickle at the back of the throat. Hay fever (*seasonal allergic rhinitis*) is commonly caused by allergens in the air – tree and grass pollens, moulds, dust, animal feathers and hairs. Some people suffer from a runny, blocked nose all the year round. This is known as *perennial allergic rhinitis* and one of the common causes is the house dust mite. Not all perennial rhinitis is caused by allergens: *vasomotor rhinitis* appears to be a fault in the nervous control of the blood supply to the nose and results in a blocked and sometimes runny nose.

● *Skin allergies* (*urticaria*)

A skin reaction can occur when something you eat disagrees with you: common allergens range from shellfish to strawberries to medicines such as aspirin. If your skin comes into contact with certain chemicals, such as household cleaners, soap powder, cosmetics or metals, these can cause rashes (*contact dermatitis*). Insect bites and stings also cause allergic reactions.

● *Asthma*

Asthma can be triggered by exposure to allergens (see page 161). Although the release of histamine plays a part in tightening the airways, other factors are involved in asthma and antihistamines are disappointing in the treatment of asthma symptoms.

● *Anaphylaxis*

Anaphylaxis or anaphylactic shock is a rare and potentially fatal allergic response and needs emergency treatment. The signs are sudden, generalised itching, rapidly followed by breathing difficulties and extremely low blood pressure. Anaphylaxis can occur as a response to certain medicines, such as antibiotics, vaccines, arthritis medicines and *hyposensitising* preparations designed to treat allergies, as well as to bee or wasp stings. The reaction is more likely to happen in someone who is already sensitive (*atopic*). The reaction may become increasingly severe with repeated exposure. If you have severe reactions to insect stings you should see your doctor to discuss the possibility of carrying an emergency supply of adrenaline during the summer months.

HOW YOU CAN HELP YOURSELF

☐ Discover the cause of your allergy and then avoid it. This may be easy if you can trace the allergen to something that you have eaten or touched, but in many cases it is quite difficult to pinpoint the cause.
☐ If you are allergic to pollens, these are hard to avoid. Sunglasses may keep some pollen out and washing your face when you come in may help.
☐ Avoid newly mown lawns or fields and stay inside as much as possible on days when there is a high pollen count.

Medicines for allergies

Allergic symptoms such as hay fever may be treated *locally* with nose sprays or eye drops or *systemically* by medicines taken into the body. Treatment will depend on whether you are mildly affected throughout the season, for only a few days a year or suffer severe symptoms during the summer months.

LOCAL PREPARATIONS

Eye drops with an antihistamine and a decongestant (**antazoline** with **xylometazoline**; brand name Otrivine-Antistin) may help allergic symptoms, but only for a short time. Nose drops and an eye preparation can be bought over the counter or your doctor may prescribe them for immediate symptom relief for a few days before medicines taken to prevent hay fever symptoms start to work.

Nasal symptoms alone are best treated with **sodium cromoglycate** or a corticosteroid in the nose during the hay fever season. Either preparation must be used regularly to prevent symptoms. Starting treatment about a month before the hay fever season will 'prime' the nose to cope better.

SODIUM CROMOGLYCATE

INTAL (for asthma) – Inhaler, breath-controlled Autohaler, dry powder inhaler (Spincaps), nebuliser solution
NALCROM (for food allergy) – Capsules

Continued over

OPTICROM (for allergic symptoms) – Eye drops, eye ointment
RYNACROM (for allergic symptoms) – Nasal drops, nasal spray

Poor choice
INTAL COMPOUND
SODIUM CROMOGLYCATE + ISOPRENALINE SULPHATE

RYNACROM COMPOUND
SODIUM CROMOGLYCATE + XYLOMETAZOLINE

Sodium cromoglycate inhibits the release of body chemicals involved in allergic reaction. It also helps to prevent narrowing of the airways caused by exercise, cold air and chemicals. Sodium cromoglycate must be taken regularly and can only prevent symptoms, not provide instant relief. It may take from a few days up to six weeks to have an effect.

Before you use this medicine

Tell your doctor if you are:
☐ pregnant or breast-feeding ☐ taking any other medicines, including vitamins and those bought over the counter.

How to use this medicine

Inhaler Use two puffs of the aerosol inhaler or one capsule in the Spinhaler four to eight times a day.
Nasal spray/drops Use one spray to each nostril four to six times daily; put two drops into each nostril six times a day. Snuff the powder from one cartridge into one nostril and repeat for the other nostril, up to four times a day.
Eye drops/ointment Apply one or two drops into each eye four times a day. Use the ointment two or three times a day. Some people prefer to use drops during the day and ointment at night.
For food allergy (with dietary restriction) Take two capsules four times daily before meals. Children take a lower dose. Powder from the capsules can be dissolved in a little very hot water and then cold water added before drinking.
Storage and disposal Capsules containing powder must be kept in a cool, dry place to stop moisture getting in. Once opened, the eye drops may become contaminated with bacteria as you use them: throw any remaining drops away after four weeks.

Over 65 No special requirements.

Interactions with other medicines

Eye drops contain a preservative, benzalkonium chloride, and should not be used with soft contact lenses. Eye ointment should not be used with contact lenses.

Unwanted effects

Likely with inhaler Throat irritation, cough; **with nasal spray** irritation of the nose and sneezing which usually lessens as you continue treatment.
Unlikely with capsules Feeling sick, skin rashes, joint pain; **with inhaler** the dry powder sometimes causes wheezing and breathlessness. If this happens, contact your doctor. Inhaling a $beta_2$-stimulant a few minutes before sodium cromoglycate may help to overcome this.

Stop taking the oral capsules if you develop a skin rash; see your doctor.

Similar preparations

TILADE MINT (for asthma) – Inhaler
NEDOCROMIL SODIUM

● *Corticosteroids*

Corticosteroids have a powerful anti-inflammatory effect. Corticosteroid nose sprays can help to control nasal symptoms of hay fever during the season. They should be started two or three weeks before the pollen season because their effect takes time to develop. They will not help with the immediate relief of hay fever symptoms. They must be used regularly, usually twice daily. **Beclomethasone** (brand name Beconase), **betamethasone** (Betnesol, Vista-Methasone), **budesonide** (Rhinocort) and **flunisolide** (Syntaris) all have similar effects on symptoms. See page 176. Corticosteroids should not be used in the eye for hay fever symptoms.

● *ANTIHISTAMINES* ●

If you have more widespread hay fever symptoms, such as itching of the mouth and ears as well as nose and eye symptoms, an antihistamine is usually helpful. An oral antihistamine can be used to treat symptoms throughout the season or an attack lasting a few days. Oral antihistamines are also used to treat allergic skin rashes, itchy skin (*pruritus*), insect bites and stings and drug allergies. Antihistamine creams or lotions applied to the skins to treat rashes, itchy skin or insect bites are not recommended because they may cause sensitivity reactions.

Widely advertised combination preparations of an antihistamine and a decongestant that are available over the counter should not be used to relieve hay fever symptoms because the decongestant is a *sympathomimetic*, a drug with adrenaline-like activity, which can cause serious unwanted effects (see 'Cold remedies', page 194).

● *Older antihistamines*

All of these have similar effects and there is no evidence that one preparation is better than another. People vary widely in their response to antihistamines, so you must find one that suits you. Most antihistamines work for a short time in the body and must be taken twice or even three or four times a day. Others, such as **promethazine**, are longer-acting and can be taken at night so that the effects last through the next day. Some antihistamines cause more drowsiness than others, but all do so to some extent. You may find that your ability to drive a car or operate machinery is impaired. Drowsiness caused by antihistamines is increased by other sedative medicines and alcohol.

Other unwanted effects include dry mouth, blurred vision and inability to pass urine, and may be troublesome for some people. Antihistamines can be bought in a pharmacy – **chlorpheniramine** and **brompheniramine** are effective and inexpensive. If you need to take an antihistamine for longer periods, such as throughout the hay fever season, your doctor can also prescribe them.

CHLORPHENIRAMINE

On prescription/from a pharmacy
CHLORPHENIRAMINE – Tablets
PIRITON – Tablets, liquid, injection

Not recommended
Over-the-counter preparations containing chlorpheniramine with a decongestant:
CONTAC 400; DRISTAN; EXPULIN; EXPURHIN; HAYMINE; MACKENZIES; SINE-OFF

Chlorpheniramine is an antihistamine which reduces allergic symptoms such as swelling, inflammation, itchiness and runny nose and eyes. It is used to treat hay fever and other forms of rhinitis, nettle rash (*urticaria*), skin rashes caused by medicines or food, itchy skin (*pruritus*) and allergic swelling (*angioedema*). The injection, on prescription only, is used for acute allergies and as a supplementary medicine for the emergency treatment of anaphylactic shock.

Before you use this medicine

Tell your doctor if you are:
☐ pregnant or breast-feeding ☐ taking any other medicines, especially a tricyclic antidepressant, a monoamine-oxidase inhibitor antidepressant or the anti-epileptic **phenytoin**, and including vitamins and those bought over the counter.

Tell your doctor if you have or have had:
☐ asthma ☐ glaucoma ☐ difficulty passing urine ☐ enlarged prostate ☐ liver disease ☐ epilepsy.

How to use this medicine

Take the tablets or syrup three or four times a day. The syrup can be given to young children, but at lower than the adult dose.

Until you know how you react to chlorpheniramine, do not drive, operate machinery or do other activities that require alertness. Avoid alcohol as chlorpheniramine enhances its effects.

If you miss a dose, take it as soon as you remember, but skip it if it is almost time for your next dose. Do not take double the dose.

Over 65 Less than the usual adult dose may be necessary. Older people are more sensitive to the unwanted effects. These include confusion, short-term memory problems and impaired attention as well as antimuscarinic effects – dry mouth, blurred vision, difficulty passing urine (especially for a man with an enlarged prostate gland), worsening of glaucoma, sexual difficulties.

Interactions with other medicines

Sedatives and anti-anxiety drugs enhance the effects of chlorpheniramine. **Antimuscarinic drugs**, such as the tricyclic antidepressants **amitriptyline** and **imipramine**, and **monoamine-oxidase inhibitors** increase the antimuscarinic effects of chlorpheniramine (see **Over 65**). **Phenytoin** (an anti-epileptic) may build up to toxic levels.

Unwanted effects

Likely Drowsiness.
Unlikely Headache, inability to concentrate, gastrointestinal disturbances – feeling or being sick, diarrhoea – dizziness, antimuscarinic effects (see **Over 65**), over-excitement in children.

If any of the unlikely effects occur and are severe, contact your doctor.

Similar preparations

On prescription/from a pharmacy

DANERAL SA – Modified-release tablets
PHENIRAMINE

DIMOTANE – Tablets, liquid, modified-release tablets
BROMPHENIRAMINE

FENOSTIL RETARD – Modified-release tablets
DIMETHINDENE

HISTRYL – Modified-release capsules
DIPHENYLPYRALINE

OPTIMINE – Tablets, liquid
AZATADINE

PERIACTIN – Tablets, liquid
CYPROHEPTADINE

PHENERGAN – Tablets, liquid, injection
PROMETHAZINE

TAVEGIL – Tablets, liquid
CLEMASTINE

THEPHORIN – Tablets
PHENINDAMINE

Prescription-only

FABAHISTIN – Tablets
MEBHYDROLIN

PRIMALAN – Tablets
MEQUITAZINE

TINSET – Tablets
OXATOMIDE

Over the counter

ALLER-EZE – Tablets
CLEMASTINE

• *Newer antihistamines*

These cause much less drowsiness than the older ones – a major advantage – but although drowsiness is rare your ability to drive a car or operate machinery may be affected. Alcohol intake should be kept low. **Astemizole** and **terfenadine** have been available for several years and both may be prescribed by your doctor or bought in small packs in a pharmacy. Astemizole takes longer to have an effect and is better for regular use throughout the season than for treating occasional symptoms. Terfenadine appears to cause few troublesome effects. The latest preparations, **acrivastine** (brand name Semprex), **cetirizine** (Zirtek) and **loratadine** (Clarityn) are equally effective, but must be prescribed.

TERFENADINE

On prescription/from a pharmacy
TRILUDAN – Tablets, high-dose tablets (Forte), liquid

From a pharmacy
SELDANE – Tablets

Terfenadine reduces allergic symptoms such as swelling, inflammation, itchiness and runny nose and eyes. It is used to treat allergic rhinitis, such as hay fever, and nettle rash (*urticaria*). It causes much less drowsiness than the older antihistamines, although a few people find sedation a problem.

Before you use this medicine

Tell your doctor if you are:
□ pregnant or breast-feeding □ taking any other medicines, including vitamins and those bought over the counter.

Tell your doctor if you have or have had:
□ poor liver function.

How to use this medicine

Take the tablets twice a day or the high-dose tablets once a day in the morning. Do not drive or do other activities that require alertness until you know how you react to terfenadine. The effects of terfenadine are not increased with small amounts of alcohol, but avoid large quantities.

Over 65 No special requirements.

Interactions with other medicines

Ketoconazole (an antifungal) interferes with the break-down of terfenadine and may cause irregular heart rhythms.

Unwanted effects

Unlikely Drowsiness, headache, hair loss.

Similar preparations

On prescription

CLARITYN – Tablets, liquid
LORATADINE

SEMPREX – Capsules
ACRIVASTINE

ZIRTEK – Tablets
CETIRIZINE

From a pharmacy

HISMANAL – Tablets, liquid (also on prescription)
ASTEMIZOLE

POLLON-EZE – Tablets
ASTEMIZOLE

• *MEDICINES FOR SEVERE HAY FEVER* •

When hay fever symptoms are severe and likely to disrupt an important occasion (such as taking an exam), a short course of a corticosteroid taken by mouth, such as **prednisolone**, may be considered by your doctor.

Hyposensitisation (also known as desensitisation or immunotherapy) may help a few people with severe symptoms that cannot be controlled by other medicines. Not everyone will be helped and people who are sensitive to a wide range of allergens will not benefit from hyposensitisation with just one preparation – containing varieties of grass pollen, for example.

Anaphylaxis, an acute and severe allergic reaction to the desensitising vaccine, can occur. The Committee on Safety of Medicines warns doctors that since 1980 in Britain, 11 people, mostly young, have died from anaphylaxis caused by allergen extract desensitising vaccines. Patients with asthma appear to be particularly sensitive. Treatment should be carried out only where there are adequate facilities for resuscitation and patients should remain under medical observation for at least two hours after the injection.

For adults with severe reactions to bee or wasp stings a course of venom injections may help.

Cough, bronchitis and emphysema

The lungs clean themselves constantly so that breathing continues efficiently. Cells lining the air passages produce mucus which traps foreign substances such as smoke, chemicals or invading organisms (bacteria or viruses). Coughing helps to remove unwanted material from the lungs. A cough is therefore a natural function with a purpose, especially a productive cough which brings up phlegm (*sputum*). A dry, irritating cough that does not bring up phlegm, a non-productive cough that may also keep you awake at night, can be a nuisance. Coughing is controlled by a signal from the brain, so a dry cough can sometimes be relieved by a medicine which calms that part of the brain.

Coughing may be a temporary nuisance or it may indicate that there is a more serious disorder of the lungs. You should consult your doctor if:

- ☐ you cough up green or yellow mucus or if it is foul-smelling
- ☐ you have a high temperature lasting a few days
- ☐ coughing or breathing in causes sharp chest pain
- ☐ you wheeze or have shortness of breath
- ☐ mucus contains blood
- ☐ a cough continues for longer than ten days.

A cough can be a symptom of a long-term condition such as asthma (see page 160), chronic bronchitis or emphysema. Chronic bronchitis is a disease in which the cells lining the air passages produce excess mucus. This leads to long-term coughing, usually producing phlegm. Emphysema is the enlargement of the air sacs (*alveoli*) beyond the air passages. The walls of the air sacs break down, leading to shortness of breath with or without cough. Sometimes there is wheezing but the narrowing of the airways is not as reversible as with asthma. The two conditions frequently overlap and may be called chronic obstructive airways disease (COAD), chronic obstructive pulmonary disease (COPD) or chronic airflow limitation (CAL). Some people may have mild chronic bronchitis and emphysema with little more than cough and phlegm but for others these diseases can become life-threatening. Chronic bronchitis and emphysema are almost always the end result of years of cigarette smoking. Pollution and occupational hazards such as dusts or chemical fumes and hereditary factors may also contribute in a small way to chronic bronchitis.

HOW YOU CAN HELP YOURSELF

☐ It is never too late to give up smoking – the condition of the lungs improves from the moment you stop.
☐ If you are overweight, lose weight. Carrying extra weight means that the heart and lungs have to work harder.
☐ Avoid smoky atmospheres and sudden changes of temperature; never go out in fog.
☐ Exercise within your capabilities. This will improve your general well-being.
☐ Always get chest infections treated promptly.

Medicines for bronchitis and emphysema

Acute bronchitis is usually a viral infection of the air passages, causing cough, yellow or green sputum and fever. The infection is self-limiting and will not respond to an antibiotic. Treatment consists of rest and drinking plenty of fluids. Chronic bronchitis may need treatment with antibiotics and some people with recurrent problems may take an antibiotic throughout the winter.

Treatment of chronic bronchitis and emphysema involves bronchodilators and corticosteroids, if there is evidence of asthma as well. In people with advanced disease corticosteroids may be given by mouth if there is good evidence that the airways still respond to steroids.

Cough medicines

● *MUCOLYTICS* ●

These contain enzymes which make mucus less sticky so that it should be easier to cough up. However, they do not seem to help people with chronic bronchitis or asthma and are not recommended. These products (**acetylcysteine**, **carbocisteine** and **methylcysteine**) are no longer available on NHS prescription except for specific conditions. Drinking extra fluids and inhaling steam is the best way to thin the mucus or sputum.

● *EXPECTORANTS* ●

A productive cough is the body's way of clearing debris from the lungs and it helps you to recover from a self-limiting condition such as a cold or flu. Expectorants are taken with the aim of thinning mucus in the lungs so that phlegm is coughed up more easily. Most expectorants are claimed to act by irritating the lining of the stomach. This causes a reflex stimulation of the nerves to the air passages in the lungs which encourages the production of mucus. This effect occurs only at high doses which would normally make you ill with nausea and vomiting. Cough medicines containing expectorants such as **ammonium chloride** and **ipecacuanha** have only small ineffective doses. Furthermore, there is no evidence that any ingredient of a cough medicine can act as an expectorant. Expectorants are of no more value than a placebo.

• *SOOTHING COUGH MEDICINES* •

These contain syrup of **glycerol** (glycerine) and may help an irritating dry cough. Your doctor can prescribe Simple Linctus BP or you can buy it cheaply over the counter. Simple Linctus Paediatric BP is particularly useful for young children, but it contains large quantities of sugar which can damage teeth. Similar remedies, such as glycerol, lemon and honey in hot water, can easily be prepared at home.

• *COUGH SUPPRESSANTS* •

These may reduce troublesome symptoms if you are kept awake at night or if your cough is interfering with normal activities. A cough suppressant does not shorten the course of colds, coughs and other respiratory infections. People with bronchitis, acute or chronic, should not take a cough suppressant because it does not help with the removal of phlegm. A cough suppressant reduces breathing control, which could be dangerous if you have asthma or chronic bronchitis.

Pholcodine, **codeine** and **dextromethorphan** are used to suppress cough but they all tend to cause constipation. Codeine and dextromethorphan are equally effective, but dextromethorphan causes fewer unwanted effects. Doctors cannot prescribe dextromethorphan on the NHS, but modified-release capsules (brand name Coughcaps) can be bought at a pharmacy. Pholcodine Linctus BP may be helpful and is inexpensive. Cough suppressants should not usually be given to children, especially those under one year old.

• *COMPOUND COUGH MEDICINES* •

These are not at all helpful in the treatment of respiratory infections and lung conditions and cannot be prescribed on the NHS.

As with most combination preparations the ingredients are often present in too low a dose for them to be effective. Many compound cough remedies are a therapeutic nonsense, with some of the ingredients acting in the opposite way to others. Manufacturers may claim that these remedies have a dual action of suppressing a cough and drying up mucus. This is unhelpful: if you have a productive cough with extra phlegm you need to remove it from your lungs by coughing, not drying it up. If the desire to cough (the cough reflex) is suppressed by another ingredient, phlegm remains on the lungs.

Other cough preparations have an unnecessary number of ingredients with similar actions. Some cough medicines contain an antihistamine which will also have a drying effect on phlegm and therefore not help you to cough it up from your lungs. For people with chronic bronchitis and emphysema an antihistamine may prevent the waste gas, carbon dioxide, leaving the lungs.

Colds

The common cold is a viral infection of the nose, throat and upper airways (upper respiratory tract). The mucous membranes become swollen and inflamed, resulting in a blocked and runny nose. Other symptoms include sneezing, sore throat, cough, mild fever and a general aching feeling.

There are a number of different cold viruses and having one cold does not give you immunity from the other viruses. A cold is spread to others by breathing out or sneezing. Colds are also spread by hands and it is a good idea to wash your hands frequently if you have a cold to prevent the virus spreading. A cold is self-limiting: it can be cured only by time. The illness has to run its course – anything from four to fourteen days. An antibiotic works against bacteria but not against viruses, least of all a cold virus. Sometimes a secondary bacterial infection may develop, such as sinusitis or an ear infection, and your doctor may then prescribe an antibiotic.

Other more serious illnesses may appear similar to a cold; you should contact your doctor if you have a high fever (above 101°F; 38·3°C) with shaking chills and you are coughing up thick phlegm, or if you have a sharp chest pain when you cough or breathe deeply.

HOW YOU CAN HELP YOURSELF

☐ Time and rest are the best healers of a common cold. If you are prone to heavy colds you may need a day in bed, but otherwise early nights are helpful.
☐ Drink plenty of fluids – at least eight to ten glasses a day.
☐ Fever is the body's way of dealing with infection, but paracetamol may help to ease aches and pains.
☐ Gently blow a blocked nose. Inhaling steam can ease congestion. Eucalyptus oil, menthol or Friar's Balsam added to a bowl of hot (not boiling) water may encourage you to inhale but does not cure the cold.
☐ A sore throat may be eased by sucking a boiled sweet or anything to promote saliva flow. Antiseptic lozenges sometimes cause irritation and sensitivity in the mouth and there is no evidence that these preparations are any more beneficial than a sweet.
☐ Gargling with warm salt water may also ease a sore throat. There is no evidence that antiseptic gargles are any more effective.
☐ A home-made drink of lemon juice, honey and warm water is also soothing.
☐ Avoid smoking.

Cold remedies

No medicine can prevent or cure a cold, but many remedies are sold for the relief of symptoms. Combination preparations – cocktails of aspirin or paracetamol with decongestants, antihistamines and expectorants – cannot be recommended and should be avoided. They cause unwanted effects and do not alter the course of the cold. A nasal decongestant, aspirin or paracetamol and a single ingredient cough syrup should be the most that is needed.

NASAL DECONGESTANTS

When you have a cold the inability to breathe through your nose is uncomfortable and can aggravate a sore throat. A nasal decongestant may lessen swelling and stuffiness in the nose. **Ephedrine** nose drops 0·5%, one or two drops in each nostril, are the mildest and can give relief for several hours. Nose drop preparations containing **xylometazoline** (brand name Otrivine), **phenylephrine** or **oxymetazoline** (Afrazine) are effective but stronger. They relieve swelling by constricting the blood vessels in the nose, but this effect can wear off, resulting in further swelling and stuffiness (rebound congestion) after a few days' use. This congestion is caused by the nose drops, not the cold.

PAIN RELIEF

Aspirin or **paracetamol** can help fever and the general aching feeling. It is important not to take more than the correct dose of paracetamol: two tablets four times a day, and no more than eight tablets in 24 hours. If you have bought an over-the-counter cold remedy containing either aspirin or paracetamol, do not take additional aspirin or paracetamol. Unbranded aspirin or paracetamol tablets are good value compared with branded products. You should not take aspirin if you have or have had a peptic ulcer.

COUGH MEDICINES

You will not need a medicine if you have a productive cough. Steam inhalations and drinking plenty of warm liquids will help to thin mucus so that it is easier to cough up from the lungs. If a dry, irritating, non-productive cough prevents you sleeping, use a single-ingredient cough suppressant such as **pholcodine**.

DECONGESTANTS

The decongestant drugs used locally in the nose are also ingredients in cold and cough remedies. When taken by mouth not only do these drugs constrict blood vessels in the nose, but they also tighten blood vessels throughout the rest of the body, causing a rise in blood pressure and an increase in heart rate. Decongestants are *sympathomimetic* drugs which mimic the effects of adrenaline. They are potentially hazardous for people with high blood pressure, heart disease (angina or coronary thrombosis), over-active thyroid (*hyperthyroidism*) and diabetes. Decongestants also enhance the effects of the antidepressant drugs monoamine-oxidase inhibitors and cause a dangerous rise in blood pressure if the two are used together. Other unwanted effects include headache, giddiness, nervousness, anxiety, palpitations, restlessness and sleeplessness. Although taking a decongestant by mouth does not cause rebound congestion in the nose, the risk of other unwanted effects is too much to make them worthwhile treatments.

You should avoid preparations containing **ephedrine**, **pseudoephedrine**, **phenylephrine** or **phenylpropanolamine** (PPA). These decongestants are also combined with antihistamines in many over-the-counter cold remedies, which may cause drowsiness and affect your ability to make decisions, drive or operate machinery.

WHAT THE LABELS REALLY MEAN

What the packet may say	What it means	One or more of these drugs will be on the label	Verdict	Non-drug alternative
'Aches, pain and fever'	painkiller	aspirin, paracetamol, ibuprofen, codeine	Relieves aches and pains, reduces fever	Stoicism is the only real alternative to using a painkiller, or you could try a hot water bottle
'To dry up a runny nose' or 'to help you sleep'	antihistamine	diphenhydramine, promethazine, pheniramine (may have prefix 'brom' or 'chlor'), triprolidine, diphenylpyraline, doxylamine	Not prove to be useful in colds. Can cause drowsiness	Just let the runny nose run its course. If it's sore, use petroleum jelly to soothe skin
'For a stuffy nose'	decongestant	*Sprays/drops*: phenylephrine, oxymetazoline, xylometazoline *Tablets/capsules*: phenylephrine, pseudophenylephrine, phenylpropanolamine, ephedrine, pseudoephedrine	Preferable in spray or drop form, but beware rebound congestion	Try inhaling hot water vapour with aromatic oils if you like
'For a chesty cough'	expectorant	ammonium chloride, guaiphenesin (or glycerol guaicolate), ipecacuanha, Gee's linctus, squill	Not recommended – efficacy doubtful	Let the cough run its course. Keep your fluid intake up. Steam inhalation may help
'For a dry or tickly cough'	suppressant	dextromethorphan pholcodine, codeine	Use sparingly if your sleep or work is being disturbed by your cough	Use sweets to soothe your throat. Menthol or camphor can help soothe a tickle

4

MIND AND NERVES

Sleeping and anxiety problems Depression
Psychotic illnesses Sickness and dizziness
Pain Migraine Epilepsy
Parkinson's disease and parkinsonism

The brain resembles a telephone junction box, with ten billion nerve cells receiving electrical and chemical impulses from all over the body. Part of the brain works out how to respond to these impulses, checking with the memory to help it decide on the action the body should take and another part controls body action. As signals come to the brain and are interpreted, the responses are sent through nerves to trigger the muscles into action. Nerve cells (*neurons*) are grouped together to form the main path that takes messages to and from the brain – the spinal cord. The spinal cord runs most of the length of the back from the bottom of the brain, inside, and protected by, the backbones. The brain and the spinal cord form the central nervous system.

Nerves that branch off from the central nervous system to the rest of the body form the peripheral nervous system. Nerves from one part of this system run to the skin and muscles while another part in the head connects the brain to the sense organs – eyes, ears, nose and taste buds.

The *autonomic* nervous system works 'automatically', to regulate the heart and circulation, breathing, digestion, the processes for removing waste from the body and the *endocrine glands*. The autonomic system works in harmony with the endocrine glands which release hormones, chemical messengers to regulate certain organs and body functions. The autonomic nervous system has two parts – the *sympathetic* and *parasympathetic* nervous systems – which work in a 'push-pull' way.

The sympathetic system stimulates a particular organ to make it work harder; the parasympathetic system dampens or inhibits activity, opposing the sympathetic system. Your daily body functions are mostly controlled by the parasympathetic system, for example food digestion and passing urine. The sympathetic system controls body functions during exercise and emotion; for example, when you are angry or frightened it makes the heart beat faster, widens the airways in the lungs, enlarges the pupils of the eyes and diverts blood flow from the intestines and skin to the muscles.

● *How nerves send messages*

Nerve messages travel to and from the brain in rapid bursts by electrical means. The minerals sodium and potassium are present everywhere in the body as tiny electrically charged particles so the inside of the nerve cell has a slight negative charge while the fluid outside is positively charged. As the nerve message approaches, the nerve cell membrane alters to change the electrical balance within the cell, allowing the transmission of the message. As the message flows on from one end of the nerve cell to the other, the balance is restored to the resting state. The whole process takes about one thousandth of a second.

The nerve cells do not actually touch each other: the message must pass across a gap (*synapse*). To bridge this gap the cell releases a chemical or *neurotransmitter* which binds on to receptor sites of nearby cells. The message is relayed by the neurotransmitter to the next cell which in turn sends the message to another nerve cell or causes activity in a muscle or organ.

The neurotransmitters in the sympathetic system are the hormones, adrenaline and noradrenaline. The activity of the sympathetic system is increased by the release of adrenaline and noradrenaline from the central part of the adrenal gland (*medulla*). These body chemicals act on alpha- and beta-receptors in the tissues. There are two types of beta-receptors – beta$_1$ in heart muscle and beta$_2$ in smooth muscle, for example muscle around the airways. Drugs that promote the release of adrenaline or noradrenaline or mimic their effects are known as *adrenergic drugs*, *adrenoceptor stimulants* or *sympathomimetics*. Drugs that oppose the sympathetic nervous system are blocking drugs, such as *beta-adrenoceptor blocking medicines* (beta blockers), *adrenergic neuron blocking drugs* or *alpha-adrenoceptor blocking drugs* (alpha blockers).

The nerves that carry messages in the parasympathetic system are *cholinergic* nerves; the chemical nerve transmitter is *acetylcholine*. The actions of acetylcholine can be increased or decreased by other chemicals or drugs. Drugs that stimulate the parasympathetic system and increase acetylcholine activity are called *cholinergic* medicines. Drugs that reduce the action of acetylcholine and the parasympathetic system are *anticholinergic* or *antimuscarinic* medicines, for example atropine and hyoscine.

The way the neurotransmitters adrenaline, noradrenaline and acetylcholine act has been known for many years and drugs to increase or oppose their effects have been developed. More recently, other neurotransmitters, their receptors and what they do in the body have been found. These neurotransmitters include dopamine and 5-hydroxytryptamine (5-HT, also called serotonin) and drugs that affect them and their receptors are among the newer medicines on the market, such as the migraine drug sumatriptan.

Sleeping and anxiety problems

• *SLEEPING PROBLEMS* •

Insomnia or the feeling of being awake for long periods at night is common: about one person in five suffers from it, although it affects women more often than men. People sleep for variable amounts of time from three to ten hours at night, with an average of seven to eight hours. The amount of sleep that each person needs varies: babies sleep a great deal; elderly people need less than the average. Many people suffer from sleeplessness or insomnia occasionally, but persistent lack of sleep can be a problem which needs sorting out. You will need to tell your doctor whether you have difficulty in getting to sleep, or whether you wake during the night or wake too early in the morning. Causes include stress and anxiety; depression; medical problems such as pain, indigestion, cough or itching; the need to pass urine; menopausal symptoms such as hot flushes and sweating; noise; and drinking tea or coffee too late in the evening. Knowing the cause of a sleeping problem is important particularly where there is an underlying medical condition, such as pain or depression, which can be treated.

A short-term sleeping problem may be related to an emotional problem and will clear up once the problem is resolved. One or two nights of broken sleep caused by noise, shift work or travel (for example 'jet lag') do not usually lead to disruption in your life, but longer periods may do so. Taking medicine for a short time may help but a long-term sleeping problem can rarely be solved by taking a sleeping tablet routinely.

• *ANXIETY* •

Anxiety is a mixture of emotional and physical symptoms, such as fear, nervousness, tension and sometimes overwhelming panic; physical signs include tense muscles, headaches, rapid heartbeat or palpitations, breathlessness, sweating, shaking, lightheadedness. The physical symptoms occur because of increased stimulation of the sympathetic nervous system and the release of adrenaline and noradrenaline. The balance of certain other chemicals in the brain may also be disturbed.

HOW YOU CAN HELP YOURSELF

☐ Avoid daytime napping or going to bed too early.
☐ Do not be determined that you *must* have a fixed number of hours sleep a night.
☐ Make sure that environmental factors such as light, heat and noise are right for you. A quiet, dark room with some ventilation promotes restful sleep.
☐ Avoid drinking stimulants such as tea, coffee or cola before bedtime; some people find that caffeine prevents sleep for six hours or more.
☐ Avoid over-the-counter medicines containing caffeine and decongestant preparations containing phenylpropanolamine. Asthma preparations containing theophylline or aminophylline are also stimulants.
☐ Avoid alcohol late at night.
☐ Make sure you establish a good bedtime routine. Have a light, bland snack or milky drink and a warm, relaxing bath.
☐ Exciting television programmes and loud noisy music before you go to bed can interfere with sleep; reading a dull book and having sex both help sleep.
☐ If you really cannot sleep it is often better to get up and do something pleasant than to lie feeling frustrated.

Stress is one of the commonest causes of anxiety. A degree of stress is important in your life to act as a springboard for action or a change of circumstances. Events such as the death of your spouse or a close friend, marriage problems, divorce, poor housing or losing your job cause a great deal of stress; if it becomes too much, symptoms of anxiety may set in. Other psychological factors are important, such as your ability to cope and your self-esteem.

Anxiety symptoms are now understood as a natural psychological reaction to social and physical problems. The best treatment is likely to be counselling in the form of explanation, reassurance and encouragement by your doctor or another suitably trained professional, such as a clinical psychologist or community psychiatric nurse or social worker.

Medicines for sleep and anxiety problems

Medicines to treat anxiety and sleeping problems are discussed together because most anti-anxiety medicines will induce sleep

HOW YOU CAN HELP YOURSELF

☐ Discuss your problems with someone; confiding in a friend, your partner or a relative may help to identify causes of anxiety and potential solutions as well as lessening the burden.
☐ Express your thoughts: try to find out what makes you anxious and make a list of your problems.
☐ Get plenty of rest and sleep if you can.
☐ Regular exercise can be very important and help to release tension; swimming is especially beneficial, particularly for older people.
☐ Yoga or relaxation classes can relieve tension; assertiveness training may also help.
☐ Eat sensibly at regular intervals; avoid drinking stimulants such as tea, coffee or cola and avoid medicines containing caffeine, phenylpropanolamine, theophylline or aminophylline.
☐ Join a self-help group: ask your doctor or local Community Health Council for addresses and phone numbers. There are groups for supporting the bereaved and ethnic and other minorities as well as groups for psychological disorders.

when given in higher doses at night and most sleeping tablets will dampen anxiety when given in lower, divided doses during the day. For example, the benzodiazepine diazepam (brand name Valium) can be used both as a tranquilliser and as a sleeping tablet, although it is more commonly used to relieve anxiety. However, a sleeping tablet should only be used when lack of sleep markedly affects your life, work or the family, and when other approaches or treatment have failed.

Anti-anxiety medicines (tranquillisers or *anxiolytics*) and sleeping tablets (sedatives or *hypnotics*) have been widely used since the 1960s when **benzodiazepines** became available. They appeared to have fewer unwanted effects than **barbiturates**, which are now rarely used for their calming and sedative effects, but see 'Benzodiazepine use', opposite. The adverse effects of barbiturates include a tendency to cause 'hangover effects' the next day and toxicity in overdose. Barbiturates also cause problems of dependence. Some barbiturates are still useful: for example phenobarbitone, which is used for the treatment of epilepsy.

Children should never be given an anti-anxiety medicine or a hypnotic unless your doctor feels there is a strong reason, such as night terrors. The antihistamine, **promethazine** (brand name Phenergan) is sometimes used and is particularly helpful for controlling itching (but not in the case of chicken pox). It acts in the body for a long time and may cause dizziness and falls the following day.

● *BENZODIAZEPINES* ●

If the balance of body chemicals is disrupted in some way, you may experience changes to your mental or physical well-being. *Gamma-aminobutyric acid* (GABA) reduces the flow of electrical impulses across nerve cells in the part of the brain where emotion is controlled. The main action of a benzodiazepine is to increase the effect of GABA, further reducing the electrical flows across cells, and so reducing feelings of anxiety and agitation and slowing mental activity. Benzodiazepines relax muscles and are particularly helpful for reducing muscle spasm, for example after sports injuries. They also have an anticonvulsant action and some are used to treat epilepsy.

● ***Benzodiazepine use***

Benzodiazepine use should be limited to the lowest possible dose for the shortest possible time. Tranquillisers and sleeping tablets must not be used indiscriminately and should be given only for short courses. They should never be given on repeat prescription without the doctor seeing the patient.

The reason is that tolerance of and dependence on the effects of benzodiazepines can occur. Tolerance means that the medicine becomes less effective even though you continue to take the same dose and can develop after 3 to 14 days of continuous use.

Physical dependence means the regular use of a substance which when stopped, especially abruptly, causes the person to develop physical symptoms of withdrawal. With benzodiazepines these include sweating, nervousness, inability to sleep, broken sleep with vivid dreams or nightmares, loss of appetite and body weight, tremor and disturbed vision. These symptoms are similar to the original complaint and may encourage further prescribing of the offending benzodiazepine. Psychological dependence, when you feel that you cannot do without the medicine often accompanies the physical problems.

When you stop taking a sleeping tablet you should expect disturbed sleep for a few nights before a normal sleep routine is re-established, but withdrawing a benzodiazepine after long-term use should be done with the help of your doctor by gradually reducing the dose over a period of time, so that withdrawal symptoms will be lessened if not eliminated. It may be helpful to keep a written record of your dose reduction schedule. Withdrawal may take months to achieve but it is better to go slowly rather than too quickly. You may have to be prepared for the withdrawal process to go on for a year or more. Joining a self-help group, where you can share your experiences and get support, may be helpful. Ask your doctor or local Community Health Council for addresses and phone numbers.

The Committee on Safety of Medicines now advises doctors that:

☐ benzodiazepines should be prescribed only for the short-term relief of anxiety that is severe, disabling or subjecting the individual to unacceptable distress

☐ it is inappropriate and unsuitable to use a benzodiazepine to treat short-term 'mild' anxiety

☐ a benzodiazepine should be used to treat sleeplessness *only* when it is severe, disabling or subjecting the individual to extreme distress.

All benzodiazepines should be avoided for the treatment of anxiety and sleeplessness whenever possible. Life events, such as family illness, bereavement, unemployment or feelings of social isolation and personal inadequacies should be managed without taking these mind-altering medicines. These problems need to be recognised, talked about and relieved without the use of medicines. Your doctor may be able to put you in contact with other professionals, such as a clinical psychologist or a counsellor. Always ask your doctor what alternatives there are to drug treatment. If you have to take a tranquilliser or hypnotic make sure it is for a short time only. Note down how you feel at the start of treatment and how you progress from day to day during the treatment.

● *Adverse effects*

Benzodiazepines have fewer unwanted effects than barbiturates and are less dangerous in overdose. Common unwanted effects include unsteadiness and drowsiness and the elderly are particularly vulnerable to them. Benzodiazepines can also cause confusion, memory loss, impaired learning ability, slurred speech, hostility and aggression.

Confusion and poor co-ordination can result in falls and fractures, especially of hips. Sleeping tablets and tranquillisers impair judgement and increase reaction time, so the ability to drive or operate machinery is affected. The daytime drowsiness or hangover effects of sleeping tablets may also impair driving on the following day. These effects are increased by alcohol and by other tranquillisers or hypnotics.

In older people the adverse effects of a benzodiazepine may be attributed to old age rather than the effects of the medicine itself.

The onset of impaired intelligence with memory loss, confusion or loss of co-ordination in a young person is likely to be attributed to the drug. The same symptoms in an older person, especially if they develop more slowly are often dismissed with the remark, 'You must expect these things at your age.' However, an older person cannot clear a drug from the body (particularly through the liver and kidneys) as rapidly as a young person and is more sensitive to adverse effects of drugs. In spite of this an older person is more likely to be given a prescription for a tranquilliser or sleeping tablets and not always at the reduced dosage recommended for elderly people. Furthermore, tranquillisers and sleeping tablets are prescribed for longer periods of time for elderly patients. Drug-induced impaired thinking and learning disability is one of the most reversible or treatable forms of mental illness. It is a by-product of the increased use of potent medicines during the last 30 years. Stopping a drug with your doctor's guidance can often be better treatment than continuing with a medicine.

A benzodiazepine usually reduces feelings of agitation and restlessness, but in some people it has the opposite effect. There have been some reports of increased hostility and aggression with effects ranging from talkativeness and excitement to aggressive and antisocial acts. American research has shown that, like alcohol, diazepam increases aggressive behaviour. Both diazepam and alcohol depress central nervous system activity and in some people this releases certain patterns of behaviour which would normally be controlled. Some people experience increased anxiety, delusions and hallucinations.

The short-acting benzodiazepine triazolam (brand name Halcion) was withdrawn from the British market in 1991. The adverse effects reported over the years had appeared more marked with triazolam than with other benzodiazepines. These included anxiety between doses and sleep disturbance on ending treatment, aggression, features of psychosis and marked memory impairment.

● *Choice of benzodiazepines*

There are over 15 benzodiazepine drugs, some marketed primarily as tranquillisers and some as hypnotics. This is a bewildering array, particularly because all of these drugs can both tranquillise and promote sleep depending on the dose taken. Calling some anti-anxiety drugs and others hypnotics has more to do with marketing than with pharmacology. However, the benzodiazepines do differ in one important respect and that is how quickly or slowly they are cleared from the body.

Longer-acting benzodiazepines, including **diazepam**, **loprazolam** and **nitrazepam**, have a prolonged action in the body and may cause residual or hangover effects, so that drowsiness persists. The effects of a longer-acting benzodiazepine accumulate so that a steady state of anxiety control and side effects such as drowsiness is reached in the body. Many benzodiazepines break down into one or more chemicals (*metabolites*) in the body and these may have further tranquillising or hypnotic effects.

Shorter-acting benzodiazepines, such as **lorezepam**, **oxazepam** and **temazepam**, pass through the body more quickly and therefore produce little or no hangover effect. However, shorter-acting benzodiazepines can cause more withdrawal problems, particularly if they are stopped abruptly. If you are taking a short-acting benzodiazepine, your doctor may transfer you to a longer-acting one to lessen the impact of withdrawal symptoms.

A short-acting benzodiazepine used as a hypnotic, such as temazepam, causes little drowsiness the next day. For anxiety diazepam is longer-acting but oxazepam is a reasonable choice because its short-acting effect means it does not accumulate in the body.

Since the Limited List was introduced in 1985 certain benzodiazepines used for sleep and anxiety problems can no longer be paid for by the NHS. Also prescribing by brand names is disallowed, so doctors must prescribe the benzodiazepines by generic name.

DIAZEPAM

VALIUM – Tablets, liquid, injection, rectal solution
DIAZEPAM

Diazepam is a long-acting benzodiazepine used for relieving severe disabling anxiety. It has a depressant effect on the part of the brain controlling emotion. Treatment should be for no more than two to four weeks. Diazepam is also used as a muscle relaxant, for relieving epileptic fits, to help withdrawal symptoms for people with acute alcohol poisoning and sometimes as premedication before operations or uncomfortable diagnostic procedures. Like all benzodiazepines, diazepam can cause tolerance, dependence and withdrawal symptoms.

Before you use this medicine

Tell your doctor if you are:
☐ pregnant or breast-feeding ☐ taking any other medicines, including vitamins and those bought over the counter.

Tell your doctor if you have or have had:
☐ liver or kidney problems ☐ mental illness or depression ☐ brief periods of not breathing during sleep (sleep apnoea) ☐ lung disease or breathing problems ☐ alcohol or drug dependence.

Do not use if you have:
☐ severe breathing problems or lung disease ☐ psychiatric disorders ☐ porphyria.

How to use this medicine

Take the tablet according to the schedule agreed with your doctor. Ask your doctor to limit the prescription to seven days of treatment and do not obtain further supplies of diazepam on a repeat prescription. It is important to see your doctor and for you both to evaluate how you feel after the course of treatment.

Do not drive a car or do other activities that require alertness until you know how you react to diazepam. Diazepam may cause drowsiness, impair judgement and increase reaction time. People who take a benzodiazepine drug are more likely to have traffic accidents. Do not take alcohol, as it increases the effects of diazepam. Do not stop taking this medicine suddenly after treatment lasting more than seven days; ask your doctor for a dosage reduction schedule that will allow you to stop gradually and prevent withdrawal symptoms. If you miss a dose, take it as soon as you remember but if it is nearly time for your next dose skip it. Do not take double the dose or more than the prescribed dose.

Over 65 Older people and those who are seriously ill or debilitated may need only half the standard adult dose or even less.

Interactions with other medicines

Always check with your doctor or pharmacist if you can take diazepam with another medicine. All drugs that have a sedative or tranquillising effect on the central nervous system will increase the effect of diazepam.

Unwanted effects

Likely Drowsiness, dizziness, lightheadedness, confusion, clumsiness, unsteadiness or falling, forgetfulness, dependence.
Rarely Headache, digestive disorders, rashes, blurred vision, low blood pressure, dry mouth, increased thirst, or unusual mouth watering, difficulty passing urine, blood disorders, jaundice, unusual excitability, hallucinations.

The unwanted effects of drowsiness and dizziness may fade as treatment continues or a lower dose may help. If you experience any of the less likely effects contact your doctor. Stop taking diazepam if you develop a skin rash.

Similar preparations

Prescribed for anxiety
CHLORDIAZEPOXIDE (LIBRIUM) – Capsules, tablets
LORAZEPAM (ATIVAN) – Tablets, injection
OXAZEPAM – Tablets

Prescribed for sleeping problems
LOPRAZOLAM – Tablets
LORMETAZEPAM – Tablets
NITRAZEPAM (MOGADON) – Tablets, liquid, capsules
TEMAZEPAM – Capsules

Not available on NHS prescription
For anxiety:
ALPRAZOLAM (XANAX); **BROMAZEPAM** (LEXOTAN); **CLOBAZAM** (FRISIUM); **CLORAZEPATE** (TRANXENE); **MEDAZEPAM** (NOBRIUM)
For sleeping problems:
FLUNITRAZEPAM (ROHYPNOL); **FLURAZEPAM** (DALMANE)

• *OTHER HYPNOTICS* •

Other hypnotics include **chloral hydrate** (brand names Welldorm; Noctec), **triclofos, chlormethiazole** (Heminevrin) and a newer preparation, **zopiclone** (Zimovane). Zopiclone is not a benzodiazepine but it acts at the same places on the nerve cell as a benzodiazepine. It should only be used for short periods and it is not certain whether tolerance and withdrawal symptoms develop with its use. Hallucinations, forgetfulness and behavioural disturbances (including aggression) have been reported occasionally. As with all hypnotics, if you take zopiclone you should not drive the day after treatment because it can cause dizziness, lightheadedness and poor co-ordination.

Alcohol cannot be recommended because it disturbs sleep later in the night. It has a diuretic (water-removing) action and causes thirst. Heavy long-term use disturbs sleep patterns and causes insomnia.

● *OTHER MEDICINES FOR ANXIETY* ●

Buspirone (brand name Buspar) is not related to the benzodiazepines and it has no muscle relaxant, hypnotic or anti-epileptic effects. Buspirone can be used for the short-term relief of anxiety, but a major disadvantage is that its effects are not felt for up to two to three weeks after starting treatment. It does not help to relieve benzodiazepine withdrawal symptoms and the benzodiazepine should be withdrawn gradually before buspirone is started. It has not yet been associated with dependence. Buspirone may cause dizziness but is unlikely to cause drowsiness, but you should not drive a car until you know how you react to it.

Meprobamate is less effective than a benzodiazepine, more hazardous in overdose and can cause dependence.

A beta blocker may be helpful if you are troubled by the physical symptoms of anxiety, such as sweating, palpitations and shaking, but it will not affect your emotions.

Depression

Depression is the most common mental disorder, affecting many thousands of people. The exact nature of the illness is poorly understood but it appears to be a blend of biochemical and psychological factors. Sad moods usually pass with time and need no medical treatment, but when the feeling does not fade it may lead to loss of interest in living and working. You may experience low self-esteem, a feeling of hopelessness, loss of appetite for food and sex and disturbed sleep. Depression may be masked by physical symptoms such as backache, headaches, dizziness, chest pains or weight loss. In severe depression you may consider taking your own life.

Social factors or events such as bereavement, losing your job or divorce can trigger depression. Feeling physically low because of a debilitating illness or the aftermath of a virus infection or continuous, nagging pain can cause depression, which is sometimes worse than the physical condition itself. You may suffer depression after childbirth, during the menopause or at a mid-life crisis. Some drugs can cause depression, for example blood pressure lowering drugs. If a depressive episode begins after the start of treatment with a new medicine, ask your doctor whether the drug could be causing the depression. When depression appears to be caused by such external factors it is called *reactive depression*.

Sometimes depression begins for no apparent reason. This is *endogenous depression*, which does not appear to have any outside trigger and may recur several times in your life. Depressive episodes may alternate with periods when you feel perfectly well (*unipolar depression*) or with periods of over-activity and with normal mood (*bipolar* or *manic depression*; see page 218). Endogenous depression may run in families.

Depression occurs in episodes and a bout may last for a few weeks or months. You may recover spontaneously but treatment with medicines and/or counselling may be needed and can help moderate to severe depressive illness. It may not be easy to help yourself when you are depressed, but some tips are given in the Box opposite.

Antidepressants

Treatment with an antidepressant medicine can help moderate to severe lingering depression. Drug treatment will not cure the underlying cause but may help you to function more normally again. A period of drug treatment may lift you sufficiently from melancholic thoughts and low self-esteem to allow you to get on with life. You may not begin to feel the beneficial effects of some medicines for 10–14 days, with full effects taking six weeks to develop. Treatment is usually needed for at least four months after the acute symptoms of depressive illness have faded. Some people may need treatment for a number of years to prevent a relapse. Your doctor should withdraw treatment very gradually over a period of four to six weeks to prevent a recurrence of symptoms and will need to see you for another three or four weeks once you have stopped your medicine altogether.

Depression is thought to be caused by a decrease in brain chemicals called neurotransmitters, such as *noradrenaline* and *5-hydroxytryptamine* (also called *serotonin*). In depression the brain cells release less of the neurotransmitters to excite neighbouring cells and stimulate activity. Antidepressants increase the amount of neurotransmitters outside brain cells, which prolongs their stimulatory effect on the brain.

– HOW YOU CAN HELP YOURSELF –

These suggestions are also useful for anyone trying to help a depressed friend or relative.

☐ Share your sadness with a friend or neighbour. Try not to bottle your feelings up.
☐ Keep a record of the pleasant things that happen to you and discuss these with someone, too. If you have no one to talk to, find out if there is a counselling service near to you or available by telephone. The Samaritans, a 24-hour listening and befriending service, have local branches throughout Britain – see your telephone directory for local numbers or ask the operator (dial 100). Organisations such as Depressives Anonymous and the British Association for Counselling have lists of self-help groups and counsellors.
☐ Do not try to overcome depression with large amounts of alcohol. Alcohol depresses brain and nervous activity and may make you even further depressed.
☐ Eat properly and try to take regular exercise – a daily walk if possible.
☐ Try to rest and sleep if possible: have a quiet time before bedtime, perhaps a warm bath to try and relax; avoid caffeine-containing drinks.
☐ If your depression seems to be lasting, see your doctor.

• *TRICYCLIC ANTIDEPRESSANTS* •

The tricyclic antidepressants, so-called because of their chemical structure, are the most widely used group of antidepressants. Your doctor is likely to try a preparation from this large group first. Some of the medicines have a more sedative effect and are helpful if you have sleeping difficulties because the single daily dose can be taken at night; these include **amitriptyline**, **dothiepin**, **doxepin** and **mianserin**. Other medicines are less sedative, for example **imipramine** and **lofepramine**, and may help if you feel lethargic. The tricyclic antidepressants are well established, relatively safe and effective at normal doses, but may cause unwanted effects such as dry mouth, blurred vision, constipation and difficulty passing urine as well as dizziness and heart problems. Some unwanted effects may fade as you continue treatment but older people are more sensitive to them. Overdosage can cause severe heart problems that need emergency treatment.

AMITRIPTYLINE

AMITRIPTYLINE – Tablets
DOMICAL – Tablets
ELAVIL – Tablets
TRYPTIZOL – Tablets, mixture, injection

Poor choice
LENTIZOL – Modified-release capsules
TRYPTIZOL – Modified-release capsules
Modified-release preparations are not necessary because the effects of ordinary tablets last long enough.

Amitriptyline is a tricyclic antidepressant which lifts mood, increases activity and improves appetite. It has a sedative effect and because it acts in the body for a long time, it can be taken at night as a single dose. Modified-release preparations are therefore unnecessary. Amitriptyline improves sleep once treatment has started but it may take two to four weeks before you feel the full antidepressive effect. It may also be used to help children over six or seven years old with bed-wetting problems, but should be used for no longer than three months. Unwanted effects can be trouble-some, especially in older people. Amitriptyline should be used with care in people with heart disease because it may cause hazardous irregular heart rhythms and heart block.

Before you use this medicine

Tell your doctor if you are:
☐ pregnant – safety of amitriptyline not established ☐ breast-feeding ☐ taking any other medicines, including vitamins and those bought over the counter.

Tell your doctor if you have or have had:
☐ diabetes ☐ heart disease, especially irregular heart rhythms ☐ epilepsy or seizures ☐ severe liver disease ☐ thyroid disease ☐ psychoses ☐ glaucoma ☐ prostate disorders.

Do not take if you have or have had:
☐ a recent heart attack ☐ heart block ☐ mania ☐ porphyria.

How to use this medicine

Take the tablet with water at night or in divided doses during the day.

Do not drive or do other activities that require alertness until you know how you react to amitriptyline. You may feel dizzy or faint when you get up from sitting or lying down, especially during the first few days of treatment. Get up slowly and stay beside the chair or bed until you are sure you are not dizzy. Avoid alcohol because it increases the sedative effects of amitriptyline.

Do not stop taking this medicine suddenly. Your doctor will give you a schedule to reduce the dose gradually if you are on long-term treatment, to prevent a recurrence of your symptoms. If you miss a dose, take it as soon as you remember. For example, if you have forgotten your night-time dose, take it the next morning if drowsiness is not a problem. Otherwise, skip it and take your next dose as usual. Do not take double doses.

Over 65 You should have a third to half the normal adult dose. Unwanted effects may be troublesome, especially antimuscarinic effects of dry mouth, blurred vision, drowsiness, constipation and difficulty passing urine, and also mental effects such as confusion, short-term memory problems, disorientation.

Interactions with other medicines

Amitriptyline interacts with many other medicines. Do not take other medicines without checking with your doctor or pharmacist. These are some important ones:

Other antidepressants Monoamine-oxidase inhibitors (MAOIs) cause excitation of the central nervous system, restlessness, high blood pressure and other signs of overactivity. They must not be taken for at least 14 days before or after another antidepressant.

Fluoxetine increases blood levels of some tricyclic antidepressants.

Anti-epileptics and tricyclic antidepressants antagonise each other's effects.

Adrenaline and adrenaline-like drugs (*sympathomimetics*) result in high blood pressure and irregular heart rhythms.

Anaesthetics Amitriptyline may need to be stopped before you have a general anaesthetic. Always tell your doctor or dentist that you take this drug.

Unwanted effects

Likely Drowsiness, dizziness, fainting, dry mouth, blurred vision, difficulty passing urine, feeling sick, constipation.

Unlikely Irregular heart rhythms, palpitations, sweating, tremor, rashes, disorientation, confusion, sexual dysfunction.

Unwanted effects may be noticed before the antidepressive effects are felt although they may fade as treatment continues. If unwanted effects are troublesome discuss with your doctor. If you have irregular heart rhythms and severe dizziness or fainting, stop taking amitriptyline and call your doctor.

Similar preparations

ALLEGRON – Tablets
NORTRIPTYLINE

ANAFRANIL – Capsules, liquid, injection
CLOMIPRAMINE

ASENDIS – Tablets
AMOXAPINE

AVENTYL – Capsules
NORTRIPTYLINE

CLOMIPRAMINE – Capsules

CONCORDIN – Tablets
PROTRIPTYLINE

DOTHIEPIN – Capsules, tablets

EVADYNE – Tablets
BUTRIPTYLINE

GAMANIL – Tablets
LOFEPRAMINE

IMIPRAMINE – Tablets

PERTOFRAN – Tablets
DESIPRAMINE

PROTHIADEN – Capsules, tablets
DOTHIEPIN

SINEQUAN – Capsules
DOXEPIN

SURMONTIL – Capsules, tablets
TRIMIPRAMINE

TOFRANIL – Tablets, liquid
IMIPRAMINE

Poor choice

ANAFRANIL SR – Modified-release tablets
CLOMIPRAMINE

LIMBITROL – combined preparation
AMITRIPTYLINE + CHLORDIAZEPOXIDE

MOTIPRESS/MOTIVAL – combined preparation
NORTRIPTYLINE + FLUPHENAZINE

TRIPTAFEN/TRIPTAFEN M – combined preparation
AMITRIPTYLINE + PERPHENAZINE

Related preparations

BOLVIDON – Tablets
MIANSERIN

LUDIOMIL – Tablets
MAPROTILINE

MIANSERIN – Tablets

MOLIPAXIN – Capsules, tablets, liquid
TRAZODONE

NORVAL – Tablets
MIANSERIN

PRONDOL – Tablets
IPRINDOLE

VIVALAN – Tablets
VILOXAZINE

Combinations of an anti-anxiety drug in one preparation, with an antidepressant such as **chlordiazepoxide** with **amitriptyline**, are not recommended. An anti-anxiety medicine is taken for a short time only while antidepressant treatment may continue for several months or more. The doses of the individual drugs cannot be adjusted in a combination preparation.

● *MONOAMINE-OXIDASE INHIBITORS (MAOIs)* ●

These have been in use for over 30 years, but doctors prescribe them less today because of their unwanted effects and interactions with other medicines, *tyramine*-containing food, beer and wine. However, they are especially helpful for anxious people with phobias or for panic attacks. MAOIs may be tried after other antidepressants, but no antidepressant should be given for at least 14 days before or after treatment with an MAOI because of the risk of toxic effects. An MAOI should not be started for five weeks after a course of fluoxetine. Combining a tricyclic antidepressant with an MAOI is no more effective than either drug used alone and can be hazardous. **Tranylcypromine** (brand name Parnate) with **clomipramine** (Anafranil) is a particularly unsafe combination.

PHENELZINE

NARDIL – Tablets

Phenelzine is a monoamine-oxidase inhibitor (MAOI) used for relieving depression particularly when anxiety and phobias are also problems. It increases the levels of neurotransmitters in the brain by blocking the enzyme which breaks them down. The full effect of phenelzine may not be felt for up to four weeks and continues for 14 days once treatment is stopped. Children should not be treated with phenelzine. The main drawback with the MAOI antidepressants is the risk of dangerous interactions with other medicines, including over-the-counter ones and with some foods and alcohol. You should always carry a treatment card with you.

Before you use this medicine

Tell your doctor if you are:
☐ pregnant or breast-feeding ☐ taking any other medicines, including vitamins and those bought over the counter.

Tell your doctor if you have or have had:
☐ diabetes mellitus ☐ heart disease ☐ epilepsy or seizures ☐ blood disorders.

Do not take if you have or have had:
☐ liver disease ☐ stroke ☐ porphyria ☐ phaeochromocytoma (a tumour causing high blood pressure).

How to use this medicine

Take the tablet three or four times daily. It may take four weeks for the full effect to develop but after this, your doctor may reduce the dose to a maintenance level.

You may feel dizzy or faint when you get up from sitting or lying down, especially during the first few days of treatment. Get up slowly and stay beside the chair or bed until you are sure you are not dizzy. Do not drive or do other activities that require alertness until you know how you react to phenelzine.

Foods containing high levels of **tyramine** must not be eaten while you are taking phenelzine or for 14 days after you have stopped treatment. These include cheese, pickled herrings, broad bean pods and meat or yeast extracts such as Marmite, Bovril and Oxo. Always carry a treatment card with you – the pharmacist will give you one with this medicine. Do not drink red wines, especially Chianti, beer or lager, including alcohol-free products.

Do not stop taking this medicine suddenly. Your doctor will give you a schedule to decrease the dose gradually to prevent withdrawal symptoms. If you miss a dose, take it as soon as you remember, but skip it if it is almost time for your next dose. Do not take double the dose.

Over 65 There is greater likelihood of adverse effects. Phenelzine should only be used if the benefits outweigh the risks.

Interactions with other medicines

Phenelzine interacts with many other medicines. Do not take any other medicines without checking with your doctor or pharmacist. The following must not be taken with phenelzine because they may cause a dangerous rise in blood pressure:

Cough and cold remedies, including nose drops, containing **ephedrine**, **pseudoephedrine**, **phenylephrine** or **phenylpropanolamine**.
Analgesics: pethidine and **morphine**.
Tricyclic antidepressants.
Levodopa, used for Parkinson's disease.

Unwanted effects

Likely Dizziness, sudden fall in blood pressure, drowsiness, weakness, fatigue, extra body fluid (*oedema*), blurred vision, dry mouth, constipation, sleeplessness.
Unlikely Headache, nervousness, sweating, rash, jaundice, difficulty passing urine, numbness or tingling of limbs, behavioural changes, euphoria, confusion, weight gain, sexual dysfunction, irregular heart rhythms.

A sudden drop in blood pressure and dizziness are common unwanted effects. If you feel unwell or develop swollen ankles while taking phenelzine, discuss the symptoms with your doctor. If you develop a severe, throbbing headache, sickness or unexplained sweating contact your doctor immediately: this may mean that your blood pressure is rising to hazardous levels.

Similar preparations

MARPLAN – Tablets
ISOCARBOXAZID

PARNATE – Tablets
TRANYLCYPROMINE

Poor choice
PARSTELIN – combined preparation
TRANYLCYPROMINE + TRIFLUOPERAZINE

• OTHER ANTIDEPRESSANTS •

Flupenthixol (brand name Fluanxol) is used for short-term treatment of depression and in low doses has fewer unwanted effects than a tricyclic antidepressant. **Fluvoxamine** (brand name Faverin), **fluoxetine** (Prozac), **sertraline** (Lustral) and **paroxetine** (Seroxat) are 5-HT blockers, also called serotonin uptake inhibitors, part of a range of medicines that work on the neurotransmitter 5-hydroxytryptamine. At present it is uncertain whether 5-HT is the main chemical involved in depression and it is clear that these newer antidepressants are no more effective than the older tricyclic type. However, they cause less drowsiness and do not cause dry mouth, blurred vision or weight gain; diarrhoea, nausea and vomiting seem to be the most common unwanted effects, but lowering the dose may ease those symptoms. Headache, anxiety and restlessness may also occur.

FLUOXETINE

▼PROZAC – Capsules

Low amounts of body chemicals for triggering brain activity (noradrenaline and 5-hydroxytryptamine – 5-HT or serotonin) are thought to cause depression. Fluoxetine is a 5-HT blocker, which prevents reabsorption of 5-HT, so that an increased amount is available to stimulate brain cells. Fluoxetine does not affect noradrenaline levels. It does not cause drowsiness and acts in the body for a long time, so a single dose can be given once a day. It causes fewer unwanted effects than tricyclic antidepressants.

Before you use this medicine

Tell your doctor if you are:
☐ pregnant ☐ breast-feeding – not usually prescribed ☐ taking any other medicines, including vitamins and those bought over the counter.

Tell your doctor if you have or have had:
☐ liver disease ☐ kidney disease (avoid fluoxetine if kidney problems are severe) ☐ epilepsy ☐ diabetes mellitus.

Do not take an MAOI for at least five weeks after stopping fluoxetine.

How to use this medicine

Take the capsule or dose prescribed by your doctor (up to four capsules daily) once a day in the morning. Do not drive or do other activities that require alertness until you know how you react to fluoxetine. If you miss a dose, take it as soon as you remember, but skip it if it is almost time for your next dose. Do not take double the dose.

Over 65 You should take no more than three capsules a day.

Interactions with other medicines

Other antidepressants The effects of MAOIs and some tricyclics are increased. MAOIs and fluoxetine should not be taken together.
Lithium Increased risk of toxicity.

Unwanted effects

Likely Feeling or being sick, diarrhoea, loss of appetite, weight loss, headache, nervousness, sleeplessness, dry mouth, dizziness, sexual dysfunction, anxiety, rash.
Unlikely Confusion, blood disorders, vaginal bleeding on stopping treatment, violent behaviour and thoughts of suicide.

At low doses unwanted effects are mild. If you develop a skin rash, stop taking fluoxetine and contact your doctor.

Similar preparations

FAVERIN – Tablets
FLUVOXAMINE

▼LUSTRAL – Tablets
SERTRALINE

▼SEROXAT – Tablets
PAROXETINE

● *STOPPING TREATMENT* ●

Unlike benzodiazepines and other tranquillisers, treatment with an antidepressant medicine does not generally cause dependence. Withdrawal symptoms may occur after stopping regular treatment suddenly, particularly with a monoamine-oxidase inhibitor, and occasionally after an older tricyclic drug. They have not been noted with newer antidepressants. Symptoms on suddenly stopping treatment include headaches, feeling and being sick, dizziness, sleeplessness, vivid dreams, anxiety and panic attacks. Your doctor will give you a schedule to withdraw treatment gradually.

● *ELECTROCONVULSIVE THERAPY* ●

Electroconvulsive therapy (ECT) may help severe acute depressive illness, particularly if someone has hallucinations, delusions, a risk of suicide and is not eating or drinking properly. ECT is usually effective and has few adverse effects, even for older people. You are given a general anaesthetic and a small current of electricity is passed through the brain, producing a mild convulsion. Recovery may take a few weeks.

Psychotic illnesses

Psychoses – mental disorders such as schizophrenia, paranoia symptoms, mania and depression – are serious illnesses. Thoughts and behaviour are disturbed in some cases for only a short time, but in others the disorders may be permanent.

Schizophrenia is an illness in which thought processes become fragmented: you lose touch with reality, often seeing or hearing things which are not really there (hallucinating) and believing things that are not true (suffering delusions). Paranoid delusions are common, for example the belief that everyone is against you. You may talk to imaginary voices and try to protect yourself from people who you believe want to harm you. You may also experience severe mood problems, such as depression, apathy, loss of emotion and difficulties relating to people.

About one person in a hundred develops schizophrenia, regardless of culture, social class or sex. It is most common in young people, especially between the ages of 15 and 45. The illness can run in families and if one of your parents has schizophrenia the risk of your developing it increases to about one in eight. However, theories that family interaction causes schizophrenia are now rejected although if you have had schizophrenic symptoms the tendency to relapse can be affected by family relationships and attitudes.

FAMILY THERAPY

If a schizophrenic's family are supportive, tolerant and keep the emotional temperature low, the person is far less likely to have a relapse than if they are critical or emotionally demanding. Of the people who return from hospital to a 'high-emotion' home, 53 per cent have a relapse during the following year. For those who return to a 'low-emotion' home, the figure is only 23 per cent.

Family therapy sessions help people adjust to the idea that their son, daughter or spouse is unlikely to regain the same levels of achievement and emotional strength that they had before they were ill. This adjustment in itself can improve the sufferer's chances.

Manic depression is a mental illness in which changes in mood are greatly exaggerated. In a mentally healthy person, your mood or state of mind may alter slightly from day to day depending on events. With manic depression episodes of deep depression may alternate with periods of normal moods and periods of elation or overactivity (*mania*). Mental illnesses also include acute states of confusion, dementia and behaviour and personality disorders.

The exact cause of psychoses is not known but it may be a blend of a number of factors including stress, heredity and brain injury. What is known is that parts of the brain become oversensitive to the brain chemical **dopamine**. This chemical is a neurotransmitter carrying messages between brain cells. In mental illness the brain cells release too much dopamine, resulting in mental overactivity. This process is thought to produce abnormal thoughts and behaviour. There may also be an imbalance in the electrical messages between the left and right sides of the brain.

Temporary psychotic symptoms can occur with drug or alcohol misuse. The abuse of mind-altering drugs such as cocaine and amphetamines can cause hallucinations and psychosis. If mental symptoms, such as hallucinations develop in older people the medicines they take or have just started should be examined. Certain prescription medicines, such as antiparkinsonian drugs, analgesics, the heart drug digoxin, beta blockers, sedatives and anti-anxiety drugs, can cause psychotic signs.

HOW YOU CAN HELP YOURSELF

Friends and relatives of a person suffering from a psychotic illness should encourage the following actions.

- ☐ Seek advice and professional help.
- ☐ Discuss treatment with your doctor.
- ☐ Take exercise or be active for a part of each day.
- ☐ Balance life between seeing people and being alone.
- ☐ Join a local help group; contact the National Schizophrenia Fellowship or National Association for Mental Health (see 'Useful addresses').

Antipsychotic medicines

Antipsychotic medicines (*neuroleptics*; also misleadingly called major tranquillisers) can help to relieve psychotic symptoms by dampening them down, but they are not cures for mental illness. Drug treatment can improve the quality of life for a mentally ill person and may prevent relapse after the illness first becomes apparent. Someone with acute schizophrenia – a dramatic crisis lasting days or weeks – generally responds to treatment better than someone who has developed the illness gradually and has chronic (long-term) symptoms. Chronic schizophrenia is usually a slow and often permanent deterioration in mental health. Although an antipsychotic medicine may be less effective in someone who is apathetic and withdrawn, drug treatment sometimes appears to have an enlivening influence. Antipsychotic drugs should not be used to treat mild cases of anxiety or depression.

Antipsychotic medicines act by interfering with the flow of nerve signals within the brain. They block dopamine receptors, places on the cell wall where dopamine locks on to the cell to produce its effect. Antipsychotics also block other receptors on cells throughout the body and therefore produce some troublesome unwanted effects.

PHENOTHIAZINES

Phenothiazines are the most commonly used antipsychotic medicines. They are all similar in effect but differ in their main actions and unwanted effects, and people have different responses to them. Your doctor will have to find the right medicine at the lowest effective dose to suit you. Taking two antipsychotic medicines is not recommended; it does not produce twice the effect or lessen unwanted effects. An acutely disturbed person needs a higher dose of medicine at first but the dose can be reduced when symptoms are controlled. Do not alter the dose or stop treatment because the illness may relapse. Your doctor will give you a schedule to withdraw treatment gradually if this seems appropriate.

Phenothiazines may be taken by mouth but they are also given by injection or long-acting *depot* injection. If you are having regular treatment, your doctor may suggest a depot injection which is given deep into a muscle at intervals of one to four weeks and releases the drug slowly into the body, so you don't have to remember to take tablets.

Unwanted effects

Extrapyramidal symptoms cause the most trouble. They cannot be predicted and depend on the dose, the type of drug and how susceptible you are to it. Antipsychotic drugs can cause several types of extrapyramidal disorders:

- **Parkinsonian symptoms** (or parkinsonism) – difficulty speaking or swallowing, loss of balance, mask-like face, muscle spasms, stiffness of the arms or legs, trembling or shaking.
- **Acute dystonia** – jaw clenching and other abnormal face, neck and body movements, unusual eye movements with eyeballs becoming fixed in one position.
- **Akathisia** – restlessness, inability to sit or stand still.
- **Tardive dyskinesia** – lip smacking, chewing movements, puf-

fing of cheeks, rapid darting tongue movements, uncontrolled movements of arms or legs.

Parkinsonian effects and akathisia may come on gradually within the first months of treatment but can be suppressed with an anti-parkinsonian medicine, such as **orphenadrine** or **benzhexol** (see page 264). Alternatively, a change of antipsychotic medicine may be needed. Acute dystonia may appear after only a few doses but can also be treated with an antiparkinsonian drug. Parkinsonian disorders disappear slowly when the drug is withdrawn, although akathisia and dystonia disappear more rapidly.

Tardive dyskinesia occurs fairly frequently, especially in older people, on long-term treatment (over one year) and at high doses. However, it can occur occasionally at low dosage after a short period of treatment. If you expericnce spontaneous or uncontrolled movements of the face, tongue, arms or legs, contact your doctor as soon as possible. It may be irreversible and result in immobility and difficulty with chewing and swallowing. Prompt detection of this unwanted effect may prevent an irreversible problem developing. Contact your doctor if you are concerned; the dose of your medicine may need to be lowered or the drug changed.

Other effects include low blood pressure, which can result in falls and accidents, and interference with the body's temperature regulation which may result in hypothermia in older people. Antimuscarinic effects can cause confusion, short-term memory problems and other mental impairment as well as dry mouth, constipation, difficulty passing urine, blurred vision, worsening of glaucoma, sexual problems and decreased sweating.

CHLORPROMAZINE

CHLORPROMAZINE – Tablets, liquid, injection, suppositories
LARGACTIL – Tablets, liquid, injection

Chlorpromazine is a phenothiazine used for treating schizophrenia and other mental illnesses, especially paranoid symptoms. It is used as a short-term measure to quieten disturbed patients. Chlorpromazine calms and sedates without impairing consciousness, but should not be regarded as a straightforward tranquilliser for use in non-psychotic people. It is also used to control nausea and sickness in people who are terminally ill. Adverse effects can be serious and troublesome.

Before you use this medicine

Tell your doctor if you are:
☐ pregnant or breast-feeding ☐ taking any other medicines, including vitamins and those bought over the counter.

Tell your doctor if you have or have had:
☐ heart or circulation problems ☐ Parkinson's disease ☐ epilepsy or seizures ☐ overactive thyroid gland ☐ glaucoma ☐ enlarged prostate or difficulty urinating ☐ liver disease.

How to use this medicine

Take the tablet with food or a full glass of water three times a day. Chlorpromazine can cause a skin rash (*contact dermatitis*); tablets should not be crushed and liquids must be handled with care. It can also cause a dry mouth; drink extra fluids to prevent dryness.

You may feel dizzy especially when you get up from sitting or lying down. Get up slowly and stand beside the chair or bed until you are sure you are not dizzy. Do not drive or do other activities that require alertness until you know how you react to chlorpromazine. Avoid alcohol as it increases the effects of chlorpromazine.

Do not stop taking chlorpromazine suddenly even if you feel well. Always discuss your treatment with the doctor who will give you a schedule to reduce the dose gradually if treatment can be stopped. If you miss a dose, take it as soon as you remember but skip it if it is almost time for your next dose. Do not take double doses.

Over 65 You should have a third to half the adult dose: older people are more susceptible to unwanted effects. You should take particular care in very hot or very cold weather because chlorpromazine affects the body's regulation of temperature. You or a relative should find out why you are being prescribed a phenothiazine. Doctors should give serious consideration to prescribing these drugs to people over 70 because of the many possible adverse effects.

Interactions with other medicines

Chlorpromazine interacts with many other medicines. Do not take other medicines without checking with your doctor or pharmacist. These are some important ones:

General anaesthetics increase the blood pressure lowering effect of chlorpromazine. If you have to have surgery tell your doctor or dentist that you take this medicine.

Anti-anxiety and sleep-inducing drugs increase drowsiness with chlorpromazine.

Antidepressants increase the anticholinergic unwanted effects of chlorpromazine, such as dry mouth, blurred vision, difficulty in passing urine and constipation.

Unwanted effects

Likely Drowsiness, lethargy, stuffy nose, dry mouth, blurred vision, dizziness, fainting, sleeplessness, agitation, weight gain, fewer periods, extrapyramidal symptoms (see below).
Unlikely Jaundice, irregular heart rhythm, blood disorders indicated by fever and sore throat, abnormal bleeding or bruising, skin rash (*contact dermatitis*); with high dosage sensitivity to light in sunny weather, eye changes.

Contact your doctor if you feel unwell on chlorpromazine but especially if you develop these extrapyramidal symptoms:

Parkinsonian symptoms Difficulty speaking or swallowing, loss of balance, mask-like face; muscle spasms; stiffness of arms and legs; trembling and shaking.
Dystonia Muscular spasms of face, neck, shoulders and body; facial distortions and grimacing; unusual eye movements when eyeballs become fixed in one position.
Akathisia Restlessness, inability to sit or stand still, pacing up and down.
Tardive dyskinesia Lip smacking, chewing movements, puffing of cheeks, darting tongue movements, uncontrolled movements of arms and legs.

Similar preparations

FENTAZIN – Tablets
PERPHENAZINE

MELLERIL – Tablets
THIORIDAZINE

MODITEN – Tablets, depot injection (Modecate)
FLUPHENAZINE

NEULACTIL – Tablets, liquid
PERICYAZINE

NOZINAN – Tablets, injection
METHOTRIMEPRAZINE

PROCHLORPERAZINE – Tablets

SPARINE – Liquid, injection
PROMAZINE

STELAZINE – Tablets, modified-release capsules, liquid, injection
TRIFLUOPERAZINE

STEMETIL – Tablets, liquid, granules, injection, suppositories
PROCHLORPERAZINE

THIORIDAZINE – Tablets

TRIFLUOPERAZINE – Tablets

Continued over

Related preparations

ANQUIL – Tablets
BENPERIDOL

CLOPIXOL – Tablets, injection, depot injection
ZUCLOPENTHIXOL

▼CLOZARIL – Tablets
CLOZAPINE

DEPIXOL – Depot injection
FLUPENTHIXOL

DOLMATIL – Tablets
SULPIRIDE

DOZIC – Liquid
HALOPERIDOL

DROLEPTAN – Tablets, liquid, injection
DROPERIDOL

HALDOL – Tablets, liquid, injection, depot injection
HALOPERIDOL

HALOPERIDOL – Tablets

INTEGRIN – Capsules, tablets
OXYPERTINE

▼LOXAPAC – Capsules
LOXAPINE

ORAP – Tablets
PIMOZIDE

PIPORTIL DEPOT – Depot injection
PIPOTHIAZINE

REDEPTIN – Depot injection
FLUSPIRILENE

▼ROXIAM – Capsules
REMOXIPRIDE

SERENACE – Capsules, tablets, liquid, injection
HALOPERIDOL

SULPITIL – Tablets
SULPIRIDE

TRIPERIDOL – Tablets
TRIFLUPERIDOL

• *LITHIUM* •

Lithium is given in cases of manic depression to reduce the intensity of the mania. An antipsychotic medicine may be given at first to relieve immediate symptoms because lithium may take three weeks to work. **Carbamazepine** (brand name Tegretol) may be useful for preventing manic depression if lithium does not help.

LITHIUM

Lithium carbonate
CAMCOLIT – Tablets, modified-release tablets

LISKONUM – Modified-release tablets

PHASAL – Modified-release tablets
PRIADEL – Modified-release tablets

Lithium citrate
LI-LIQUID — Liquid
LITAREX – Modified-release tablets
PRIADEL – Liquid

Lithium is used for preventing and treating mania, manic depression and recurrent depression. It lessens the intensity and frequency of mood swings. The decision to start treatment with lithium has to be carefully considered because there is a narrow range between a helpful and a harmful dose. Treatment is usually started by a hospital specialist and blood levels of the drug must be measured regularly so that the dose can be tailored to your needs. Treatment may be for a period of up to five years, or even longer. Lithium can cause serious adverse effects and medical help must be sought immediately if they occur.

Before you use this medicine

Tell your doctor if you are:
☐ pregnant – do not become pregnant without talking to your doctor because lithium can affect the foetus ☐ breast-feeding ☐ on a low-salt diet ☐ taking any other medicines, including vitamins and those bought over the counter.

Tell your doctor if you have or have had:
☐ heart or circulation problems ☐ kidney disease ☐ myasthenia gravis ☐ overactive thyroid.

How to use this medicine

Take the tablet with plenty of water as a single dose or in divided doses exactly as directed by your doctor. Swallow each tablet whole, especially modified-release tablets. Try to take the dose at the same time each day. It may be several days and up to three weeks before you can tell whether the drug is working.

Different preparations vary in how much lithium reaches the blood. Never accept a different preparation from the one you have, unless your doctor specifically prescribes it. Ask the pharmacist to give you a treatment card with information about lithium and space to note the brand name, or use medicines worksheet.

Lithium blood levels are affected by the amount of sodium in your body. Be especially careful to keep your salt and fluid intake constant. Drink more fluids during hot weather or illness such as diarrhoea. Do not drive or do other activities that require alertness until you know how you react to lithium. Alcohol can enhance the sedative effects of lithium.

Do not stop taking this medicine suddenly as your condition may worsen. Your doctor will give you a schedule to reduce the dose of lithium gradually. If you are taking lithium three times a day and miss a dose, skip it and then take the next dose as usual. If you are taking lithium once a day and miss a dose, take it as soon as you remember, but skip it if it is less than eight hours until your next scheduled dose. Do not take double doses.

See your doctor regularly to make sure lithium is working. You will need regular blood tests and a check to see that you are not developing unwanted effects. You will also need periodic tests for thyroid, kidney and heart function.

Over 65 You need less than the normal adult dose; older people are more sensitive to the effects of lithium.

Interactions with other medicines

Lithium interacts with many other medicines. Do not take other medicines, including those bought over the counter, without checking with your doctor or pharmacist.
Aspirin-like analgesics and other NSAIDs may increase the risk of lithium toxicity.
Blood pressure lowering drugs: ACE inhibitors may increase lithium toxicity.
Methyldopa may cause nerve damage.
Diuretics increased risk of lithium toxicity, especially with thiazide diuretics.
Antidepressants: fluoxetine, **fluvoxamine, paroxetine** and **sertraline** increase the risk of toxic effects on the nervous system.
Sumatriptan Increased risk of toxic effects on nervous system.

Unwanted effects

Likely Feeling sick, diarrhoea, fine tremor of the hands, dizziness, muscle weakness.
Unlikely Drowsiness, lethargy, blurred vision, weight gain, oedema, skin rash.

If you develop any symptoms of toxicity, stop taking lithium and contact your doctor immediately.
Early signs Diarrhoea, feeling or being sick, loss of appetite, muscle weakness, drowsiness, slurred speech, trembling.
Late signs Blurred vision, giddiness, clumsiness, confusion, coarse tremor, trembling.

Sickness and dizziness

Feeling sick (nausea) and being sick (vomiting) are common symptoms of a variety of disorders. Vomiting is one of the ways that the body gets rid of harmful substances, as in the case of food poisoning, but it may also be a sign of disease. Causes of sickness include gastroenteritis, bacterial and viral infections, hormonal changes during pregnancy, diabetes, motion sickness, Ménière's disease, vertigo and unwanted effects of medicines.

Vomiting is a reflex action in response to stimulation of the *vomiting centre* in the brain. The vomiting centre can receive signals from the stomach and intestines, from the inner ear and from the brain. Another part of the brain, the *chemoreceptor trigger zone*, which is thought to be sensitive to foreign substances in the blood, can also stimulate the vomiting centre. Medicines to prevent or control sickness seem to suppress the stimulus to vomit. Treatment of vomiting depends on its cause.

Giddiness is described clinically as vertigo – a condition in which you feel that either you or the room is spinning. You may lose balance and feel or be sick. The inner ear controls balance and responds to changes in bodily movements and if it is damaged through illness, such as infection, your balance may be affected. Sudden attacks of vertigo, associated with hearing loss and noises in the ear (*tinnitus*), occur in a wide variety of disorders of the inner ear. When there appears to be no direct cause of the condition, the disorder is known as Ménière's disease.

A dizzy feeling (a swimming, lightheaded feeling) can also be caused by anxiety, lack of food when blood-sugar is low and overbreathing (*hyperventilation*). If you stand up or lift your head up quickly when your blood pressure is low, you may feel dizzy or faint (*postural hypotension*).

Medicines for sickness and dizziness

The choice of medicine depends on the cause of sickness. Sometimes a medicine is unnecessary because the body may be reacting to an infection, such as food poisoning. Taking a medicine to stop sickness (an anti-emetic) can delay the removal of bacteria and toxins from the body. An anti-emetic may mask diagnosis or a medicine's unwanted effect, when lowering the dose or stopping the drug would be better treatment.

HOW YOU CAN HELP YOURSELF

☐ If you have vomited, drink fluids to replace those lost from the body. The rehydration solution of glucose and salt used for diarrhoea is ideal (see page 82). If vomiting occurs over a few days, for example as a result of gastroenteritis, rehydration is important and food should be avoided until vomiting has stopped. Re-introduce food gradually.
☐ If you are liable to travel sickness, find a medicine that suits you to take before you travel. Avoid overindulging in food and drink before the journey; find a good position on an aeroplane, stay on deck on a boat and look out of the window in a car. Avoid reading in the car – children are particularly liable to feel sick doing this. Take something to drink and/or suck, such as bottled water and some glucose sweets.
☐ If you are sick during pregnancy, eat a little food before you get up in the morning and take small amounts frequently throughout the day.
☐ Eat meals regularly if lack of food makes you dizzy; carry glucose sweets as a standby.
☐ If you feel dizzy after resting, get up slowly from sitting or lying down and stay beside the chair or bed until you are sure you are not dizzy. If you have been lying down, hang your legs over the side of the bed for a few minutes then get up slowly.

Contact your doctor:
☐ if you have severe vomiting for 24 hours
☐ if you have taken a medicine for sickness and it is not having any effect after two days
☐ if a young child has diarrhoea and vomiting with a temperature
☐ if you are vomiting and feeling very ill
☐ if you vomit after a head injury.

• *MOTION SICKNESS* •

The most effective drug for preventing motion or travel sickness on short journeys is **hyoscine** (related to atropine). It should be taken about half an hour before travelling and is effective for around four hours. You can take another dose after six to eight hours, but no more than three doses in 24 hours. Remedies to prevent travel sickness, such as Kwells, can be bought from a pharmacy. Children under the age of four years should not take a hyoscine-containing preparation, but older children can take a lower dose than adults – Joy-Rides or Kwells Junior, for example. Unwanted effects include drowsiness, dizziness, dry mouth, blurred vision and difficulty passing urine. Hyoscine can cause troublesome visual disturbances; you should avoid activities such as driving until vision has recovered. You should not take hyoscine if you have glaucoma.

Hyoscine can also be applied to the skin as a plaster (brand name Scopoderm), which for longer protection, for instance on sailing voyages, may be more convenient than taking tablets. Unwanted effects are similar. Doctors can prescribe the plasters but you cannot buy them over the counter.

Antihistamines such as **cinnarizine** (brand names Stugeron; Marzine RF), **dimenhydrinate** (Dramamine), **meclozine** (Sea-Legs) and **promethazine** (Phenergan; Avomine) are slightly less effective than hyoscine, but unwanted effects are fewer. Promethazine and dimenhydrinate cause greater drowsiness than the others. **Cyclizine** has also been used for preventing travel sickness; drowsiness is the main unwanted effect, but it can also cause dry mouth and blurred vision.

Alcohol and other medicines that affect the brain, such as tranquillisers and antidepressants, should not be taken with hyoscine or an antihistamine. Both hyoscine and antihistamines commonly cause drowsiness and interfere with your ability to drive or operate machinery. Alcohol increases this effect.

• *VERTIGO* •

Giddiness and sickness associated with Ménière's disease and middle-ear disorders may sometimes be helped by hyoscine, an antihistamine or a phenothiazine (for example **prochlorperazine**; brand name Stemetil). **Betahistine** (brand name Serc) and **cinnarizine** have been used specifically for Ménière's disease but have no advantage over other antihistamines or a phenothiazine. In acute attacks **cyclizine**, **prochlorperazine** or **thiethylperazine** (brand name Torecan) may be given by injection or by suppository.

Vague symptoms of dizziness which often afflict older people need investigation rather than long-term treatment with prochlorperazine. Many medicines cause dizziness as an unwanted effect, for example the heart drug digoxin and diuretics, and altering the dose of these can stop the dizziness. Prochlorperazine can cause *extrapyramidal* effects (see page 220) especially in older people and when treatment is prolonged.

• *VOMITING DURING PREGNANCY* •

It is quite usual to feel sick or to be sick during the first three months of pregnancy, but this gradually fades and does not need drug treatment. Occasionally vomiting may be severe and your doctor may prescribe an antihistamine or a phenothiazine for a short period. If vomiting continues you may need to see a specialist.

• *UNDERLYING DISORDERS* •

Some medicines, such as opioid analgesics, general anaesthetics and anticancer drugs, some diseases and radiotherapy can cause nausea and vomiting. A phenothiazine, in low dose, is the recommended drug for preventing and treating this sort of sickness. **Metoclopramide** is another effective anti-emetic which acts on the gut as well as on the brain to stop vomiting. Like the phenothiazines, metoclopramide may cause extrapyramidal effects, usually uncontrolled movement of the neck, face, tongue and eyes (*dystonia*), especially in children and young people. It is therefore given to people under 20 only when vomiting is severe. **Domperidone** is similar to metoclopramide but is less likely to cause drowsiness and dystonia and can be used in younger people. **Nabilone** (brand name Cesamet) is a synthetic medicine derived from cannabis which helps to relieve sickness caused by anticancer drugs, except when high doses of the platinum containing drug cisplatin are used.

Ondansetron (brand name Zofran) is a new type of anti-emetic which does help prevent nausea and vomiting induced by cisplatin. It is one of the new class of drugs that affects the neurotransmitter 5-hydroxytryptamine (5-HT). 5-HT activity in the small intestine and in the brain appears to trigger nausea and vomiting and ondansetron blocks these stimuli. Unwanted effects include headache and constipation or diarrhoea. **Granisetron** (brand name Kytril) is similar to ondansetron.

METOCLOPRAMIDE

METOCLOPRAMIDE – Tablets, liquid, injection
MAXOLON – Tablets, liquid, injection

Antimigraine preparations
MIGRAVESS – Tablets
METOCLOPRAMIDE + ASPIRIN
PARAMAX – Tablets, soluble powder
METOCLOPRAMIDE + PARACETAMOL

Poor choice
Modified-release preparations:
GASTROBID CONTINUS; GASTROMAX; MAXOLON SR

Metoclopramide is used in adults to relieve nausea and vomiting caused by digestive disorders and anticancer treatment. It blocks dopamine receptors in the intestines and in the vomiting centre in the brain. Metoclopramide may also help non-ulcer dyspepsia and oesophageal reflux because it acts on the gut, speeding the stomach contents along the intestines. Metoclopramide's anti-emetic and stomach-emptying effect may also help in migraine attacks, although absorption of low doses taken by mouth is variable. The combined preparations with aspirin and paracetamol are likely to provide variable benefit. Metoclopramide in modified-release preparations is absorbed too slowly to help with nausea and vomiting. Metoclopramide is also used after operations to restore gastric activity and in some diagnostic procedures.

Before you use this medicine

Tell your doctor if you are:
☐ pregnant or breast-feeding ☐ taking any other medicines, including vitamins and those bought over the counter.

Tell your doctor if you have or have had:
☐ liver or kidney disease ☐ porphyria ☐ phaeochromocytoma (a tumour causing high blood pressure) ☐ epilepsy

How to use this medicine

Take the tablet three times a day. Tablets should not be used for children under 15, but a liquid preparation can be used – this must be measured accurately to get the exact dose for the weight of the child.

Do not drive or do other activities that require alertness until you know how you react to metoclopramide. Avoid alcohol because it works against metoclopramide's actions and enhances drowsiness.

If you miss a dose, take it as soon as you remember. If the next dose is due within two hours, take the missed dose immediately and skip the next one.

Over 65 Usually you need less than the normal adult dose. Prolonged treatment has caused extrapyramidal effects. Your doctor should review treatment regularly.

Interactions with other medicines

Metoclopramide can interact with any other medicine that has a sedative effect on the central nervous system, such as tranquillisers.

Hyoscine and atropine-like drugs antagonise metoclopramide's effect on the stomach and gut.

Unwanted effects

Unlikely Extrapyramidal symptoms (see page 220) such as dystonia (in children and young adults it is **likely**) and tardive dyskinesia (after prolonged treatment, mainly affecting elderly people); drowsiness, restlessness, diarrhoea.

Metoclopramide causes few problems in adults. If extrapyramidal symptoms develop in people under 20 or over 65, stop metoclopramide and contact your doctor immediately.

Similar preparations

MOTILIUM – Tablets, liquid, suppositories
DOMPERIDONE

Pain

Pain is a symptom not a disease. It is an unpleasant sensory and emotional experience associated with actual or likely damage to the body. You learn the nature of pain from early childhood, for example when falling over as a toddler and cutting a knee. When the body is hurt nerve endings detect the damage and relay impulses to the brain via the central nervous system. Your brain registers pain and the need to act to avoid further damage. However, pain is not always associated with damage to the body; there may be a psychological cause.

You and your doctor or dentist should try to discover the underlying cause of pain. Understanding what causes your pain can help you cope with it: when you see a cut finger and know how it happened you attend to the physical damage first and then cope mentally with the sensation of pain afterwards, but it is much harder to understand pain from within the body, whether it is backache or a symptom of a disease. Anxiety and depression lessen your tolerance of pain. If pain becomes a worry or a nagging fear then you must see your doctor.

Treating the underlying cause generally relieves pain, so a pain-relieving medicine (*analgesic*) may not always be needed; treatment with another type of medicine or other pain-relief technique may be better. Your doctor may prescribe a combination of medicines, one to relieve the underlying cause and one to tackle pain. The intensity with which pain is felt varies from person to person, so the amount of pain relief needed for any problem varies. Alternatives to analgesics include heat (massaging a pulled muscle, for example) or cold (for burns); rest or exercise; acupuncture; nerve stimulation; manipulation or chiropractic; meditation; and hypnosis.

– HOW YOU CAN HELP YOURSELF –

☐ Use simple local treatments where relevant – ice packs or cold compresses for sports injuries; heat (hot water bottle, infra red lamp or massage) for pulled muscles or stiffness.
☐ Rest if possible to help the injured part relax.
☐ Exercise gently and within the capability of the damaged part to strengthen the injured muscles and tissue.
☐ Keep a small supply of pain-relief medicines in the house, one for adult use and one for children. Do not use more than the recommended dose.
☐ If you are still in pain and simple remedies have not helped after 48 hours, see your doctor.

Severe pain:
☐ Work with your doctor to try to establish the cause of pain, describing accurately where the pain is and how severe you think it is.
☐ You are the authority on your pain and only you can feel it; do not be afraid to ask for pain relief. Suffering pain after an operation, however minor, is unnecessary and may slow your recovery.
☐ If you have continuous pain you should have regular doses of a pain-relieving medicine to prevent pain breaking through.
☐ Your doctor may be able to refer you to a pain-relief clinic if you have severe intractable pain.

Analgesics

There are two main types of pain-relieving medicine: *non-opioid analgesics* such as **aspirin** and **paracetamol** and *opioid analgesics (narcotics)* such as **morphine**. Non-opioid medicines are helpful for headaches and muscular pain, stopping the transmission of pain stimuli in nerve endings at the site of pain. Opioid analgesics are used for moderate to severe pain. They act directly on the brain, altering your perception of pain.

• NON-OPIOID ANALGESICS •

Aspirin is the analgesic of choice for headache, sore throat, muscular pains and period pains, as long as you can tolerate its irritant effect on the stomach. It brings the body temperature down and reduces inflammation. Aspirin blocks the effect of *prostaglandins* – body chemicals that contribute to pain and swelling, which are released when tissue is damaged. Taken regularly, aspirin can relieve the pain and swelling in rheumatoid arthritis, although more effective drugs now exist.

Aspirin is an excellent pain reliever except that many people find that it upsets their stomach. It may irritate the stomach lining and sometimes cause ulceration and bleeding. Taking aspirin after food helps to reduce this effect and there are also aspirin preparations which are specially formulated to lessen the problem: a tablet with *enteric coating* is designed to release aspirin in the small intestine but it takes time to work, so it is not suitable for immediate pain relief, say for a headache. It may be helpful for relieving long-lasting pain, for example at night. Dispersible aspirin tablets can be dissolved in a little water and taken as a liquid; aspirin in liquid form is absorbed more quickly into the bloodstream from the digestive system. Pain relief is faster, but dispersible aspirin does not protect the stomach from the irritant effects of aspirin.

Paracetamol is similar in analgesic effect to aspirin but it does not reduce inflammation. It appears to act centrally on the brain and does not irritate the stomach. There is a range of liquid paracetamol preparations which are suitable for treating children with minor illnesses and for reducing fever.

• *Toxic effects of aspirin and paracetamol*

Although aspirin and paracetamol are found in ordinary, everyday medicines used for the relief of minor aches and pains, both can be toxic if more than the recommended dose is taken. Always check the label of compound preparations, such as cold remedies and analgesics or ask the pharmacist about the contents of prescription medicines. Never take more than one type of pain- or cold-relief preparation at any one time and always follow the instructions on how much to take and how often. Plain aspirin or paracetamol sold generically give the clearest indication of the ingredients and dosage of the preparation.

You should take no more than 12 aspirin tablets of 300mg strength a day, at intervals of at least four hours. If you need to use aspirin for more than a few days, you should see your doctor. Regular use of even smaller doses of aspirin may cause stomach upsets and bleeding. You should take no more than eight paracetamol tablets of 500mg strength a day, at intervals of at least four hours. If you need to take eight tablets of paracetamol every day for more than a few days, see your doctor.

An overdose of aspirin or paracetamol needs immediate and urgent medical attention. Signs of too high a dose of aspirin include noises or ringing in the ears (*tinnitus*), deafness, overbreathing, high body temperature and sweating, thirst, stomach pain and vomiting. Signs of too high a dose of paracetamol are not very obvious, but there may be some nausea and vomiting at first. However, an overdose of paracetamol causes severe liver damage which may be fatal unless you have immediate treatment in hospital. Both aspirin and paracetamol can also cause kidney damage.

ASPIRIN IS NOT FOR CHILDREN

Aspirin should not be given to children under 12 for treating minor illnesses. A rare but potentially fatal illness involving the brain and liver (Reye's syndrome) has been linked to aspirin usage in children, particularly those with a viral infection. Aspirin may occasionally be used to treat children with juvenile rheumatoid arthritis (Still's disease) under the guidance of a specialist. Paracetamol is an effective alternative treatment for relieving the pain and fever of minor complaints for children under 12.

ASPIRIN

On prescription/over the counter
ASPIRIN – Tablets, soluble tablets
CAPRIN – Enteric-coated tablets
LABOPRIN DL – Soluble powder (buffered) (not on prescription)
NU-SEALS ASPIRIN – Enteric-coated tablets
PALAPRIN FORTE – Tablets (buffered)
Many branded pain-relievers are aspirin preparations: check the ingredients and the dose

Antimigraine preparation
MIGRAVESS – Tablets
ASPIRIN + METOCLOPRAMIDE

Poor choice
Combination preparations (on prescription):
ASPAV; **CO-CODAPRIN** (with **CODEINE**) – also from a pharmacy; DOLOXENE COMPOUND; EQUAGESIC

Aspirin (*acetylsalicylic acid*) is a non-opioid analgesic for headache, muscular injuries and period pains. It blocks the effects of *prostaglandins* which are released when body tissue is injured. Aspirin is also used in small doses to prevent blood clots after heart attacks or strokes and may be useful for preventing heart attacks in people at serious risk. Irritation of the stomach is the main unwanted effect; buffered and enteric-coated preparations deliver the aspirin in a less irritant form, but some do not act as quickly as simple preparations. Aspirin should not be given to children under 12 except under medical guidance, because a rare, but often fatal, disorder, Reye's syndrome, has been linked to its use.

Before you use this medicine

Tell your doctor if you are:
☐ pregnant – avoid aspirin particularly in the last week of pregnancy ☐ breast-feeding – avoid aspirin ☐ taking any other medicines, including vitamins and those bought over the counter.

Tell your doctor if you have or have had:
☐ asthma ☐ allergies ☐ nasal polyps ☐ a previous reaction to aspirin or a non-steroidal anti-inflammatory drug such as ibuprofen ☐ blood-clotting disorders ☐ kidney or liver disease – avoid aspirin if severe ☐ anaemia.

Do not take if you have or have had:
☐ a stomach or duodenal ulcer ☐ haemophilia ☐ gout.

How to use this medicine

Take the tablets every four or more hours if needed with milk or water at or just after meals. Do not take aspirin more often than every four hours. If you are treating yourself do not take regular doses of aspirin for more than two days without contacting your doctor. If you are taking a high dose of aspirin for long periods, see your doctor for regular checks. Avoid alcohol because it increases the risk of gastric or intestinal bleeding.

If you are going to have surgery, regular treatment with aspirin should be stopped about five days beforehand. Aspirin interferes with your ability to stop bleeding.

Storage Keep aspirin tablets in a cool dry place. Do not use if the tablets smell of vinegar, look mottled or are crumbling. Renew stocks of aspirin for household use once a year.

Over 65 You may need less than the normal adult dose.

Interactions with other medicines

Aspirin interacts with several other medicines. Do not take other medicines without checking with your doctor or pharmacist. These are the important interactions:
Anticoagulants Increased risk of bleeding.
NSAIDs Increased risk of stomach irritation.

Unwanted effects

Likely Heartburn, indigestion, feeling sick, stomach pain, abnormal weakness.
Unlikely Skin rash, itching, wheezing, chest tightness, trouble breathing, gastrointestinal bleeding.

Unwanted effects are generally mild and infrequent but stomach irritation and bleeding can occur. Vomiting bloody or coffee ground-like matter or black, tarry stools are signs of serious gastrointestinal bleeding and you should contact your doctor. Some people are hypersensitive to the effects of aspirin: if a skin rash develops or you have wheezing or difficulty breathing, stop taking aspirin and contact your doctor immediately.

Similar preparations

BENORAL – Tablets, granules, liquid
BENORYLATE

BENORYLATE – Tablets, liquid

DISALCID – Capsules
SALICYLATE

TRILISATE – Tablets
SALICYLATE

PARACETAMOL

Over the counter/on prescription
PARACETAMOL – Tablets, soluble tablets, liquid, suppositories
Brands include:
ALVEDON; CALPOL; DISPROL; PALDESIC

Continued over

PAMETON – Tablets (protect the liver from overdose)
PARACETAMOL + METHIONINE

Antimigraine preparation

PARAMAX – Tablets, soluble powder
PARACETAMOL + METOCLOPRAMIDE

Poor choice

Combined preparations (on prescription):
CO-CODAMOL (with **CODEINE**) – Low dose of opioid (also from a pharmacy); **CO-DYDRAMOL** (with **DIHYDROCODEINE**) – Low dose of opioid; **CO-PROXAMOL** (with **DEXTROPROPOXYPHENE**) – Low dose of both drugs

Paracetamol relieves mild to moderate pain such as headache and reduces fever. Unlike aspirin it does not reduce swelling and stiffness. It can be used by children for relieving fever and pain. As it does not cause stomach irritation, people with a stomach ulcer can take paracetamol. People allergic to aspirin can usually take paracetamol. Paracetamol is a safe and effective analgesic provided the dosage instructions are followed carefully. In overdose it can cause fatal liver and kidney damage.

Before you use this medicine

Tell your doctor if you are:
☐ pregnant or breast-feeding ☐ taking any other medicines, including vitamins and those bought over the counter.

Tell your doctor if you have or have had:
☐ liver or kidney disease ☐ alcohol dependence.

How to use this medicine

Take two tablets every four to six hours if needed. Do not take more often than every four hours. Do not take more than eight tablets in 24 hours. Children older than three months may be given paracetamol. If you have a baby under three months your doctor may recommend paracetamol after immunisation, but otherwise do not give it to this age group.

If you are a moderate to heavy regular drinker, routine use of paracetamol carries a risk of liver damage.

If you are treating yourself with paracetamol, contact your doctor if you have a fever that lasts for more than three days or if your symptoms do not improve.

Over 65 Paracetamol is a suitable analgesic for self-treatment. If you have liver or kidney disease you may need less than the normal adult dose.

Interactions with other medicines

Check with your doctor or pharmacist that paracetamol does not interact with any medicine you are already taking.
Anticoagulants The dose may need adjusting if paracetamol is taken frequently.

Unwanted effects

Unlikely Skin rash, blood disorders, acute pancreatitis.

Unwanted effects are rare when paracetamol is taken as recommended. Immediate medical attention must be sought if you suspect an overdose whether by design or accident. Families with an unstable teenager or a depressed person in the house may wish to buy **paracetamol + methionine** (brand name Pameton) to have as the analgesic in the medicine cupboard instead of other aspirin or paracetamol products. Methionine helps to prevent liver damage caused by an overdose of paracetamol.

● *Other non-opioid analgesics*

Benorylate, a derivative of aspirin and paracetamol, is mostly used to relieve pain and swelling in arthritic conditions. If you take benorylate it is very important not to take other aspirin- or paracetamol-containing preparations with it.

Ibuprofen and other non-steroidal anti-inflammatory drugs (NSAIDs) are related to aspirin and, like aspirin, they are irritant to the stomach. Although mainly used to relieve the pain and inflammation of arthritic diseases they are useful pain-relievers for a variety of conditions, for example period pains or sports injuries. They are useful for long-term conditions, for example bone pain where bones have tumour deposits in them. They may also be useful for relieving pain after surgery and may reduce the need for opioid analgesics.

Diclofenac is used by injection or suppository to relieve the acute and excruciating pain of renal colic.

● *COMBINED ANALGESIC PREPARATIONS* ●

Many preparations combine paracetamol, aspirin or paracetamol with one of the weaker opioid analgesics (see page 242). When pain is inadequately controlled with aspirin or paracetamol alone, it seems logical to combine one or other with a stronger analgesic. Yet there is little evidence that combined analgesics are more effective than either drug given alone. The doses of the two analgesics are fixed in a combined preparation and the dose of the opioid analgesic is often too small to be felt. Preparations containing higher doses of opioids with paracetamol (Fortagesic, Remedeine, Solpadol, Tylex) may be more effective, but it is questionable whether the paracetamol is still needed. Combinations of aspirin or paracetamol with dextropropoxyphene are less suitable because the drugs act in the body for different lengths of time. Dihydrocodeine and dextropropoxyphene reduce breathing and make treatment of overdoses of combined analgesics complicated.

Some pain-relief preparations contain other ingredients such as caffeine, an antihistamine or a muscle relaxant. However, such ingredients add nothing to the pain-relieving properties of an analgesic. Caffeine may aggravate the gastric irritation caused by aspirin. High doses or stopping caffeine may cause headaches.

The names of compound analgesics, both generic and brand, do not reveal the ingredients of the preparations. This information has to be carefully looked for on the label of products bought over the counter, although some packs now declare 'contains paracetamol'. The labels on dispensed medicines should now say whether the product contains paracetamol but will not do so for other analgesics. Always check the ingredients of a pain-relief product with the pharmacist. *Acetylsalicylic acid* is another name for aspirin which you may come across and all salicylates are similar to aspirin. If you take a combined analgesic you should not take any other type of pain-relief product with it. It is usually best to find a single-ingredient preparation that suits you for occasional pain relief and stick to the product. If pain relief is inadequate with paracetamol or aspirin, discuss other methods of pain relief with your doctor.

● *OPIOID ANALGESICS* ●

Morphine and related drugs are extracted from the head of the opium poppy. The opioids, also called narcotic analgesics, relieve moderate to severe pain, particularly pain after surgery and the pain of terminal illnesses such as cancer. They act directly on the areas of the brain where pain is perceived. They also block the flow of pain signals.

Morphine is the most valuable opioid analgesic for relieving severe pain and is the standard against which other opioids are compared. In addition to relieving pain morphine also causes euphoria, a sense of well-being, and mental detachment. Other related analgesics include **diamorphine** (heroin), **methadone**

WHAT'S IN PAIN-RELIEVERS?

Analgesic ingredients of branded pain-relievers sold over the counter and in pharmacies.

Aspirin
ANADIN
ASKIT
ASPRO
ASPRO CLEAR
BAYER
BEECHAMS POWDERS
BEECHAMS POWDERS TABLETS
CAPRIN
MRS CULLEN'S
DISPRIN
FEMIGRAINE (with antihistamine)
FYNNON
SOLMIN
PHENSIC
TOPTABS

Paracetamol
ANADIN PARACETAMOL
ASPRO PARACLEAR
BEECHAMS POWDERS CAPSULES (with decongestant)
CAFADOL
CALPOL
CUPANOL
DEWITT'S
DISPROL
DOAN'S
ELKAMOL
FANALGIC
HEDEX
MIRADOL
PALDESIC
PANADOL
PANALEVE
PARACETS
PARAMIN
SALZONE
TRAMIL

Ibuprofen
ANADIN IBUPROFEN
CUPROFEN
IBRUFHALAL
INOVEN
LIBROFEM
MIGRAFEN
NOVAPRIN
NUROFEN
PACIFENE
PHOR PAIN
PROFLEX
RELCOFEN

Aspirin + paracetamol
ANADIN EXTRA
BANIMAX
DISPRIN EXTRA
NURSE SYKES
POWERIN
VEGANIN (with codeine)

Aspirin + codeine
ANTOIN
CODIS
COJENE
HYPON

Paracetamol + codeine
CALPOL EXTRA
CODA-MED
CODANIN
E.P.
PANADEINE CO
PANEREL
PARACODOL
PARAMOL (*dihydrocodeine*)
PROPAIN (with antihistamine)
SOLPADEINE
SYNDOL (with antihistamine)

and **pethidine**. Opioid analgesics all have similar actions and effects although they differ in when and for how long they work and whether they can be taken by mouth or by another method such as injection. People vary in their response to them. They have similar unwanted effects, the most common being nausea and vomiting, drowsiness and constipation. Adverse effects include depressed breathing and low blood pressure. Drowsiness may affect the performance of skilled tasks, such as driving, and the effects of alcohol are enhanced.

High doses of morphine or any other opioid analgesic lead to breathing difficulties, narrowing of the pupil to pinpoint size and even coma. **Naloxone**, a drug that blocks the effects of morphine can be given by injection to reverse morphine poisoning.

The use of opioid analgesics has to be strictly controlled because of their tendency to cause dependence (addiction). But when morphine or related medicines are used medically for the control of acute pain the risk of dependence is small.

● *Weaker opioid analgesics*

Dihydrocodeine, **codeine** and **dextropropoxyphene** are used to relieve mild to moderate pain, but codeine and dihydrocodeine both cause constipation and are not suitable for long-term use. Dextropropoxyphene is slightly less effective than codeine and is mostly used in combination preparations.

MORPHINE

MORPHINE – Liquid, injection, suppositories
MST CONTINUS – Modified-release tablets
ORAMORPH – Liquid
SEVREDOL – Tablets, suppositories
SRM RHOTARD – Modified-release tablets

With anti-emetic
CYCLIMORPH – Injection
MORPHINE + CYCLIZINE

Poor choice
NEPENTHE – No advantage over morphine and risk of overdosage
MIXED OPIUM ALKALOIDS

Morphine – the main active ingredient of opium – is an opioid analgesic used to relieve severe pain caused by surgery, heart attack or injury and is most valuable in controlling pain in terminal illnesses such as cancer. Morphine acts on the brain and alters your perception of pain. It makes you drowsy, lightheaded and less anxious. Tolerance and dependence may occur, but short courses of morphine do not usually cause dependence and the drug can be stopped or gradually withdrawn without problems.

Before you use this medicine

Tell your doctor if you are:
☐ pregnant – morphine is not usually prescribed ☐ breast-feeding – usual doses are unlikely to affect the baby, but discuss with your doctor ☐ taking any other medicines, including vitamins and those bought over the counter.

Tell your doctor if you have or have had:
☐ brain disease or head injury – morphine should not be used ☐ heart and circulatory disorders, including low blood pressure ☐ asthma, emphysema, bronchitis or lung disease ☐ underactive thyroid gland ☐ kidney or liver disease.

How to use this medicine

Take the tablet or liquid or use suppositories regularly every four hours for serious constant pain. Modified-release tablets should be taken every 12 hours.

You may feel dizzy or faint when you get up from sitting or lying down, especially during the first few days of treatment. Get up slowly and stay beside the chair or bed until you are sure you are not dizzy. Do not drive or do other activities that require alertness until you know how you react to morphine. Avoid alcohol as it will make you more drowsy.

If you miss a dose take it as soon as possible, but skip it if it is almost time for the next dose. Do not take double the dose. If you have been taking morphine for more than a few weeks, do not stop taking it suddenly. Ask your doctor to give you a schedule to reduce the dose gradually. If you take morphine for a short period you can stop the drug as soon as you no longer need pain relief.

Over 65 The dose of morphine varies from person to person but you may need less than the standard adult dose, especially if you have poor kidney function.

Interactions with other medicines

Morphine will enhance the sedative effects of all drugs acting on the brain such as **tranquillisers**, **antidepressants**, **sleep-inducing drugs**, **antihistamines** and **antipsychotics**.
Antidepressants, especially monoamine-oxidase inhibitors affect the brain, causing either excitation or depression with high blood pressure or low blood pressure.

Unwanted effects

Likely Feeling or being sick, drowsiness, dizziness, confusion, lightheadedness, constipation.
Unlikely Breathing difficulties, sudden drop in blood pressure, dry mouth, difficulty passing urine, sweating, palpitations, hallucinations, mood changes, skin rash, itching.

Feeling or being sick and constipation are common unwanted effects which may be alleviated with other medicines. Call the doctor immediately if someone has slow and troubled breathing, severe drowsiness or loss of consciousness.

Similar preparations

DIAMORPHINE (HEROIN) – Tablets, liquid, injection

DICONAL – Tablets (with anti-emetic)
DIPIPANONE + CYCLIZINE

MEPTID – Tablets, injection
MEPTAZINOL

METHADONE – Liquid

NARPHEN – Tablets
PHENAZOCINE

NUBAIN – Injection
NALBUPHINE

PALFIUM – Tablets, injection, suppositories
DEXTROMORAMIDE

PETHIDINE – Tablets, injection

PHYSEPTONE – Tablets, injection
METHADONE

Migraine

Migraine is a recurring severe headache, usually affecting the front of the head on only one side, although both sides may be painful. Before the pain begins you may have warning signs (*aura*) when you see flashing lights, bright or coloured lines or even lose sight temporarily; you may experience 'pins and needles' in the arms or legs; occasionally speech may be affected. These symptoms disappear as the headache develops, and as it comes on you may feel or be sick, lose your appetite and want to avoid light or some sounds or smells. About one person in five has aura before a migraine attack and the pain can affect both sides of the head. All types of migraine, with or without aura, can be very painful and debilitating.

At least one in ten adults in Britain has migraine attacks, yet the exact cause of these severe headaches is unknown. Migraine may be caused by the action of neurotransmitters, such as *5-hydroxytryptamine* (*serotonin*), on blood vessels surrounding the brain and scalp. The blood vessels surrounding the brain may tighten, triggering the warning signs, followed by blood vessels in the scalp widening and causing the severe throbbing headache. The headache may last for several hours, or even days. A number of factors or 'triggers' are known to set off migraine, including:

☐ Physical factors – exercise, too much sleep, hormonal changes before a period, pains in the head, neck, teeth, eyes and sinuses
☐ Psychological factors – stress, shock, anxiety and worry
☐ Nutritional factors – chocolate, alcohol, fish and cheese or hunger due to missed meals
☐ Medical factors – the oral contraceptive pill
☐ Environmental factors – loud noises, strong smells and bright lights.

Most migraine sufferers have their first attack before the age of 20. Some people have only two or three attacks during a lifetime, but others may have two a week. Women are two to three times more likely to have migraine attacks than men. This may be associated with hormonal changes during the menstrual cycle. Attacks may start during puberty and continue until or after the menopause. It is unusual to have the first one after the age of 40, but not unknown. Migraine attacks can suddenly stop at any time and generally become less frequent and severe with age.

There is some evidence that migraine runs in families, but there is no typical sufferer. Children can also have migraine attacks – around three or four out of every hundred are likely to be sick and have severe stomach cramps and headache – but migraine is very rare in children under the age of five.

● *Cluster headache*

Cluster headache is a very severe headache occurring usually on one side of the head. This type of headache mainly affects men and is quite distinct from migraine. Headaches occur daily and last from half an hour to two hours in clusters of four to sixteen weeks. The pain is aching, boring or stabbing and often occurs at night an hour or so after sleep. It may recur in the daytime and often at the same time – it is sometimes called 'alarm-clock headache'.

HOW YOU CAN HELP YOURSELF

☐ Identify your trigger factors so that you can avoid them whenever possible.
☐ Keep a diary and note any likely triggers; after an attack jot down:
☐ the time you got out of bed that day ☐ the time the attack started and how long it lasted ☐ any medicines you took, the dose and time taken ☐ the way your migraine developed ☐ food and drink ☐ work and social activities ☐ your mood ☐ any unusual events or news ☐ extra travel or exercise ☐ the stage of your menstrual cycle.
☐ Always keep a supply of medicine such as aspirin or paracetamol immediately to hand. Take an analgesic at the first signs of a migraine, before the headache develops.
☐ Rest or lie down. Many sufferers have to lie in a quiet, darkened room until the attack is over; others may be able to carry on working, but should still rest after an attack.
☐ See your doctor if your migraine attacks change in severity or frequency; severe headaches can be caused by other conditions such as high blood pressure.
☐ Find out about migraine. British Migraine Association and The Migraine Trust can help (see 'Useful addresses').

Medicines for migraine

There are medicines for treating an acute attack but if you get frequent migraine attacks you may need a preventive drug.

• *ACUTE MIGRAINE ATTACK* •

Most migraine headaches respond to an analgesic such as **paracetamol** or **aspirin** (not for children under 12) taken as soon as you notice warning signs or other features of an imminent attack. The digestive system slows down during a migraine attack so that aspirin or paracetamol may not be absorbed in time to be effective. A soluble (dispersible) or effervescent pain-relief preparation can help to overcome this. Combined preparations of aspirin or paracetamol with another analgesic or an antihistamine (for example Migraleve) are no more effective than an analgesic used on its own.

The anti-emetic **metoclopramide** is used to speed up stomach emptying and the absorption of the analgesic. A single dose can be taken as symptoms start and before the analgesic. There are combination preparations of aspirin or paracetamol with metoclopramide but the dose of metoclopramide is low and its effect unpredictable. These combination preparations (brand names Migravess; Paramax) are unlikely to be as effective as the two drugs taken separately.

Ergotamine, a derivative of ergot – a mould that grows on rye – may be prescribed if you do not respond to an analgesic. It relieves migraine headache by narrowing the blood vessels in the scalp, but does not improve visual and other warning signs and may make vomiting worse. If vomiting is severe you may need a **phenothiazine** anti-emetic by injection or suppository. Ergotamine should not be given to children under 12 years.

Sumatriptan (brand name Imigran) is a new antimigraine medicine that can relieve migraine attacks or cluster headache. It can be given by injection just under the skin for rapid relief, or taken in tablet form. Sumatriptan is chemically related to the body's neurotransmitter 5-hydroxytryptamine (serotonin) and acts at 5-HT receptors.

ERGOTAMINE

CAFERGOT – Tablets, suppositories (with caffeine)
LINGRAINE – Tablets
MEDIHALER-ERGOTAMINE – Aerosol inhaler

Poor choice
MIGRIL
ERGOTAMINE + CYCLIZINE + CAFFEINE

Ergotamine is used for relieving migraine which is not helped by analgesics such as aspirin or paracetamol. It narrows the dilated arteries in the scalp, which are thought to be the cause of severe headache. Ergotamine should be taken as early as possible in an attack because once headache and nausea are established, ergotamine may itself cause vomiting. Caffeine probably enhances the absorption of ergotamine and is combined with it in tablets and suppositories. Ergotamine must not be taken regularly for preventing migraine. It narrows blood vessels elsewhere in the body and can dangerously reduce the blood supply to hands and feet. It should not be given to children under 12.

Before you use this medicine

Tell your doctor if you are:

☐ pregnant or breast-feeding – you should not take ergotamine

☐ taking any other medicines, including vitamins and those bought over the counter.

Tell your doctor if you have or have had:
☐ circulatory problems, such as peripheral vascular disease or Raynaud's disease ☐ heart disease ☐ kidney or liver disease ☐ infection ☐ high blood pressure ☐ overactive thyroid gland ☐ porphyria.

You should not take ergotamine if you have any of these problems.

How to use this medicine

Ergotamine must be used very carefully and it is important not to take too much in too short a time. Stop taking ergotamine immediately if you develop numbness or tingling of the fingers or toes.
Ergotamine 2mg tablets (Lingraine) Dissolve one tablet under the tongue. If necessary another tablet may be taken in half to one hour, but take no more than three tablets in 24 hours. Take no more than six tablets a week.
Ergotamine 1mg + caffeine tablets (Cafergot) Take one or two tablets at the first sign of attack, but no more than four tablets in 24 hours. Do not repeat treatment in less than four days. Take no more than ten tablets a week.
Ergotamine 2mg + caffeine suppositories (Cafergot) One suppository is usually sufficient, but use no more than two suppositories in 24 hours. Use no more than five suppositories a week.
Ergotamine 360 micrograms inhaler (Medihaler-Ergotamine) Shake the container and inhale one metered dose. Repeat if necessary after five minutes. The full effect should be felt within 15 minutes. Take no more than six inhalations in 24 hours. Take no more than 15 inhalations a week.

Over 65 Ergotamine may aggravate heart and circulatory problems. Do not take it if you have kidney or liver disease.

Interactions with other medicines

Beta blockers increase ergotamine's narrowing effect on the blood vessels.
Erythromycin Increased likelihood of ergotamine's unwanted effects.

Unwanted effects

Likely Feeling or being sick, headache, stomach or abdominal pains.
Unlikely Muscle pain and weakness, numbness or tingling in fingers, arms, toes and feet.

Repeated high dosage may cause symptoms of overdosage: nausea, vomiting, drowsiness, confusion, dizziness, thirst and tingling and numbness in the fingers and toes.

Similar preparations

Poor choice
DIHYDERGOT
DIHYDROERGOTAMINE MESYLATE

SUMATRIPTAN

▼IMIGRAN – Tablets, injection

Sumatriptan is used for relieving attacks of migraine with or without aura. The injection can also be used for treating cluster headache. Sumatriptan should not be used for preventing migraine or cluster headache. It is chemically similar to the body's neurotransmitter 5-hydroxytryptamine and acts at 5-HT receptors. Sumatriptan appears to prevent the widening of certain blood vessels, which is thought to cause migraine. The injection begins to act after ten to fifteen minutes, the tablets within half an hour.

Before you use this medicine

Tell your doctor if you are:
☐ pregnant – as yet there is limited experience of the effects of sumatriptan on the foetus ☐ breast-feeding – sumatriptan passes into breast milk but there is no information on its effects on the baby; discuss with your doctor ☐ taking any other medicines, including vitamins and those bought over the counter.

Tell your doctor if you have or have had:
☐ ischaemic heart disease ☐ angina (Prinzmetal's variety) ☐ uncontrolled high blood pressure ☐ heart attack ☐ poor kidney or liver function.

Do not use if you:
are taking an MAOI antidepressant or one of the newer antidepressants that affects 5-HT receptors – fluvoxamine, fluoxetine, sertraline or paroxetine.

How to use this medicine

Tablets Swallow one tablet whole with water. If this dose gives some relief but the migraine returns, take another tablet. Take no more than three tablets in 24 hours. If the first tablet gives no relief there is no point in taking a second dose for the same attack.
Injection Sumatriptan is injected just under the skin, usually the outside of the thigh, as early as possible in an attack. Detailed instructions are provided. The recommended dose is one injection, but a further dose may be used if necessary one hour or more after the first dose. The maximum dose is two injections in 24 hours.

Do not drive or do other activities that require alertness until you know how you react to sumatriptan. Avoid alcohol in a migraine attack. Sumatriptan does not appear to interact with alcohol.

Over 65 Until there is more information sumatriptan is not recommended for people over 65.

Interactions with other medicines

Ergotamine and sumatriptan should not be used together as they add to each other's effects on the nervous system.
Lithium Increased risk of toxicity.

Unwanted effects

These are mostly mild to moderate and pass off.
Likely Slight but fleeting pain at the injection site; sensations of tingling, heat, heaviness, pressure or tightness in any part of the body (especially the chest); flushing, dizziness; weakness.
Unlikely Feeling or being sick, increase in blood pressure which wears off.

● PREVENTING MIGRAINE ●

If you have migraine attacks often you should try to find out what factors might provoke them. For example, some women taking the combined oral contraceptive 'pill' may find migraine gets worse. If you have migraine with visual disturbances or if your attacks worsen when you start the oral contraceptive, you should change to another form of contraception. However, some women experience fewer migraine attacks when they start oral contraception.

Pizotifen (brand name Sanomigran) is an antihistamine and a 5-HT blocker which gives some protection against both types of migraine (with and without warning signs) and cluster headache. It may cause drowsiness but can be given as a single dose at night to lessen this problem. It may also cause weight gain, dry mouth and occasionally nausea and dizziness.

A beta blocker may be used twice or three times a day or a longer-acting preparation taken once a day. **Propranolol** is most commonly used, but it should not be taken with ergotamine. Occasionally a tricyclic antidepressant may be helpful, even if you are not suffering from depression.

Clonidine (brand name Dixarit) and **methysergide** (Deseril) are less effective than other medicines for preventing migraine and methysergide has unpleasant unwanted effects.

Epilepsy

An epileptic seizure (fit or convulsion are other common terms) occurs when the normal co-ordinated electrical activity of the brain's nerve cells is disrupted. The chaotic discharge of electrical activity usually results in loss of control over muscle and body movements and/or perceptual changes in the mind. An *electro-encephalogram* (EEG) can assess the brain's electrical activity and can occasionally help to establish whether or not you have epilepsy, but is particularly helpful in deciding what type of epilepsy may be occurring. Sometimes an EEG may be normal in between seizures in someone with epilepsy and abnormal in a person who has not had a seizure. Having one isolated epileptic seizure does not mean you have a *tendency* to epilepsy. Each person has a different threshold above which a seizure may occur and the threshold varies from time to time, depending on the stimulus or provocation. For most people that threshold is never reached, but for someone with a low threshold or tolerance to abnormal, electrical activity in the brain any of a number of stimuli may trigger seizures.

Epilepsy may start as a result of injury to the brain caused by infection, stroke or an accident. Long-term abuse of alcohol may result in seizures which may continue even if you stop drinking. Seizures sometimes occur with acute (one-off) excessive alcohol intake or as a result of drug toxicity. In some people no obvious cause can be identified. However, there may be any number of factors that precipitate a seizure and these vary from person to person. Common examples include lack of sleep, lack of food, menstruation, flashing bright lights and repetitive patterns on a floor or wall. Seizures may occur in young children with a high temperature and these are known as *febrile convulsions*. Epilepsy is generally not inherited, but a history of epilepsy in both parents' families does increase the likelihood of a tendency to epilepsy.

● *TYPES OF SEIZURE* ●

Tonic-clonic (*grand mal*) seizures are generalised convulsions characterised by electrical disturbance across the whole brain. You may have a warning sensation or aura, such as flashing lights, a smell or taste, before the body becomes rigid and you suddenly lose consciousness. The chest muscles contract, forcing air through the larynx and causing an involuntary grunt or cry. Limbs jerk as muscles contract and relax in a disordered way. Sometimes you lose bladder control or foam at the mouth or bite your tongue. The seizure usually lasts for only a few minutes and afterwards you may have a headache, feel dazed and exhausted. A prolonged attack as seizures follow each other without stopping is called *status epilepticus*.

Partial (*focal*) seizures occur in one part of the brain but may sometimes become generalised. Partial seizures vary from person to person. They may start with muscle contractions or unusual sensations at one point of the body such as the mouth, a finger or a toe and then spread without your losing consciousness. You may experience loss of speech, confusion and involuntary movements, and may not remember what has happened.

Absence (*petit mal*) seizures commonly occur in children and may be mistaken for daydreaming. An absence attack is brief and lasts only a second or two. The child loses consciousness for a moment and appears to go blank, stares and may flutter the eyelids. Sometimes body movements occur, such as dropping the head forwards.

HOW YOU CAN HELP YOURSELF

☐ Keep a record of your attacks and the circumstances in which they occur – this information will be very helpful to your doctor.
☐ If you take an antiepileptic medicine, take it regularly. It may take you and your doctor some months to establish the best treatment plan. Keep a note of unwanted effects and discuss them with the doctor.
☐ Wear an identification bracelet or carry a card with details of your medicines.
☐ Get information and advice from one of the organisations concerned with epilepsy, such as the British Epilepsy Association or the National Society for Epilepsy (see 'Useful addresses').
☐ If there are trigger factors that precipitate your seizures, try to avoid them. Keep a record of events leading up to attacks – the trigger factors may become apparent.
☐ Lead a healthy life, eating, exercising and sleeping regularly. You can safely participate in most activities except climbing and underwater diving.
☐ Avoid alcohol: it may interfere with your medicine or may start an attack.
☐ If you drive, you must inform the DVLC (Driver and Vehicle Licencing Centre) of your epilepsy. Generally you are allowed to drive a car, but not heavy goods or public service vehicles, if you have had a seizure-free period of two years or if you have only had attacks while asleep over a three-year period.

• *HOW TO HELP* •

• *Tonic-clonic seizures*

Note the time as soon as a fit begins and clear a space around the person having the seizure. Cushion the head and loosen clothes; remove glasses, false teeth (if this is easily done) and any sharp objects in the vicinity. Do not move the person having the seizure or force anything between his or her teeth. Do not try to rouse the person or to make him or her drink anything.

As soon as the seizure begins to settle, turn the person on one side to keep the airways open. As the person begins to recover, offer reassurance and talk quietly until full recovery.

Only seek medical assistance if the seizure lasts longer than five minutes or if one seizure follows another without the person regaining consciousness.

Partial seizures

These seizures do not require medical attention. The person having the seizure may wander around with a blank expression and should be accompanied to make sure he or she is safe. Do not interfere or attempt to stop the seizure, but talk calmly after the seizure to provide reassurance.

Febrile convulsions

Some children have a seizure only when they develop a high temperature. A febrile convulsion is a seizure that occurs in a child aged between 3 months and 5 years with a fever, but without any evident underlying cause. As a parent you may be very frightened by your child having a febrile convulsion, but most seizures are brief and there is no lasting problem. You can take some measures to help. Place the child on his or her side to keep the airway open. There is no need to intervene unless the convulsions last longer than 15 minutes. Seek medical help if the convulsions last longer than 15 minutes or if your child is under 18 months.

Reduce the child's temperature by removing clothing, sponging with tepid water and gentle fanning. Paracetamol elixir for children may help to reduce the fever.

If your child has a tendency to have febrile convulsions, your doctor may teach you how to use rectal diazepam solution in an emergency.

Antiepileptic medicines

Your doctor will look for any underlying disorder that might cause seizures and try to identify any trigger factors. Treatment with an antiepileptic medicine will not usually be started after just one seizure. If you have recurrent seizures, an antiepileptic medicine can prevent attacks, allow you to lead a normal life with few restraints and reduce the risk of brain damage which may occur with frequent, uncontrolled convulsions. Antiepileptics act on the brain to increase the seizure threshold and to prevent the spread of abnormal brain activity. The choice of medicine depends on the type of epilepsy and also on your age and response to treatment.

Medicines used for tonic-clonic and partial seizures include **phenytoin** (brand name Epanutin), **carbamazepine** (Tegretol) and **sodium valproate** (Epilim). Phenytoin is effective in both types of seizures but the range between an effective dose and one which causes adverse effects is narrow. Blood levels of the drug may have to be measured to help with dosage adjustment. Carbamazepine has a wider therapeutic range than phenytoin and fewer unwanted effects than either phenytoin or **phenobarbitone** (see below). Most unwanted effects are dose-related, but if the dose is established, your doctor may alter the time when you take carbamazepine to reduce unwanted effects. Sodium valproate is effective for controlling tonic-clonic seizures as well as other forms of epilepsy. Occasionally it affects the liver so that tests for liver function may be necessary before and once in a while during treatment.

The barbiturates **phenobarbitone** and **primidone** (brand name Mysoline) are also used but cause drowsiness. Primidone (and another barbiturate, **methylphenobarbitone**) is largely broken down to phenobarbitone in the body, so it is not logical to take primidone and phenobarbitone together. Other less-used medicines include **clonazepam** (brand name Rivotril) and **clobazam** (both benzodiazepines) and **acetazolamide**. The benzodiazepines are most effective at the start of treatment, but tolerance to their effects appears as treatment continues. **Vigabatrin** (brand name Sabril) is a new antiepileptic which may be useful for someone who has chronic epilepsy, either added to existing treatment or in place of other medicines. Unwanted effects include drowsiness, dizziness and irritability.

Ethosuximide (brand names Zarontin and Emeside) and **sodium valproate** are used for treating absence seizures.

Most people are treated with one medicine, but it may take time to establish which drug suits you best. Treatment is started with a low dose and gradually increased until seizures are controlled or unwanted effects develop. You may need to have blood tests to help to establish the dosage. A second medicine should only be added if seizures continue; a few people seem to need more than one drug. Treatment aims to keep you seizure-free and if you have a period of a few years without a seizure, your doctor may consider withdrawing treatment very gradually over at least six months. Whether it will be possible to withdraw treatment depends on your age, how many attacks you have had and over what period, and whether you want to drive. Never stop taking an antiepileptic without consulting your doctor – gradual dose reduction under supervision is essential.

● *Pregnancy and breast-feeding*

Congenital abnormalities, such as cleft lip and palate occur in seven per cent of babies born to mothers with epilepsy who are taking antiepileptic drugs. This is about two to three times more common than in babies born to other mothers. Genetic and other factors may contribute, but drug treatment may be responsible for the excess of abnormalities. No antiepileptic drug is completely free from the risk of causing abnormalities.

Women taking sodium valproate during the first three months of pregnancy are at increased risk of having a baby with spina bifida. This incidence is around one per cent, about 50 times the normal rate. If you take an antiepileptic medicine and want to start a family you should consult your doctor long before trying to become pregnant. You may wish to discuss whether to change from an antiepileptic that suits you or accept the small risk of spina bifida and the possible need for termination. Checks during the first three months of pregnancy will be essential.

Breast-feeding is possible with all the antiepileptic medicines taken in normal dosage, with the exception of barbiturates such as phenobarbitone.

Status epilepticus

Status epilepticus is a medical emergency and is treated with **diazepam** or **clonazepam**, given intravenously. These benzodiazepines must be used cautiously because they can cause breathing difficulties. Diazepam can be given by rectal solution. Other drugs that are sometimes used include **chlormethiazole**, **phenytoin** and **paraldehyde**.

PHENYTOIN

PHENYTOIN – Tablets
EPANUTIN – Capsules, chewable tablets, liquid, injection

Phenytoin is an antiepileptic which stabilises a person's seizure threshold and prevents the spread of abnormal electrical activity across the brain. It is used for all forms of epilepsy, especially tonic-clonic seizures and partial seizures. Phenytoin injection is also used to control status epilepticus. The range between the desired effects and adverse ones is narrow and blood levels of the drug often need to be measured to establish dosage. Some adverse effects may be troublesome, especially for young people, such as acne, hairiness and overgrowth of the gums.

Before you use this medicine

Tell your doctor if you are:
☐ pregnant or breast-feeding ☐ taking any other medicines,

including the oral contraceptive 'pill', vitamins – especially those containing folic acid – and others bought over the counter.

Tell your doctor if you have or have had:
☐ kidney or liver problems ☐ diabetes ☐ porphyria ☐ alcohol dependence.

How to use this medicine

Take the tablet or capsule with plenty of water, with or after food. Phenytoin can be taken as a single dose once a day or in two doses. Eat plenty of fresh, green vegetables because folic acid deficiency may occur with long-term treatment.

Do not drive or do other activities that require alertness until you know how you react to phenytoin. You may not be allowed to drive a car at all. Avoid alcohol as it interferes with phenytoin.

Do not stop taking this medicine suddenly as seizures may recur. Discuss the possibility of stopping treatment with your doctor. You will need a gradual reduction of dosage over a period of time. Do not withdraw treatment without medical guidance. If you miss a dose take it as soon as you remember. Do not change brands of phenytoin or dosage forms without checking with your doctor. Different brands of phenytoin produce different blood levels.

Over 65 If you are taking other medicines check that interactions do not occur.

Interactions with other medicines

Phenytoin interacts with many other medicines. Do not take other medicines without checking with your doctor or pharmacist. Medicines may increase or decrease phenytoin blood levels, so the dosage of phenytoin may need adjusting.

Phenytoin's effects are increased by:
Other antiepileptics
Analgesics and antirheumatics – aspirin, azapropazone, phenylbutazone and sulphinpyrazone
Anti-arrhythmic heart drug – amiodarone
Anti-infectives – chloramphenicol, isoniazid, co-trimoxazole, trimethoprim and metronidazole
Antifungals – fluconazole, ketoconazole and miconazole
Ulcer-healing drugs – cimetidine and omeprazole
Alcohol dependence treatment – disulfiram.

Folic acid is likely to be depleted even further when phenytoin is taken with antimalarial drugs containing pyrimethamine (brand names Fansidar; Maloprim), the antibacterial co-trimoxazole or the immunosuppressant methotrexate.

Phenytoin may reduce the effectiveness of:
Oral contraceptives (the 'pill')
Tricyclic antidepressants
Anti-arrhythmic drugs – disopyramide, mexiletine and quinidine
Corticosteroids.

Unwanted effects

Likely Feeling or being sick, confusion, headache, nervousness, sleeplessness, dizziness, tremor.
Unlikely Weakness or numbness of feet or legs, dyskinesia (see page 220), acne, hairiness, fever, mood changes, clumsiness or unsteadiness, unusual bleeding or bruising, bleeding and overgrown gums, skin rashes.

Likely unwanted effects may fade as treatment continues. If they are troublesome discuss with your doctor. If a skin rash develops contact your doctor. Signs of overdosage include blurred vision, clumsiness or unsteadiness, slurred speech, confusion, uncontrolled eye movements. Contact your doctor immediately if these occur.

Parkinson's disease and parkinsonism

Parkinson's disease is a degenerative condition of the nervous system in which voluntary movement is disturbed. The most noticeable features of the disease are slowness of movement (*bradykinesia*), tremor – shaking and a rhythmic rolling movement in the fingers – difficulty starting to walk and stopping once walking, stiffness and muscle rigidity. Tremor is often first noticed by others. Other signs include the face becoming blank and mask-like and the voice soft and monotonous. People with the disease may have one or more of the symptoms and in different proportions. The condition is progressive and some sufferers are eventually disabled by it. However, for many people medical treatment can dampen symptoms for many years, allowing them to lead full lives.

HOW YOU CAN HELP YOURSELF

- ☐ In the early stages of Parkinson's disease, often before drug treatment is needed, regular moderate exercise may help.
- ☐ Learn what your capabilities and energy levels are; plan your day around your best times.
- ☐ Find out whether other treatments would help, such as physiotherapy, speech therapy or occupational therapy.
- ☐ Find out about equipment which could help you to get around or you could use at home, such as special utensils and hand rails in the bathroom and toilet. The Disabled Living Foundation produces information and has a centre where equipment can be tried out, but not purchased. See 'Useful addresses'. The local branch of the British Red Cross Society may also be able to help with equipment. See the Phone Book for your nearest branch.
- ☐ Get advice on shoes and clothing which are easy to put on and take off.
- ☐ Get more information from the Parkinson's Disease Society. See 'Useful addresses'.

Nerve cells in part of the brain responsible for controlling movement, the *basal ganglia*, lose supplies of the body chemical **dopamine**. Dopamine and another body chemical, **acetylcholine**, are neurotransmitters, which help to relay messages along the nerves which control movement. The control of movement is finely balanced between sets of nerves which respond to one of the two chemicals. When dopamine supplies are reduced, an imbalance between the two chemical transmitter systems, *cholinergic* and *dopaminergic*, occurs in the brain. The resulting imbalance means that the basal ganglia are unable to modify the nerve messages to the muscles, which leads to rigid joints, slow movements and tremor.

The exact cause of Parkinson's disease is unknown. It is rare in under 40 year olds, but both sexes and all races are affected. The rate at which the disease progresses varies considerably.

Parkinsonian symptoms (*parkinsonism*) can be caused by drug treatment; for example by antipsychotic medicines such as chlorpromazine. These unwanted effects usually improve when the dose is reduced or the drug is stopped. Other causes of parkinsonism include brain damage and narrowed blood vessels in the brain.

Medicines for Parkinson's disease

Medicines can help to relieve the symptoms of Parkinson's disease, but cannot cure it. Medicines cannot halt the degeneration of brain cells or permanently restore the chemical imbalance. There are two main groups: those that boost dopamine levels in the brain and those that reduce acetylcholine action.

• *BOOSTING DOPAMINE ACTIVITY* •

Levodopa is the most commonly used medicine; it is the chemical which brain cells convert into dopamine. Dopamine is not effective as a medicine because it is not absorbed very well from the digestive system, nor can it pass from the bloodstream into the brain, where it is needed. Levodopa replenishes dopamine in the brain and in particular helps to improve difficulty in starting movement, slow walking and rigidity. However, a large proportion of the drug is broken down in the body before it ever reaches the brain. To overcome this levodopa is usually given with **carbidopa** or **benserazide**, drugs that block the breakdown of levodopa in the body, but do not themselves enter the brain.

Levodopa can produce a range of unwanted effects such as nausea, vomiting and a sudden drop in blood pressure, sleeplessness, vivid dreams and changes to the mental state, including hallucinations. When it is given with carbidopa or benserazide, levodopa can be given in much smaller doses so that adverse effects are minimised. These are worthwhile combination preparations where a fixed dose of each drug is contained in one formulation. The combination of carbidopa + levodopa has the generic name of **co-careldopa** (brand name Sinemet) while benserazide + levodopa is known as **co-beneldopa** (Madopar).

Levodopa treatment is started with a low dose. High doses do not always increase the benefit and risk producing adverse effects. During the first 6–18 months of levodopa treatment you may slowly improve, perhaps for up to two years. After that time the benefit from levodopa treatment wanes because the disease progresses and possibly because drug levels in the brain fluctuate. Former disabilities may return insidiously, new ones appear and unwanted effects of levodopa may increase. This long-term levodopa syndrome includes abnormal involuntary movements, 'end-of-dose' deterioration – when effective treatment is limited to three or four hours – and the 'on-off' phenomenon (see Box). There may also be changes to the mental state, such as hallucinations, confusion and psychotic behaviour. Sometimes drug treatment causes these changes but dementia may also be part of the underlying disorder. There is evidence that high doses of levodopa cause its advantages to wear off faster. Depression is also common in Parkinson's disease.

SWITCHING ON AND OFF

As time goes on you may start to experience fluctuations or swings between mobility and immobility – a kind of 'on-off' phenomenon. 'On' periods are the relatively normal times when the medicines are working. 'Off' periods are times when you are immobile, stiff, rigid, tremulous and sometimes in pain. Your voice may be slurred or inaudible, and you may perspire profusely. You also have 'over-stimulated' periods due to excess stimulation by the medicines. When this happens, you have no control over your body: you writhe and make involuntary movements.

Swings between these extremes may occur with little or no warning and sometimes frequently throughout the day – as if the mains switch is repeatedly being thrown. It can be terrifying for you and your carer.

Selegiline (brand name Eldepryl) is used with levodopa to reduce 'end-of-dose' deterioration. More recently early treatment with selegiline has been shown to delay the need to start levodopa in some patients and possibly to slow progression of the disease. It is a *monoamine-oxidase-B* inhibitor which prevents the breakdown of dopamine in the brain. The dietary restrictions needed with *monoamine-oxidase-A* antidepressants (see page 214) are not necessary.

LEVODOPA

BROCADOPA – Capsules
LARODOPA – Tablets
MADOPAR – Capsules, soluble tablets, modified-release capsules
CO-BENELDOPA

SINEMET – Tablets, modified-release tablets
CO-CARELDOPA

Levodopa is the chemical the body converts to dopamine, the neurotransmitter that is lacking in the brain of someone with Parkinson's disease. Levodopa is an effective antiparkinsonian drug but higher and higher doses have to be given to maintain an effect. Unwanted effects such as abnormal movements, nausea and vomiting then become a problem. Carbidopa and benserazide stop levodopa being converted into dopamine in the body instead of the brain, thereby increasing brain-dopamine levels: the combination preparations, co-careldopa and co-beneldopa enable a lower dose of levodopa to be given. Unwanted effects are also reduced.

Before you use this medicine

Tell your doctor if you are:
☐ pregnant or breast-feeding ☐ taking any other medicines, including vitamins and those bought over the counter.

Tell your doctor if you have or have had:
☐ lung disease or bronchial asthma ☐ heart or circulation problems ☐ diabetes ☐ overactive thyroid gland ☐ glaucoma ☐ peptic ulcer ☐ skin cancer ☐ kidney or liver disease ☐ psychiatric illness.

How to use this medicine

Take the tablet or capsule after meals to minimise stomach upsets. Dosage has to be tailored to each person. Your doctor will start you with a low dose, gradually increasing the dosage until improvement or unwanted effects occur. Large amounts of **pyridoxine** (vitamin B_6) reduce the effect of levodopa, so do not take vitamin supplements containing B_6. This is not such a problem with the combination preparations, co-beneldopa or co-careldopa.

You may feel dizzy or faint when you get up from sitting or lying down, especially during the first few days of treatment. Get up slowly and stay beside the chair or bed until you are sure you are not dizzy. Do not drive or do other activities that require alertness until you know how you react to levodopa. Alcohol in small amounts may be acceptable.

Do not stop taking this medicine suddenly as this will lead to a return of the disease symptoms. Discuss any problems with the medicine with your doctor. If you miss a dose, take it as soon as you remember; but delay or omit the next dose. Do not take double the dose.

Over 65 You may be more susceptible to unwanted effects, especially a sudden drop in blood pressure when getting up from sitting or lying down. Combination preparations minimise unwanted effects.

Interactions with other medicines

Anaesthetics increase risk of irregular heart rhythm.
Antidepressants – monoamine-oxidase inhibitors produce a dangerous rise in blood pressure with levodopa.
Antipsychotics and some benzodiazepines may interfere with levodopa. Antipsychotics should not be given with levodopa unless carefully supervised.

Unwanted effects

Likely Abnormal body movements, feeling or being sick, loss of appetite, sleeplessness, agitation, nervousness, sudden drop in blood pressure (postural hypotension), palpitations and irregular heart rhythm.
Unlikely Mood changes, aggressive behaviour, depression, drowsiness, headache, unusual tiredness or weakness.

Reddish discoloration of urine and other body fluids such as sweat may occur but is nothing to worry about. Discuss all levodopa's unwanted effects with your doctor.

Another group of medicines, the **dopamine agonists**, act by stimulating surviving dopamine receptors in the brain. These are **bromocriptine** (brand name Parlodel), **lysuride** (Revanil) and **pergolide** (Celance). Although a dopamine agonist can be used on its own, it has no advantages over levodopa. It is usually tried after levodopa treatment and when added to co-beneldopa or co-careldopa may help in the late stages of the disease. Unwanted effects such as feeling or being sick can be a problem. Tolerance to these effects may develop, but if they persist an anti-emetic such as **domperidone** may help. All the dopamine agonists can cause psychiatric problems such as hallucinations, confusion and paranoia. Relatives and helpers should note any mood changes or aggressive behaviour, even the start of mild disturbances, and discuss them with the doctor.

Amantadine (brand name Symmetrel) has modest antiparkinsonian effects and may help if you have not responded to levodopa. It may help mild slowness of movement (bradykinesia), rigidity and tremor but tolerance of its effects occurs.

• *DECREASING ACETYLCHOLINE ACTIVITY* •

The other approach to relieving symptoms of Parkinson's disease is to dampen cholinergic activity in the brain. This allows a better balance between the dopaminergic and cholinergic systems. Drugs which oppose the actions of cholinergic nerves have been used for many years and were the mainstay of treatment before levodopa was introduced in the late 1960s. Their effects are modest but they help muscle rigidity and tremor. They can reduce excessive salivation which results in dribbling and drooling. An antimuscarinic drug may be used alone in mild cases of the disease or in combination with levodopa, as the drugs work well together.

The most commonly used medicines are **orphenadrine** (brand names Disipal; Biorphen) and **benzhexol** (Artane; Bentex; Broflex). Others include **benztropine** (Cogentin), **procyclidine** (Kemadrin; Arpicolin), **biperiden** (Akineton) and **methixene** (Tremonil). There is no important difference between these preparations but some people appear to tolerate one preparation better than another. Doses may be taken before meals if dry mouth is a problem, or after food if the particular drug upsets the stomach. Apart from the common anticholinergic unwanted effects of constipation, difficulty in passing urine and visual disturbances, these drugs can impair memory and cause nightmares and confusion, especially if someone has dementia.

These drugs can also lessen the symptoms of drug-induced parkinsonism, for example with phenothiazines or other antipsychotic medicines. They should not be taken routinely with an antipsychotic medicine unless parkinsonism develops. *Tardive dyskinesia* (see page 220) is not improved.

5

INFECTIONS

Bacterial infections Cystitis
Fungal infections Viruses
Protozoa Worms

Micro-organisms are all around us and some of them, given the right conditions, can cause disease. There are four main groups of disease-causing micro-organisms: *bacteria*, *viruses*, *fungi* and *protozoa*. Very few of the organisms in these groups are harmful. Many live side by side with humans without generating disease. Some bacteria and fungi co-exist happily with people, living on skin or other areas of the body, such as the bowel, and stop harmful organisms getting a hold. The body's immune system protects you from constant invasion by harmful organisms, commonly known as germs.

In the body germs are usually killed before they multiply to large numbers and cause disease. Blood contains various types of white cells responsible for killing germs, which are carried to the site of infection. It also produces antibodies specific to the invading organism. Antibodies and special white cells remain in the bloodstream so that the next time the organism enters the body, they recognise it and disarm it. This process builds up the body's immunity, but white blood cells are sometimes overwhelmed by an invading germ or the immune system may be destroyed (as in AIDS), allowing a disease to take hold. Symptoms of infection can be confined to one part of the body, such as urine or the lungs, or extended throughout the body, as in the case of chicken pox or septicaemia.

Disease is also caused by other organisms or parasites which depend for part of their life cycle on an animal or human host, and sometimes both. Examples include viruses, worms (helminths) such as tapeworm, malaria, scabies and lice.

● *The body's defences*

The body is under constant attack from organisms but it is reasonably well defended. Invading organisms enter the body by several routes:

□ **Nose** As you breathe in through your nose you take in micro-organisms. The inside of the nose is lined with a layer of cells (*membrane*) covered in very fine projections (*cilia*). Mucus produced by the nasal membranes traps germs and foreign particles. The cilia move the foreign bodies along the membranes to the throat where they are swallowed; alternatively they may be sneezed out.

☐ **Mouth** Micro-organisms enter the body when you breathe in through your mouth and in food and drink. Stomach juices contain hydrochloric acid and kill many germs that can cause gastroenteritis.

☐ **Eyes** When you sleep or blink the eyes are cleaned by liquid from the tear glands; tears can kill some germs.

☐ **Skin** is a natural barrier to micro-organisms. However, they can enter through cuts, scratches and when the skin is pierced by a disease-carrying insect such as a mosquito. Bacteria causing boils and acne can enter through hair follicles.

☐ **Vagina and urinary tract** The vagina is naturally acidic, which kills many germs. Urine washes bacteria out of the bladder and urethra.

● *HOW INFECTION IS SPREAD* ●

Infection is illness or disease that is spread from person to person. Infection results when, for instance, a virus entering the nose attacks and damages some of the cilia, allowing the organism to get into your body. Once you are infected with the organism the virus is carried on drops of liquid in your breath to another person (droplet infection).

Micro-organisms can also transfer from one person to another on direct physical contact. For example, the cold virus can be passed on with a hand shake. The cold-sore virus *herpes* can be transferred by direct contact or from sharing the same article, such as a toothbrush, with someone with an active cold sore. Some diseases can be passed from one person to another through sexual intercourse. Genital contact also allows pubic lice to transfer from an infected person to another.

Many types of food are ideal breeding grounds for micro-organisms, particularly bacteria. Water can carry infections especially where there is no clean water supply or sewage system. Cholera is passed on this way, for example.

Flies, fleas and mosquitos are among the animals that pass on disease. They convey the infecting organism from one host to another. For example, malaria is caused by species of the protozoan *Plasmodium*, which depends on a female mosquito for part of its life-cycle and a human for the other part. The mosquito passes on the protozoan in saliva when it bites a human. Other blood-sucking animals such as fleas transmit disease. Bubonic plague was carried from rats to humans by fleas. In warm countries flies

HOW YOU CAN HELP YOURSELF

Many infections cannot be avoided but you can cut down the risk.
- ☐ Always wash hands after going to the toilet or changing a nappy and immediately before eating.
- ☐ Store food at recommended temperatures and take note of 'Use by' or 'Best before' dates. Keep raw and cooked food covered and on separate shelves.
- ☐ Prepare food hygienically: wash your hands before preparing a meal.
- ☐ Cook food thoroughly, especially ready-prepared meals.
- ☐ Avoid passing colds on – do not go to work if the cold is heavy; wash your hands after blowing your nose.
- ☐ Do not share towels, toothbrushes, swimwear or underwear.
- ☐ Use a condom for sex, to prevent the transmission of diseases such as gonorrhoea, syphilis, genital warts, herpes, chlamydia and AIDS.

acquire germs on their feet or from dirty places such as rubbish dumps which they pass on to food.

Bacterial infections

Infections are common even though the body defences and the immune system are protective. However, doctors are finding that the strength or virulence of bacteria has changed and some infections are not as dangerous as they used to be. A healthy body can often control and overcome infections naturally with time. It is only when the defence systems break down or harmful micro-organisms overwhelm you that treatment may be needed. The most frequently infected parts of the body are the respiratory system, the digestive system, skin and the bladder and urinary tract.

Bacteria multiply very rapidly and may release poisons (toxins) that damage body cells. You may have a high temperature and feel unwell. Bacteria may stay at one site in the body or spread throughout the body in the bloodstream.

Antibacterial medicines

A *bactericidal* drug kills the invading organism; a *bacteriostatic* drug stops the multiplication of bacteria. Both types of antibacterial drugs are also known as *antibiotics*. An antibiotic is usually given to treat an infection, but may also be given to prevent one. For example, if you have an artificial heart valve and need to have routine surgery, you will be given antibiotic cover before you have the operation. Each year around half the British population visits the doctor for the treatment of infections. Apart from prescribing an antibacterial medicine your doctor may advise some simple pain relief and rest. Your doctor may be able to guess the type of bacteria involved or may need it to be identified in a laboratory in order to select the appropriate antibiotic for your illness. In practice this is difficult because laboratory testing takes time, so the doctor may decide to prescribe a *broad-spectrum* antibiotic – one that affects a wide range of bacterial species – while waiting for the results of tests. Treatment may be switched to another antibiotic in the light of the laboratory results.

Many infections, particularly of the upper respiratory tract, are caused by viruses and not by bacteria. An antibacterial drug is ineffective against a virus. Sometimes no specific organism can be identified in apparent infections, for example an upset stomach (gastroenteritis). However, your doctor may prescribe an antibacterial medicine even if it is not possible to tell at once if bacteria are responsible. Bacteria which have not previously grown and caused infection are constantly being discovered. When prescribing an antibiotic (or choosing to avoid using one) the doctor has to consider your resistance to infection, the severity of your illness, where the infection is and the likely organism causing the problem. Other important factors are your age, ethnic origin and history of allergies, the state of your kidney and liver function and if you are a woman, whether you are pregnant, breast-feeding or taking an oral contraceptive.

Don't expect your doctor to give you an antibiotic automatically: you may not need one. If you take an antibiotic, don't stop taking it until the course is complete, even if you feel better. Don't be tempted to take the few left over from a previous prescription for a new problem without talking to your doctor and don't give your antibiotics to anyone else in the family or your friends.

● *UNWANTED EFFECTS* ●

Most antibiotics prescribed by your GP are unlikely to cause many serious unwanted effects. Common unwanted effects include feeling sick (nausea) and diarrhoea, but these are not allergic reactions. Most antibiotics are either broken down in the liver or leave the body via the kidneys. If you have reduced liver or kidney function you are more liable to unwanted effects, especially if you are over 65.

● *Allergy*

Rashes may occur, not always at the start of treatment and sometimes after stopping the medicine. The most serious unwanted effect, especially of the **penicillin** group is severe allergic reaction (*anaphylaxis*), which affects around one person in 5000 and is very occasionally fatal. If you are allergic to penicillin, you will be allergic to all the medicines in the penicillin group. **Cephalosporin** antibiotics are similar to the penicillins and about ten per cent of patients who are sensitive to penicillin will also react to them. You must always tell the doctor, particularly someone you have not consulted before, if you have had a severe reaction to an antibiotic – keep a note of its name on a medicines worksheet. It is important not to say you are allergic if an antibiotic made you feel sick or have diarrhoea.

● *Interaction with oral contraceptives*

The effectiveness of the oral contraceptive may be reduced. **Rifampicin** and the antifungal drug **griseofulvin** certainly reduce the activity of all oral contraceptives and additional precautions are needed if you are taking either drug. Diarrhoea caused by an antibiotic may disrupt the absorption of an oral contraceptive. Women should follow the advice for a missed pill or use another contraceptive measure.

● *Upsetting the flora*

Sometimes antibiotic treatment may upset the natural balance of micro-organisms in your body, especially if you have a long course of treatment, affecting the organisms which co-exist with the body, living in or on it without causing harm. For example, antibiotics can kill off the bacteria that check the growth of *Candida albicans*, a yeast which normally lives in or on the body without harming you. If the yeast, a member of the fungus family, grows unchecked, it also causes infection, with symptoms of soreness and irritation (thrush) in the mouth, throat, gullet and vagina.

● *Pseudomembranous colitis*

Antibiotic treatment occasionally leads to the overgrowth of one type of bacterium (*Clostridium difficile*) which is not killed by the antibiotic. These bacteria release a toxin that causes *pseudomembranous colitis*, unremitting diarrhoea which can be fatal in elderly people. This complication can occur with cephalosporins, penicillins and erythromycin, but is most common with **clindamycin** and **lincomycin**. If you develop diarrhoea while taking either of these, stop treatment immediately and contact your doctor. These antibiotics have limited uses because of this potentially serious unwanted effect.

● *BACTERIAL RESISTANCE* ●

Bacteria live life at a pace: they are born, grow up and multiply in the space of a few hours and can change and adapt to a new environment. Bacteria develop ways to avoid the effects of antibiotics, either by adapting their growth and reproductive cycles or by producing an enzyme to neutralise the antibiotic. Not all bacteria causing an infection are necessarily killed during a course of antibiotic treatment and the ones that survive eventually become the dominant strain by a process of natural selection. When penicillin was first introduced it was a powerful killer of *Staphylococcus aureus*, a bacterium causing skin infections. After 20 years of treatment, penicillin was no longer effective against almost all strains of staphylococcus because the bacteria had developed an enzyme to counter the effects of penicillin. A new antibiotic, **methicillin**, was developed and was successful at first. Gradually methicillin-resistant strains developed to produce a 'super staph'. Even with the development of new antibiotics, bacteria continue to find ways to become resistant to treatment.

Antibiotics must be used only when they are really needed. Sensitivity testing to find out which antibiotic will be most effective against a particular bacterium is important. If you have an established bacterial infection, the benefits of using an antibiotic to treat it far outweigh the risks of not taking the antibiotic. However, using an antibiotic to treat a viral infection, such as a cold or influenza is a misuse of an antibiotic because antibiotics act against bacteria and will not help infections caused by viruses. If you take an antibiotic, it may make you more susceptible to further bacterial infection and other unwanted effects of an antibiotic.

GROUPS OF ANTIBIOTICS

Many antibiotics have been developed from moulds and fungi. Penicillin was the first antibiotic developed from a mould, *Penicillium notatum*, some years after Alexander Fleming noticed that the mould, which had accidently contaminated some culture dishes, inhibited the growth of bacteria. There are now many different types of penicillin, some capable of eliminating a wide range of bacteria, while others have a more specific action. Over the years many more antibacterial drugs have been discovered and developed. Most are produced synthetically in the laboratory and the search for new antibiotics in attempt to counteract bacterial resistance continues.

Antibacterial medicines are classified into several groups: **penicillins**, **cephalosporins**, **tetracyclines**, **erythromycinol, sulphonamides** and **trimethoprim**, **quinolones** and **metronidazole**.

AMOXYCILLIN

AMOXYCILLIN – Capsules, liquid
AMOXIL – Capsules, soluble tablets, chewable tablets (Fiztabs), liquid, soluble powder, injection
FLEMOXIN SOLUTAB – Soluble tablets

Co-amoxiclav
AUGMENTIN – Tablets, soluble tablets, liquid, injection
AMOXYCILLIN + CLAVULANIC ACID

The addition of clavulanic acid makes amoxycillin effective against more infections.

Amoxycillin is a member of the penicillin group used for a wide range of bacterial infections of the ear, chest and bladder. Some bladder and urinary tract infections can be treated with a three-day course of amoxycillin. It is also used for the treatment of gonorrhoea and for preventing heart inflammation due to infection in dental and surgical procedures. Amoxycillin is similar to an older penicillin, ampicillin, but is better absorbed and can be taken with food. A blotchy skin rash is a common unwanted effect, but this is not necessarily an allergic reaction. Rash almost always occurs in people with glandular fever. These penicillins should not be used for treating a sore throat until the cause is known.

Before you use this medicine

Tell your doctor if you are:
☐ pregnant or breast-feeding ☐ taking any other medicines, including vitamins and those bought over the counter.

Tell your doctor if you have or have had:
☐ a rash or allergy to a penicillin or cephalosporin antibiotic ☐ glandular fever.

How to use this medicine

Take the capsules regularly three times a day or as prescribed. Liquid preparations should be shaken thoroughly before use. You can take amoxycillin with or after food if necessary.

Always take all the amoxycillin prescribed for you, even if you feel better before the prescription is finished. If you stop too soon, your symptoms may come back. If you miss a dose, take it as soon as you remember, but skip it if it is almost time for your next dose. Do not take double the dose. Small amounts of alcohol should not be a problem. Amoxycillin and alcohol do not interact, but an infection means that your body needs rest and recuperation.

Liquid preparations should be stored in a refrigerator, but not frozen.

Over 65 No special requirements.

Interactions with other medicines

Oral contraceptives may not be as effective and there may be breakthrough bleeding. Discuss this with your doctor.

Unwanted effects

Likely Loose stools, diarrhoea, skin rashes (hives or itching).
Unlikely Feeling or being sick, sore mouth and tongue, weakness or tiredness.

Unwanted effects are usually mild. Rashes are more likely with long or repeated courses. If you develop a rash or severe diarrhoea contact your doctor. If you have a severe allergic reaction (wheezing, swollen mouth and tongue, itching) stop taking amoxycillin and call your doctor immediately.

Similar preparations

AMBAXIN – Tablets
BACAMPICILLIN

AMPICILLIN – Capsules, liquid

AMPICLOX – Liquid, injection
AMPICILLIN + CLOXACILLIN

CO-FLUAMPICIL – Capsules
AMPICILLIN + FLUCLOXACILLIN

▼DICAPEN – Injection
AMPICILLIN + SULBACTAM

MAGNAPEN – Capsules, liquid, injection
CO-FLUAMPICIL

MIRAXID – Tablets, liquid
PIVAMPICILLIN + PIVMECILLINAM

PENBRITIN – Capsules, liquid, injection
AMPICILLIN

PONDOCILLIN – Tablets, liquid, soluble powder
PIVAMPICILLIN

PONDOCILLIN PLUS – Tablets
PIVAMPICILLIN + PIVMECILLINAM

▼UNASYN – Tablets, injection
AMPICILLIN + SULBACTAM

VIDOPEN – Injection
AMPICILLIN

CEPHALEXIN

CEPHALEXIN –Capsules, tablets, liquid
CEPOREX – Capsules, tablets, liquid, drops
KEFLEX – Capsules, tablets, liquid

Cephalexin is a broad-spectrum cephalosporin-type antibiotic. Cephalosporins are related to penicillins and have a similar range of action, although this varies for individual cephalosporins. About one person in ten who are sensitive to penicillin will also react to a cephalosporin.

Cephalexin is useful for treating bladder infections which have not responded to other drugs or during pregnancy. It may also be used for skin and infected wounds or deep cuts, although other antibiotics are more suitable.

Before you use this medicine

Tell your doctor if you are:
☐ pregnant or breast-feeding ☐ taking any other medicines, including vitamins and those bought over the counter.

Tell your doctor if you have had:

☐ an allergic reaction to a cephalosporin or penicillin.

How to use this medicine

Take the tablet or capsule every six hours or you may be able to take a higher dose every eight hours. Shake liquid preparations thoroughly before use. You can take cephalexin before food.

Always take all the cephalexin prescribed for you, even if you feel better before the prescription is finished. If you stop too soon, your symptoms may recur. If you miss a dose, take it as soon as you remember, but skip it if it is almost time for your next dose. Do not take double the dose.

Small amounts of alcohol should not be a problem. Cephalexin and alcohol do not interact but an infection means that your body needs rest and recuperation.

Syrup preparations and drops should be stored in a refrigerator, but not frozen.

Over 65 If you have severe kidney problems, you may need less than the standard adult dose.

Interactions with other medicines

Oral contraceptives may not be as effective and there may be breakthrough bleeding. Discuss this with your doctor.

Unwanted effects

Likely Mild diarrhoea, feeling or being sick.
Unlikely Sore mouth or tongue, itching in the genital or rectal area, fever, rash.

Unwanted effects are usually mild and fade as you continue treatment. If you develop a rash or severe diarrhoea contact your doctor. If you have a severe allergic reaction (wheezing, swollen mouth and tongue, itching) stop taking cephalexin and call your doctor immediately.

Similar preparations

BAXAN – Capsules, liquid
CEFADROXIL

DISTACLOR – Capsules, liquid
CEFACLOR

▼SUPRAX – Tablets, liquid
CEFIXIME

VELOSEF – Capsules, liquid, injection
CEPHRADINE

ZINNAT – Tablets, liquid, powder
CEFUROXIME

TETRACYCLINE

On prescription
TETRACYCLINE – Tablets
ACHROMYCIN – Capsules, tablets, eye/ear ointment, injection
PANMYCIN – Capsules
SUSTAMYCIN – Capsules
TETRABID-ORGANON – Capsules
TETRACHEL – Capsules, tablets
TOPICYCLINE – Skin preparation for acne

Combination preparations
DETECLO – Tablets
TETRACYCLINE + CHLORTETRACYCLINE + DEMECLOCYCLINE

MYSTECLIN – Poor choice
TETRACYCLINE + NYSTATIN

Tetracycline is a broad-spectrum antibiotic which has been widely used, although increasing bacterial resistance has now limited its effectiveness. It is used for the long-term treatment of acne, either by mouth or applied directly on to the skin. Tetracycline is also especially useful for treating *Chlamydia* infections such as inflammation of the urinary tract (*urethritis*), pelvic inflammatory disease, certain types of respiratory disease, Lyme disease (a protozoal infection) and sometimes skin infections or pneumonia.

Tetracycline may cause stomach upsets and overgrowth of the fungus *Candida*. Tetracycline combines with calcium in the body and is laid down in growing bones and teeth of unborn babies and young children. This causes yellow-brown staining not just of the milk teeth, but also of the permanent teeth. **Tetracycline should not be given to pregnant women and children under the age of 12.**

Before you use this medicine

Tell your doctor if you are:
☐ breast-feeding – tetracycline is best avoided ☐ taking any other medicines, including vitamins and those bought over the counter.

Tell your doctor if you have or have had:
☐ poor liver or kidney function ☐ allergic reaction to a tetracycline antibiotic.

Do not use tetracycline:
☐ if you are pregnant ☐ for children under 12 years ☐ if you have severe kidney disease ☐ if you have systemic lupus erythematosus.

How to use this medicine

By mouth Take the dose every six or twelve hours with a full glass of water, one hour before meals or two hours afterwards. Avoid taking milk, dairy products and any other medicine, especially antacids, calcium and iron preparations, for an hour before or two hours after tetracycline as they prevent absorption.
On the skin for acne Apply to clean skin twice daily. Other local preparations are used for skin, ear and eye infections.

Always take all the tetracycline prescribed for you, even if you feel better before the prescription is finished. If you stop too soon, your symptoms may come back. If you miss a dose, take it as soon as you remember, but skip it if it is almost time for your next dose.
Alcohol in small amounts should not be a problem.

If you have poor kidney function a tetracycline antibiotic can damage the kidneys further. **Doxycycline** and **minocycline** are less harmful to the kidneys. If you have severe kidney disease you should not take tetracycline. If you have liver disease you may need a lower dose of tetracycline. Injectable tetracycline is more likely to impair liver function further.

Over 65 As kidney function decreases with age, tetracycline should be used with care.

Interactions with other medicines

Calcium, antacids and dairy products reduce the absorption and therefore the effectiveness of tetracyclines.
Iron and zinc salts reduce tetracycline absorption and vice versa.
Oral contraceptives may not be as effective. Discuss this with your doctor.
Oral anticoagulants such as warfarin Tetracycline may increase the risk of bleeding.

Unwanted effects

Likely Feeling or being sick, diarrhoea.
Unlikely Increased sensitivity to the sun (increased sunburn), sore mouth or tongue or itching in the genital or rectal area due to candidal overgrowth.

Contact your doctor if diarrhoea or stomach upsets are severe. Stop taking tetracycline and contact your doctor if you have a skin reaction or severe itching and soreness.

Similar preparations

AUREOMYCIN – Capsules
CHLORTETRACYCLINE

DALACIN T – Skin preparation for acne
CLINDAMYCIN

DOXYCYCLINE – Capsules

IMPERACIN – Tablets
OXYTETRACYCLINE

LEDERMYCIN – Capsules
DEMECLOCYCLINE

MINOCIN – Tablets
MINOCYCLINE

NORDOX – Capsules
DOXYCYCLINE

OXYTETRACYCLINE – Tablets

TERRAMYCIN – Capsules, tablets
OXYTETRACYCLINE

TETRALYSAL 300 – Tablets
LYMECYCLINE

VIBRAMYCIN – Capsules, soluble tablets
DOXYCYCLINE

ERYTHROMYCIN

ERYTHROMYCIN – Tablets
ARPIMYCIN – Liquid
ERYCEN – Tablets
ERYMAX – Capsules
ERYTHROCIN – Tablets, injection
ERYTHROMID – Tablets
ERYTHROPED – Liquid, soluble granules, tablets
ILOSONE – Tablets, capsules, liquid
STIEMYCIN – Skin preparation for acne
ZINERYT – Skin preparation for acne

Erythromycin is used in a similar way to penicillin, although it does not affect an identical range of bacteria. It is widely used and people who are allergic to penicillins or must avoid tetracycline can take erythromycin safely. Erythromycin is used for treating middle ear, throat and chest infections in children, sinusitis and sometimes pneumonia. Intestinal infections caused by *Campylobacter* bacteria may be treated with erythromycin. It is also used for treating certain sexually transmitted diseases. It may also be given to prevent the spread of whooping cough or diphtheria. Erythromycin is also used for the long-term treatment of acne and skin infections either by mouth or applied directly to the skin.

Before you use this medicine

Tell your doctor if you are:
☐ pregnant or breast-feeding ☐ taking any other medicines, including vitamins and those bought over the counter.

Tell your doctor if you have or have had:
☐ an allergic reaction to erythromycin ☐ liver disease or poor kidney function.

How to use this medicine

By mouth Take the tablet or capsule every six hours with a full glass of water, before or with meals. For the long-term treatment of acne you may have to take erythromycin twice or three times a day. The granules should be dispersed in 100ml (4fl. oz) of water before swallowing. The liquid should be shaken thoroughly before use.
On the skin for acne Apply to clean skin twice daily.

Always take all the erythromycin prescribed for you, even if you feel better before the prescription is finished. If you stop too soon, your symptoms may come back. If you miss a dose, take it as soon as you remember, but skip it if it is almost time for your next dose.

Alcohol in small amounts should not be a problem. Erythromycin and alcohol do not interact but an infection means that your body needs rest and recuperation.

Liquid preparations should be stored in a refrigerator, but not frozen.

Over 65 No special requirements.

Interactions with other medicines

Disopyramide, a medicine for irregular heart rhythms – erythromycin increases the risk of toxicity.
Oral anticoagulants such as warfarin Erythromycin may increase the risk of bleeding.
Carbamazepine, an antiepileptic – increased blood levels when used with erythromycin.
Cyclosporin, used to suppress immune responses – increased blood levels when used with erythromycin.
Theophylline, used for asthma – erythromycin increases blood levels and the risk of toxicity.

Unwanted effects

Likely Feeling or being sick, abdominal pain, diarrhoea with high doses.
Less likely Deafness, itching, jaundice, skin rashes.

Contact your doctor if you feel sick while taking erythromycin: a lower dose or a change of antibiotic may avoid this. (**Clarithromycin**, a new, closely related drug, causes less stomach upset.) Some infections must be treated with a high dose. Deafness is reversible on stopping treatment and is usually associated with doses over 4 grams a day. Erythromycin taken for longer than 14 days, and especially erythromycin estolate ((Ilosone) may occasionally cause jaundice which clears up on stopping treatment.

Similar preparations

▼KLARICID – Tablets
CLARITHROMYCIN

▼ZITHROMAX – Capsules, liquid
AZITHROMYCIN

● *SULPHONAMIDES AND TRIMETHOPRIM* ●

The sulphonamides are bacteriostatic antibacterials which originated from the dye industry in the 1930s. **Sulphanilamide** from the red dye *prontosil rubra* was the first to be found to have antibacterial activity. The sulphonamides have been widely used for many years, but with increasing bacterial resistance to their effects, they are seldom used and have been replaced by more active and less toxic antibiotics.

Co-trimoxazole is a combination of **trimethoprim** and the sulphonamide **sulphamethoxazole**, but its useful effects are almost all produced by trimethoprim. Like all sulphonamides, sulphamethoxazole causes unwanted effects, some severe, such as blood disorders and the Stevens-Johnson syndrome – a condition of the skin and mucous membranes with swelling, blistering and ulcers, which is sometimes fatal. There have been recent reports of deaths of people over the age of 65 treated with co-trimoxazole and this is probably due to sulphamethoxazole. Co-trimoxazole is not an ideal drug for older people and should only be used when there is no alternative. It is used in high doses for treating the pneumonia *Pneumocystis carinii* and in lower doses for preventing it in patients who have had transplants or who have AIDS. The sulphonamide component may be particularly important with this infection.

Co-trimoxazole is being used less now because of the increase in bacterial resistance and its adverse effects. **Trimethoprim** on its own may be used for bladder and chest infections. Other sulphonamides include **sulfametopyrazine** (brand name Kelfizine W), **sulphadiazine** and **sulphadimidine**.

TRIMETHOPRIM

TRIMETHOPRIM – Tablets
IPRAL – Tablets
MONOTRIM – Tablets, liquid, injection
SYRAPRIM – Tablets, injection
TRIMOGAL – Tablets
TRIMOPAN – Tablets, liquid

Trimethoprim is an antibacterial drug used for treating and preventing bladder (urinary tract) infections, chest infections such as a flare up in chronic bronchitis, prostate infections and sometimes salmonella infections. It is also a component of co-trimoxazole. Trimethoprim alone causes fewer unwanted effects than co-trimoxazole and it is worth asking if it would be a suitable alternative if co-trimoxazole is prescribed.

Before you use this medicine

Tell your doctor if you are:
□ pregnant – trimethoprim should be avoided (also in babies under 2 months old) □ breast-feeding □ taking any other medicines, including vitamins and those bought over the counter.

Tell your doctor if you have or have had:
□ sensitivity to trimethoprim □ folic acid deficiency or any other blood disorder □ kidney or liver disease.

How to use this medicine

Take the tablets every 12 hours. You may be able to take the dose once a day if you are taking trimethoprim to prevent recurrent bladder or kidney infections. Trimethoprim can be taken with food and this may help if the drug irritates your stomach. Small amounts of alcohol should not be a problem. Trimethoprim and alcohol do not interact but an infection means that your body needs rest and recuperation.

Always take all the trimethoprim prescribed for you, even if you feel better before the prescription is finished. If you stop too soon, your symptoms may come back. If you miss a dose, take it as soon as you remember. If you are taking trimethoprim twice a day, take the dose you missed and wait about six hours before taking the next dose. For once-a-day trimethoprim, take the dose you missed and wait about 12 hours before the next one.

Over 65 No special requirements.

Interactions with other medicines

Oral anticoagulants such as warfarin The risk of bleeding may be increased.
Oral antidiabetics (sulphonylureas) The effects are enhanced by trimethoprim.

Unwanted effects

Likely Feeling or being sick, rash and itching.
Unlikely Blood disorders.

Trimethoprim usually causes no unwanted effects. If stomach upsets or skin reactions are severe, contact your doctor. If you are on long-term treatment with trimethoprim, you may need periodic blood tests.

CIPROFLOXACIN

CIPROXIN – Tablets, injection

Ciprofloxacin is an antimicrobial of the quinolone group, a relative of an early drug called nalidixic acid. It is active against a wide range of bacteria and chlamydia and is used for infections of the respiratory system, urinary tracts and digestive system. Ciprofloxacin is also used for treating septicaemia and gonorrhoea if the bacteria are sensitive to its effects. It should be reserved for treating infections caused by micro-organisms resistant to standard medicines.

Before you use this medicine

Tell your doctor if you are:
☐ pregnant ☐ breast-feeding – not usually prescribed ☐ taking any other medicines, including vitamins and those bought over the counter.

Tell your doctor if you have or have had:
☐ sensitivity to ciprofloxacin or other quinolones ☐ poor kidney function ☐ excessive alkalinity of the urine ☐ epilepsy or other central nervous system disorders ☐ deficiency of the enzyme glucose-6-phosphate dehydrogenase.

Ciprofloxacin is not recommended for children or growing teenagers, except where the benefit outweighs the risk. Studies have shown damage to weight-bearing joints in animals and this is a potential risk in humans.

How to use this medicine

Take the tablets, usually twice daily, with a glassful of water. Drink plenty of fluids during treatment with ciprofloxacin to avoid crystals forming in the urine. Avoid taking ciprofloxacin at the same time of day as indigestion remedies because they affect its absorption.

Do not drive or do other activities that require alertness until you know how you react to ciprofloxacin. Avoid alcohol because ciprofloxacin enhances its effects.

Always take all the ciprofloxacin prescribed for you, even if you feel better before the prescription is finished. If you stop too soon, your symptoms may come back. If you miss a dose, take it as soon as you remember, but skip it if it is almost time for your next dose.

Over 65 No special requirements.

Interactions with other medicines

Theophylline, used to treat asthma – ciprofloxacin prolongs and increases the blood levels of theophylline causing toxicity. If you have to use the two drugs together, your doctor should reduce the dose of theophylline. Blood tests to measure the level of theophylline may be necessary.
Anticoagulants such as warfarin The risk of bleeding is increased.

Unwanted effects

Likely Feeling or being sick, diarrhoea, indigestion, abdominal pain, headache, restlessness, dizziness, rash, itching.
Unlikely Tremor, confusion, convulsions, hallucinations, blurred vision, muscle and joint pain, sensitivity to sunlight (*photosensitivity*), hives, blood disorders, jaundice.

Ciprofloxacin is generally well tolerated. Contact your doctor if any unwanted effects are troublesome.

Similar preparations

CINOBAC – Capsules
CINOXACIN

COMPRECIN – Tablets
ENOXACIN

ERADACIN – Capsules
ACROSOXACIN

MICTRAL – Soluble granules
NALIDIXIC ACID

NALIDIXIC ACID – Tablets

NEGRAM – Tablets, liquid
NALIDIXIC ACID

▼NOROXIN – Eye drops
NORFLOXACIN

▼TARIVID – Tablets, injection
OFLOXACIN

URIBEN – Liquid
NALIDIXIC ACID

▼UTINOR – Tablets
NORFLOXACIN

Cystitis

Cystitis is inflammation of the bladder, usually involving painful passing of urine caused by infection. The kidneys or bloodstream may be infected by the infection spreading upwards from the bladder. You may pass urine frequently or uncontrollably and sometimes urine is blood-stained. The tube leading down from the bladder to outside the body (the urethra) usually becomes inflamed first, causing urination to sting. The bladder may also be inflamed, causing a dull ache in the lower part of the abdomen. Sometimes the kidneys are involved, which you feel as a dull backache. You may have a fever.

Cystitis is much more common in women than men. When it occurs in men, especially middle-aged or older, there is frequently an underlying disorder, such as enlargement of the prostate or a bladder tumour. Children who get cystitis should see a doctor.

Cystitis is more difficult to spot in children under two because the symptoms – loss of appetite, being sick, diarrhoea, drowsiness and fever – are similar to other childhood conditions. It can make older children wet the bed. Cystitis in children is usually a sign that there is something wrong with the kidneys and may lead to permanent kidney damage. If cystitis keeps coming back, you must see your doctor.

HOW YOU CAN HELP YOURSELF

☐ Drink at least three to four pints of liquid a day – more if the weather is hot. This helps to flush out bacteria.
☐ If you find you get cystitis after drinking coffee, tea or alcohol try diluting them – or avoid them altogether.
☐ Pass urine when you need to. Holding on can encourage an attack of cystitis.
☐ After passing urine count to twenty and then see if any more will come, but don't strain.
☐ If you are a woman who gets cystitis after sexual intercourse, it will help to pass water and wash your genitals and anus before and after sex. A man can also help by washing his penis before and after intercourse. Women who suffer from soreness and bruising may find it helps to use a lubricating jelly during intercourse. You can buy this from a pharmacy.
☐ Wash your genital area morning and night; and always wipe the anus from front to back. This helps to prevent any of the bacteria from the genitals or anus reaching the urethra and causing infection.
☐ Avoid using bubble bath or bath gels if you find they irritate your skin. Do not use perfumed soap, deodorants, talcum powder or antiseptics on the genital area.
☐ Avoid wearing tight trousers or nylon pants or tights. They can create a warm moist environment which helps bacteria to breed. Cotton pants allow the skin to breathe.

Medicines for cystitis

Self-treatment can be very helpful, for example with **sodium bicarbonate** which makes the urine more alkaline. Preparations available from a pharmacy include **sodium** or **potassium citrate**. For example, sodium citrate as a powder to make into a liquid (brand names Cymalon; Cystemme) and potassium citrate

THREE-HOUR REMEDY

1. Mix a teaspoon of sodium bicarbonate (bicarbonate of soda) in a pint of water and drink it immediately. Water is best, but if you can't stomach it try another bland liquid like weak tea, milk or weak orange squash.

The water helps flush out the bacteria in your bladder. Bicarbonate of soda has the same effect as products sold by pharmacists for cystitis. It makes your urine less acidic, which hinders the growth of bacteria. After a time the urine doesn't sting so much when you pass it.

If you have high blood pressure or heart trouble you should talk to your doctor before taking bicarbonate of soda.

2. Get two hot water bottles ready – one for your lower back and the other for between your thighs. Wrap them in towels so they won't burn you. Hot water bottles should not be used by children or people over 65.

3. If you are in pain take one or two pain relievers.

4. Go to bed or put your feet up. Take your hot water bottles, bicarbonate of soda, a large jug of water and a glass.

5. Drink a half pint of water every twenty minutes. After an hour (that is, after every third drink), drink a pint of water and bicarbonate of soda, mixed as before.

6. Keep relaxing and drinking water (as in step 5) for a total of three hours.

Do not take bicarbonate of soda for more than three hours.

If you still have cystitis after a day or two, take a sample of urine and get it analysed as soon as possible. Collect the sample after you have passed the first spurt of urine and keep it in a cool place until you take it to your doctor.

as a liquid (Potassium Citrate Mixture BP) or as effervescent tablets (brand name Effercitrate). You should see your doctor if cystitis continues for more than two days or you have recurrent attacks. If you have blood in your urine, a temperature, backache or you are pregnant, you should see your doctor at once, without trying the self-help remedy. Blood in the urine usually means that bacteria are attacking the lining of the urethra.

Bacteria are responsible for around half the cases of cystitis. They live harmlessly in the bowel and around the anus, but in the urethra or bladder can cause infection and inflammation. The openings of the urethra and anus are closer together in a woman than in a man and the urethra is shorter. It is therefore easier for bacteria to contaminate the urethra and reach the bladder in a woman. This is why cystitis is more common in women than men. Vaginal candidiasis and other sexually transmitted diseases such as chlamydia can also produce cystitis-like symptoms.

Your doctor will usually prescribe an antibiotic, such as **ampicillin**, **amoxycillin** or **trimethoprim** for five to seven days. However, bacterial resistance is becoming more of a problem, especially to ampicillin. Your doctor may ask you for a urine sample so that the choice of antibiotic can be checked if the first one does not work.

Fungal infections

There are around a hundred thousand different kinds of fungi in the world, growing on all kinds of plants and animals and their derivatives. They are prolific and many are able to live either as parasites or to co-exist happily with their host, depending on the food supply and local conditions. One of the common fungi associated with humans is *Candida albicans*, a simple yeast. *Aspergillus* is another fungus that can cause allergies or infections. Some fungal infections involve the skin and other parts of the body, such as ringworm (*Tinea*) infections of the scalp, nails and skin.

● *CANDIDA ALBICANS* ●

Candida lives on the skin and in the mouth, the gut and the vagina without causing any harm until its living conditions are changed. Taking an antibiotic by mouth changes the composition of microorganisms in the digestive system, killing harmless bacteria that keep candida under control and allowing it to proliferate unchecked. Fungal infection often begins when the body's resistance is lowered in some way. An antibiotic is taken when the body is already under attack by bacteria. Other conditions such as pregnancy and illnesses such as diabetes, cancer or AIDS alter the body's natural resistance and immunity to infection with fungi as well as bacteria. The oral contraceptive or prolonged treatment with a corticosteroid may also predispose the body to candidal infection.

Symptoms of candida infection are patchy white spots (thrush), usually in the mouth or vagina. The mouth is a common site of infection and in babies it may be hard to distinguish candida from milk curds. Older people who wear dentures are also candidates for fungal mouth infections. A baby's nappy rash may become infected with candida. In women the vulva and vagina are common sites of infection and also the skin under the breasts and other areas of skin folds. Nipple infection can occur if you are breast-feeding.

In uncircumcised men, the area under the foreskin is liable to candidal infection. Candida infection can occur without the presence of other predisposing factors, such as antibiotic treatment or a weakened immune system that allows the fungus to flourish.

HOW YOU CAN HELP YOURSELF

□ Cleanliness is essential and it is important to keep potential areas of infection dry and cool. Take care with drying skin folds and creases and use a light dusting of a non-perfumed talcum powder to absorb remaining moisture.
□ Avoid using perfumed soaps and irritant bath additives.
□ Avoid tight-fitting clothes such as jeans or tights.
□ Wear natural fabrics, rather than nylon, next to your skin to allow it to breathe.
□ Do not share towels, swimwear, underwear or toothbrushes. Candida and other infections can be spread this way.
□ Use a condom for sex if your partner has recently had candida infection.
□ If you wear dentures, keep them and your mouth clean. Watch out for the slightest sign of infection, such as redness and soreness at the corners of the mouth, which should be treated.
□ Change babies' nappies regularly and clean the nappy area well with warm water. Dry thoroughly and leave the area exposed to the air whenever practical. Avoid tight-fitting plastic pants.
□ Sterilise teats and bottles before putting them into the baby's mouth and avoid putting sugary solutions in bottles.

● *TINEA* ●

Tinea species commonly cause fungal infections of the scalp (*Tinea capitis*), the nail (*Tinea unguium*), on the body (*Tinea corporis*), of the feet (athlete's foot – *Tinea pedis*) and in the groin area (*Tinea cruris*). These ringworm infections can be passed from human to human, from animal to human and from soil to human.

Antifungal medicines

Fungal infections generally need treatment because they rarely clear up alone. Most antifungal drugs affect the cell wall of the fungus allowing the cell contents to leak out; the cell then dies.

• *CANDIDA* •

Candidal skin infections are treated locally with an *imidazole* cream or lotion form or another antifungal preparation such as **nystatin**. In the mouth, lozenges or pastilles of **amphotericin** or nystatin may be sucked. Babies can be treated with amphotericin or nystatin suspension or **miconazole** gel. Treatment should continue for 48 hours after the infection appears to have cleared.

Vaginal and vulval infections are treated with pessaries and cream. Nystatin is a well-established treatment but must be used for a fortnight whereas imadazole antifungal preparations can be given in shorter courses and are equally effective. Vaginal preparations of imidazoles are becoming available from pharmacies for treating uncomplicated vaginal candidiasis. This is an important advance for female consumers.

Recurrent infection is common if the course of treatment is not completed, but may also be due to underlying causes, such as long-term antibiotic treatment (see pages 286–7). Your doctor may need to take swabs for culture. Your partner should wear a condom during sexual intercourse and use an antifungal cream while you are being treated.

You may need to take a course of nystatin tablets or one of the newer *triazole* antifungal drugs – **fluconazole** (brand name Diflucan) or **itraconazole** (Sporanox) – to clear the gut and bowel of infection. Recurrent vaginal candidiasis may need treating with one of these drugs, but they cannot be used during pregnancy.

Severe fungal infections within the body (systemic infections) need treatment either with an antifungal by injection into the veins or by mouth. Systemic fungal infections may need weeks of treatment, usually in hospital, especially if the immune system is damaged. *Aspergillosis* and *cryptococcal* infection are particularly difficult to treat.

MICONAZOLE

DAKTARIN – Tablets, mouth gel (also from a pharmacy), vaginal preparations (GYNO-DAKTARIN), injection
MONISTAT – Vaginal cream

With a corticosteroid
DAKTACORT – Skin preparations for eczema, etc.
MICONAZOLE + HYDROCORTISONE

Miconazole is a broad-spectrum imidazole antifungal drug which acts against yeasts such as candida. Miconazole tablets or gel are used for treating and preventing fungal infections of the mouth, throat and gut. Miconazole can be used on the skin to treat candida infections such as nappy rash. Pessaries, tampons and creams are available for use in the vagina, and there is a high-dose pessary for use as a single-dose treatment.

Before you use this medicine

Tell your doctor if you are:
☐ pregnant or breast-feeding ☐ taking any other medicines, including vitamins and those bought over the counter.

Tell your doctor if you have or have had:
☐ sensitivity to miconazole.

How to use this medicine

Tablets or gel Take four times a day after meals for ten days or for up to two days after the symptoms have cleared. The oral gel should be put directly on to the affected areas with a clean finger and kept in the mouth for as long as possible.
Skin Apply to the affected area, rub in gently.
Vagina Insert the cream or pessaries at night high into the vagina. Miconazole tampons are used in the morning and evening for five days. The single-dose pessary is inserted into the vagina at night. A constituent of the pessaries may damage the rubber of diaphragms and condoms.

Always take or use all the miconazole prescribed for you, even if you feel better before the prescription is finished. If you stop too soon, your symptoms may come back. If you miss a dose, take or use it as soon as you remember, but skip it if it is almost time for the next dose.

Over 65 No special requirements.

Unwanted effects

Unlikely with tablets or gel Mild digestive system disturbances; **with skin and vaginal preparations** irritation, occasionally local sensitivity reaction – if this occurs, discontinue treatment and contact your doctor.

Similar preparations

CANESTEN – Skin and vaginal preparations
CLOTRIMAZOLE

CANESTEN 10% VC–Cream (from pharmacies)
CLOTRIMAZOLE

DIFLUCAN – Capsules, liquid, injection
FLUCONAZOLE

ECOSTATIN – Skin and vaginal preparations
ECONAZOLE

EXELDERM – Skin preparations
SULCONAZOLE

NIZORAL – Tablets, liquid, skin and vaginal preparations
KETOCONAZOLE

NYSTAN – skin, vaginal and mouth preparations
NYSTATIN

PEVARYL – Skin preparations, vaginal preparations (GYNO-PEVARYL)
ECONAZOLE

SPORANOX – Capsules
ITRACONAZOLE

TRAVOGYN – Vaginal preparations
ISOCONAZOLE

TROSYL – Nail solution; cream (from pharmacies)
TIOCONAZOLE

● *TINEA* ●

Mild ringworm infections, for example athlete's foot – scaling and itching between the toes – can be treated locally with ointment or powder. **Compound benzoic acid** ointment (Whitfield's ointment) remains a cheap and effective preparation for treating patches of ringworm on the body and between the toes. The *imidazole* antifungal skin preparations, such as **clotrimazole**, **econazole** and **miconazole**, are used. **Tolnaftate** (brand names Timoped, Tineafax, Tinaderm and Mycil) and the **undecenoates** (Mycota) are less helpful for treating infections.

More severe and widespread ringworm infections of the nails and scalp usually need treatment by mouth with an antifungal drug. Nail infections, especially on toenails, are difficult to treat and may need local treatment as well. Treatment may have to be continued for weeks or months. Griseofulvin has been widely used, but treatment is not always successful and it can cause unwanted effects. A newer product, **terbinafine** (brand name Lamisil), which is taken by mouth, seems promising for fungal infections, but experience wih the drug is still limited. **Amorolfine** (Loceryl) is a new antifungal lacquer for painting on infected nails, but it is not clear whether the drug is effective without additional treatment by mouth. The product is applied once a week for six months.

GRISEOFULVIN

FULCIN – Tablets, liquid
GRISOVIN – Tablets

Griseofulvin is an antifungal drug used for treating fungal infections of the skin, scalp, hair or nails, such as ringworm. It gets into keratin – an ingredient of skin, hair and nails – enabling newly formed keratin to resist attack by the fungi. As the new keratin develops, the old infected keratin is shed. Treatment must be continued for weeks and sometimes months.

Before you use this medicine

Tell your doctor if you are:
☐ breast-feeding ☐ taking any other medicines, including vitamins and those bought over the counter.

Tell your doctor if you have or have had:
☐ poor liver function ☐ systemic lupus erythematosus ☐ sensitivity to griseofulvin.

Do not take griseofulvin:
☐ if you are pregnant ☐ if you have porphyria ☐ if you have severe liver disease.

How to use this medicine

Take the tablets or liquid once or twice daily after food. Divided doses may be more effective if you respond poorly to treatment: tablets or liquid may be taken four times a day.

Always take all the griseofulvin prescribed for you, even if the infection appears to have cleared up. If you stop too soon, your symptoms may come back. For hair or skin you may need at least four week's treatment while toe- or fingernails may need six to nine months' treatment. You should continue with treatment for at least two weeks after all the signs of infection have disappeared.

Reservoirs of infection may remain in clothing, footwear, and bedding, so general measures of care and hygiene are important. Pets can carry infection, too.

Do not drive or do other activities that require alertness until you know how you react to griseofulvin. Avoid alcohol – the effects are enhanced by griseofulvin.

If you miss a dose, take it as soon as you remember. If it is nearly time for your next dose, skip the missed dose and take the next one as usual.

Over 65 No special dose requirements unless liver function is poor.

Interactions with other medicines

Oral anticoagulants such as warfarin Effects reduced by griseofulvin.
Oral contraceptives Effects reduced by griseofulvin and pregnancies have occurred, so additional contraceptive measures may be necessary. Discuss this with your doctor.
Phenobarbitone, an antiepileptic, lessens the effectiveness of griseofulvin treatment.

Unwanted effects

Likely Headache, feeling or being sick.
Unlikely Rashes, drowsiness, dizziness.

Unwanted effects with griseofulvin are uncommon. There have been occasional reports of increased sensitivity to light, the arthritis-like condition systemic lupus erythematosus and blood disorders.

Viruses

Viruses are much smaller than bacteria and depend on living cells for their survival. A virus penetrates a cell and then uses the cell's DNA (basic cell matter which carries genetic codes) to multiply and spread to other cells. As new viruses are released the body's cell dies and the viruses go on to infect other cells. There are many different types of virus, from the common cold and influenza to German measles and other childhood infections such as chicken pox, measles and mumps. Infections of the throat, lungs and digestive system are often caused by viruses. Individual viral infections cause a variety of symptoms with differing degrees of severity; for example, some strains of the influenza virus may produce severe symptoms and cause an epidemic.

Antiviral medicines

Treatment of viral infections with specific antiviral medicines is difficult because the virus gets right into and sometimes becomes a permanent part of the body's cells. The ideal antiviral drug should kill the virus within the cell or prevent it from multiplying without harming the human cell. Only a few antiviral drugs have been developed and they sometimes have unpleasant and toxic unwanted effects. Some potentially serious viral illnesses are avoided by immunisation, for example German measles and polio. Antibiotics are of no use in the treatment of viral infections.

Fortunately, many viral infections clear up spontaneously as the body's immune system overcomes them. Symptoms of infection can be eased with bed rest and a medicine for pain relief and lowering temperature. Antiviral medicines are really only used with any success against diseases caused by the herpes virus – *Herpes simplex* (cold sores and genital herpes) and *Herpes zoster* (chicken pox and shingles) – and in the treatment of the human immunodeficiency virus (HIV).

Acyclovir (brand name Zovirax) is active against herpes, but does not rid the body of the virus. Treatment must be started at the first sign of infection, for example within 48 hours of the appearance of a shingles rash. In people with a weakened immune system chicken pox and shingles are life-threatening diseases; acyclovir can be life-saving and is usually given by injection in hospital. Acyclovir is also given by mouth to prevent herpes infections and to prevent recurrences of infections.

Shingles is an infection caused by the chicken pox virus (*herpes zoster*). After you have had chicken pox, the virus lies in the nerves of the body inactive for many years. Sometimes the virus will suddenly become active and spread down the nerve causing a painful, itchy rash in the area of the nerve. Occasionally a nerve of the face and eye is affected; chicken pox blisters may develop on the cornea. Shingles can be very painful and the pain can continue after the rash has gone. Acyclovir by mouth helps to shorten the length of time of pain slightly, but does not affect the painful episodes after the illness (*post-herpetic neuralgia*). However, acyclovir does lessen the complications of herpes zoster in the eye.

Cold sores and genital herpes can be treated with acyclovir cream applied to the affected areas, but it should not be used inside the mouth, in the vagina or in the eye. Acyclovir tablets may be needed for acute herpes simplex infections of the genital area. An eye ointment is used for herpes simplex of the eye.

Zidovudine (brand name Retrovir) is not a cure for AIDS but may delay progression of the disease. It inhibits HIV but does not rid the body of it. Zidovudine can be used for people with serious symptoms of HIV. It lessens the incidence and severity of opportunistic infections, such as *Pneumocystis pneumonia* and other complications. People who are HIV antibody positive but without symptoms may also be given the drug to stop the progression of the virus and so prolong survival. Unwanted effects include severe headache, feeling or being sick, sleeplessness, muscle pains, stomach pains, numbness or tingling of the nerves, rashes and fever. The drug causes blood disorders and needs careful monitoring.

Protozoa

Protozoa are microscopic single-celled organisms. They are abundant creatures, mostly found in soil and water and some can exist for years in cyst form, resistant to temperature and climatic changes. Some can be passed to humans through contaminated food or water. Protozoal diseases can also be spread by sexual contact and through insect bites or by other animal carriers. Diseases caused by protozoans include *amoebic dysentery* (a severe bowel infection), *trichomoniasis* (predominantly a vaginal infection), *giardiasis* (a bowel infection), *cryptosporidiosis* (which causes severe diarrhoea) and *malaria*. Protozoal infections are sometimes difficult to cure and must always be treated promptly. The antimicrobial drug, **metronidizole** is used for treating amoebic dysentery, trichomonal infections and giardiasis.

METRONIDAZOLE

METRONIDAZOLE – Tablets
ELYZOL – Suppositories
FLAGYL – Tablets, liquid, injection, suppositories, skin preparation
METROGEL/METROTOP – Skin preparations
ZADSTAT – Suppositories

With antifungal
FLAGYL COMPAK – Tablets and pessaries in pack
METRONIDAZOLE + NYSTATIN

Metronidazole is an antimicrobial drug active against a variety of bacterial infections and protozoa. It is used for treating protozoal diseases including some vaginal infections, amoebic dysentery and giardiasis. It is also used to treat or prevent infections following surgery and is effective in treating pseudomembranous colitis. Infections of the gums and other dental infections succumb to metronidazole treatment and it is also useful for infected tumours, leg ulcers, pressure sores and rosacea (a type of acne).

Before you use this medicine

Tell your doctor if you are:
☐ pregnant or breast-feeding ☐ taking any other medicines, including vitamins and those bought over the counter.

Tell your doctor if you have or have had:
☐ severe liver disease ☐ sensitivity to metronidazole ☐ a central nervous system disorder, for example epilepsy.

How to use this medicine

Swallow the tablets whole with water, generally three times daily during or after meals. Treatment usually lasts for five to ten days. The liquid should be taken at least one hour before a meal.

Always take all the metronidazole prescribed for you, even if you feel better before the prescription is finished. If you stop too soon, your symptoms may come back. A course of metronidazole should not last more than ten days. If you miss a dose take it as soon as you remember. If your next dose is due within two hours, take it and skip the next dose.

Do not drink alcohol. Metronidazole with alcohol may cause headache, stomach cramps, nausea, vomiting, flushing.

Over 65 No special dose requirements.

Interactions with other medicines

Oral anticoagulants such as warfarin Blood-thinning effects may be increased.
Antiepileptic drugs Metronidazole increases blood levels of **phenytoin. Phenobarbitone** reduces the blood levels of metronidazole.

Unwanted effects

Likely Feeling sick, digestive disorders, unpleasant taste in mouth, furred tongue, rashes, swollen face and tongue. Metronidazole may darken your urine, but this is usual.
Less likely Drowsiness, headache, dizziness, unsteadiness, itching.

Serious adverse effects rarely occur with standard courses. During prolonged treatment, numbness or tingling of the hands and feet, seizures and blood disorders have been reported. If you feel unwell whilst taking metronidazole, contact your doctor.

Similar preparations

FASIGYN – Tablets
TINIDAZOLE

NAXOGIN 500 – Tablets
NIMORAZOLE

MALARIA

The most important and serious protozoal infection is malaria, which is transmitted to man by the female mosquito. Malaria symptoms include aching joints, soaring temperatures, shivering, vomiting and delirium. In extreme cases, malaria can lead to coma and death. Each year there are over two thousand cases of malaria in Britain, including a number of deaths; all are caught abroad. Regions where malaria is endemic include Africa, the Middle East, parts of Asia, Pacific islands and Latin America. The risk varies within regions and with the seasons.

There are medicines for preventing malaria as well as for treating it. Chloroquine has been used for many years, but some species of the protozoa are now resistant to it. Other medicines include **halofantrine** (brand name Halfan), **mefloquine** (Lariam), **primaquine**, **proguanil** (Paludrine), **pyrimethamine** + **sulfadoxine** (Fansidar), **pyrimethamine** + **dapsone** (Maloprim) and **quinine**.

The recommendations for medicines to prevent malaria are constantly being updated because of the changing patterns of resistance. Always ask your doctor and pharmacist for the latest advice if you are preparing to visit a country where there is a risk of malaria. They have access to advice about where malaria has developed resistance to antimalarial medicines. You can also get advice from the Malaria Reference Laboratory and a number of other agencies (see 'Useful addresses'). Prevention with a recommended antimalarial is important and must be started one week before travel and continued for at least four weeks after leaving the risk area. Personal protection against mosquito bites, including the use of mosquito nets, insect repellents and adequate clothing is also essential.

Worms

Worms (*helminths*) are parasites that live part of their life in a human and part in another animal. Many worm infestations are spread in contaminated food carrying the eggs or young worms (*larvae*), because it is inadequately cooked or washed. Some, for example the hookworm, get into the body through the skin. Many worms live in the intestine, attaching themselves to the gut wall, such as the tapeworm which feeds off the intestinal contents or the hookworm which feeds off the blood supply.

Some worms cause general signs of unhealthiness whilst others cause a great deal of harm. These infections need treatment, but often occur in Third World countries where treatment may not always be possible. Fortunately, the threadworm, the most common parasitic worm in Britain, causes only mild symptoms of itching, but nevertheless should be treated. Anthelmintic medicines are often specific for the particular worm, so your doctor should identify the parasite before treatment.

Anthelmintic treatments

Threadworm commonly affects young children because the eggs are easily spread by sucking unwashed fingers or eating food with unwashed hands. The eggs can survive in sandpits, modelling clay, and in soil. Once inside the body, the eggs develop in the upper intestines and then the adult female worm passes out to the skin around the anus where it lays eggs during the night. This causes itching and if the area is scratched, the eggs are transferred back into the body via unwashed fingers and nails. Washing hands and scrubbing nails before eating and after each visit to the toilet is therefore essential to break the chain of infection. Washing the bottom first thing in the morning will help to remove the eggs laid at night.

Threadworm infections can be treated with either **mebendazole** (brand names Vermox; Ovex), **piperazine** or **pyrantel** (Combantrin). Mebendazole is effective in a single dose, but cannot be given to children under two. Treatment may have to be repeated after two or three weeks. All members of a household should be treated at the same time, whether or not they have symptoms, to ensure that the cycle of infection is broken.

PIPERAZINE

From a pharmacy
ECTODYNE – Liquid
WORMEX – Liquid

With a laxative
PRIPSEN – Soluble powder
PIPERAZINE + SENNA

Piperazine is an anthelmintic medicine used for treating threadworm (pinworm) and roundworm. It paralyses the worms in the intestines and these are then passed out with the faeces. Pripsen contains a laxative, senna, to hasten the worms' removal from the intestine. Threadworm infection may be treated with a daily dose for seven days or a larger, single dose. Treatment may be repeated after a week or a fortnight, depending on the product recommendations. All members of the family should be treated to eliminate possible sources of infection. Cleanliness is essential to break the chain of infection.

Before you use this medicine

Tell your doctor if you are:
☐ pregnant – avoid piperazine, but discuss with your doctor ☐ breast-feeding – discuss with your doctor or pharmacist ☐ taking any other medicines, including vitamins and those bought over the counter.

Tell your doctor if you have or have had:
☐ liver or kidney problems ☐ epilepsy ☐ chronic disease of the nervous system.

Do not take if you have:
☐ severe liver disease ☐ epilepsy.

How to use this medicine

Threadworm The dose depends on the age and approximate weight of each person. Soluble powder stirred into milk or water should be drunk immediately. Repeat the dosage after fourteen days.
Roundworm A large single dose taken in the morning is usually effective.

Until you know how you react to piperazine, do not drive or do other activities that require alertness. Piperazine may occasionally cause dizziness and loss of co-ordination.

Over 65 No special dose requirements.

Unwanted effects

Unlikely Feeling or being sick, diarrhoea, stomach pains, colic, headache, dizziness, skin rash, loss of co-ordination ('worm wobble'), drowsiness, confusion.

If any unwanted effects are severe contact your doctor. Stop taking piperazine if you get a rash.

6

HORMONES

Diabetes Thyroid disorders
Adrenal disorders Corticosteroids
Sex hormone deficiencies

Many of the body's functions are regulated by chemical messengers or *hormones* produced by a number of *glands* and other structures throughout the body. This is known as the **endocrine system**. Each gland produces one or more hormones to control a particular aspect of body function. Growth, sexual development and the body's control of nutrition and responses to stress are all regulated by hormones. For example, the *pancreas*, situated under the stomach next to the duodenum, produces **insulin**, which plays a key role in regulating the way the body uses carbohydrate, fat and protein. The *thyroid gland* in the neck regulates the body's *metabolism* – the chemical processes which keep the body working, for example by breaking down substances to release energy. The *adrenal glands* located on top of the kidneys produce **corticosteroids** which regulate the body's response to stress and injury and the balance of mineral salts and water. The overall functioning of the endocrine system is controlled by the *pituitary gland* in the brain.

The pituitary gland controls and regulates growth, metabolism, sexual development and reproduction through its hormones, which are responsible for activating the hormones of the other endocrine glands. The pituitary gland is partly controlled by a part of the brain called the *hypothalamus* which produces its own hormones to stimulate the pituitary. The hormones in the bloodstream feed back to regulate the pituitary and the hypothalamus. There is a continuous ebb and flow of hormones with the delicate balance maintained by the pituitary gland.

The hormone balance can be disrupted at a particular endocrine gland, for instance if the gland becomes diseased and malfunctions, or the flow of hormones secreted in the brain in the hypothalamus and the pituitary, can be disturbed. Most hormones are released from birth onwards but the amount varies according to the body's requirements. Other hormones are produced at particular times, for example the growth hormone during childhood and teenage years and sex hormones from the start of puberty.

Diabetes

Diabetes mellitus (or 'sugar diabetes') is not a single disease, but a condition where the breakdown of sugars and starches (*carbohydrates*) in the body is permanently disordered due to lack of **insulin**. In a normal body, carbohydrates are broken down in the intestines to simple sugars, mostly **glucose**, which are then absorbed into the bloodstream. Insulin, a hormone produced by the pancreas gland is responsible for controlling glucose output from the liver and for transporting glucose in the blood into the body's cells. Glucose within the cells is a source of energy for the body's muscles and organs.

If you have no insulin, or too little for it to be effective, glucose cannot enter the cells and remains in the bloodstream. Blood-glucose reaches a level at which the kidneys cannot hold back the glucose and it spills into the urine. The body's cells are then starved of energy and may switch to burning fats and proteins as an energy source. When the body uses glucose for energy, the waste products are carbon dioxide and water. When fat is burnt, it produces *ketoacids* and other chemicals which can harm the body. The signs of *ketoacidosis* include feeling or being sick, weakness, stomach pains, thirst and dehydration. You also pass large quantities of urine and *ketones* from the breakdown of fats make the breath smell of fruit. Untreated, these symptoms can lead to coma and death.

Diabetes needs careful treatment and complications may occur in some people. This is usually related to how long you have had the disease and how well it has been controlled. Diabetes shortens life-expectancy and puts people at increased risk of heart disease, blindness, stroke, circulatory disorders, nerve damage leading to impotence, infections and kidney disease. After 30 years of diabetes, around a quarter of diabetics develop kidney disease and need dialysis or a kidney transplant. Around eight per cent of diabetics go blind after 30 years with the disease.

One to two per cent of the British population have diabetes and it appears to be getting more common, especially in teenagers and younger children. A study has found that the national incidence in children for the years 1988–89 is nearly double that of 15 years ago.

Insulin-dependent diabetes (type 1) occurs when there is almost complete lack of insulin production. This affects young people most often but can occur at any age. Regular injections of insulin are essential to maintain health. **Non insulin-dependent diabetes (type 2)** develops when the pancreas cannot produce enough insulin or the body cannot use it efficiently. This occurs more often in middle aged and older people, particularly people who are overweight; it is treated by diet and medicines taken by mouth to stimulate extra insulin production, although insulin treatment may also be necessary.

• *INSULIN-DEPENDENT DIABETES* •

This usually occurs in young people under the age of 35 and most commonly between the ages of 10 and 16. There appears to be a peak at 12 years, when a large number of hormonal changes take place in the body at the beginning of puberty. The insulin-making cells in the pancreas are destroyed by the body's own immune system, which has been triggered into action – possibly by a virus infection. Researchers are not entirely sure why the condition develops. Some cases appear to be hereditary.

Signs of insulin failure may develop swiftly with lethargy, sickness, general ill health and weight loss, thirst, dehydration and a need to pass more urine. Most children developing diabetes will need life-long treatment with insulin to avoid the symptoms of ketoacidosis. Much progress has been made in the management of diabetes and patients now work closely with a medical team to maintain quality of life and achieve the best possible control of blood-sugar levels and other aspects of metabolism, avoiding disabling periods of low blood-sugar (*hypoglycaemia*) and preventing complications.

• *Management*

The pancreas releases insulin into the bloodstream around the clock, adjusting levels according to the amount of glucose in the blood. When insulin production is reduced, it is easy enough to replace the body's internal insulin with an external source, but it is difficult to copy the body's fluctuations and the exact insulin requirements. You must plan what you are going to eat every day and calculate the carbohydrate content of your food. You can then work out approximately how much insulin you need to counter the high blood-sugar levels normally produced after eating.

Diet, particularly controlling the daily intake of carbohydrate, is very important. You have to take in enough carbohydrate to allow normal growth and development, but you must not become overweight. Your daily carbohydrate intake should be spread throughout the day and portions can be moved from one meal to another to achieve the best control of blood-sugar levels. Insulin requirements vary, so the amount you need has to be carefully determined. Usually a mixture of short-acting and longer-acting insulin is given: the long-acting insulin provides a background level while the short-acting preparation

HOW YOU CAN HELP YOURSELF

□ Learn to monitor your health and the control of diabetes. You will need to see your doctor or specialist nurse routinely even if you are managing treatment well.
□ Measure your blood or urine levels of sugar. This is an important indicator of how well carbohydrate is controlled in the body. Insulin-dependent diabetics should measure blood glucose because it gives a better idea of body sugar levels. Measuring urine levels of glucose is not such an accurate reflection of sugar levels because glucose only spills into urine when there is too much in blood. Ideally the urine should always be free of glucose.
□ Try not to let diabetes interfere with your lifestyle. Get to know your capabilities and limitations; for example, extra carbohydrate may be needed before exercise. Talk to your doctor about the quality of your life.
□ Diet is important in both types of diabetes; you should eat sensibly and regularly. You should not avoid carbohydrate completely, but you should refrain from eating large quantities of rapidly absorbed carbohydrate alone, except small amounts in emergencies for a 'hypo'. You do not need to eat special, expensive diabetic foods; you can easily buy low-calorie drinks and foods. Eat plenty of high-fibre foods and avoid fat.
□ Always carry glucose tablets, a sugary drink or chocolate or some other snack to relieve 'hypo' symptoms.
□ Carry a card or an identity bracelet to tell passers-by that you are an insulin-dependent diabetic, just in case you have a severe 'hypo' and lose consciousness. Note the type of insulin and dose.
□ Join a self-help group. For example, the British Diabetic Association has local branches and information on many aspects of diabetes (see 'Useful addresses').
□ Avoid smoking: diabetics can suffer from circulatory disorders, narrowed blood vessels and sometimes gangrene. Smoking adds to these effects.
□ Exercise regularly and within your capabilities. You may need to adjust your insulin dosage when you try a new activity.
□ Foot care is particularly important. You should inspect your feet regularly for signs of sores, ulcers and infection. Wear well-fitting shoes and never walk barefoot. Discuss any problems with the doctor, nurse or chiropodist.

boosts insulin after meals to deal with the additional blood-sugar.

Balancing the dose of insulin is quite a skill. Too little insulin means too much sugar remains in the blood and signs of ketoacidosis may reappear. Too much insulin and the blood-sugar will be lowered too far causing *hypoglycaemia* – a 'hypo'. Signs of low blood-sugar range from irritability, bad temper and poor judgement to confusion, sweating, faintness and loss of consciousness which can happen suddenly and without warning. Blood-sugar levels must be restored as soon as possible by taking some form of sugar or glucose immediately.

● *NON INSULIN-DEPENDENT DIABETES* ●

This form of diabetes (type 2) often develops gradually, usually in people over the age of 40. It is more common than insulin-dependent diabetes and may affect as many as one in 25 people over the age of 65 in Britain. It commonly runs in families, often occurring in overweight people. Non insulin-dependent diabetes, also known as 'maturity onset' diabetes, does not need treatment with daily injections of insulin. The body still produces insulin but in too small an amount to be effective, or the cells cannot use insulin efficiently. The upset in body chemistry is less than with type 1 and you may not know that you have the condition until it is detected at a health check-up when urine is tested routinely for the presence of sugar. Early signs of this type of diabetes include thirst, increased eating and drinking (especially of sweet drinks), tiredness and getting up at night to pass urine. You may also lose weight and *Candida*, normally a harmless body fungus, may grow out of control and cause infection, especially in the vagina or penis.

The illness *chronic pancreatitis* and certain medicines can both trigger non insulin-dependent diabetes. Drugs such as corticosteroids and diuretics (**thiazides** and the **frusemide** group) may cause diabetes because they oppose the effect of the body's own insulin. If you take one of these medicines, you should tell any new doctor what you are taking. The prescription may need to be stopped or changed.

● *Management*

As with insulin-dependent diabetes, treatment aims to relieve the immediate symptoms and to prevent long-term complications, especially heart disease, circulatory disorders and nerve damage. The first approach to treatment is weight reduction if you are overweight and changes to your diet if you do not have a weight problem. It may be unnecessary to take a medicine to control non-insulin dependent diabetes because diet is often all that is needed to control high blood-sugar. You should eat carbohydrate in the form of potatoes, bread or beans and cut back on fatty foods and sugar-laden foods and drinks. If diet does not control blood-sugar, you may have to take an antidiabetic medicine by mouth, but diet will still be an important part of treatment.

HOW YOU CAN HELP YOURSELF

The pointers to self-management of non-insulin dependent diabetes are much the same as those for the insulin-dependent type. The important points to think about are:

- ☐ change your diet
- ☐ avoid being overweight
- ☐ take regular exercise
- ☐ avoid smoking
- ☐ monitor your blood-sugar levels or test your urine regularly and keep a written record of the result
- ☐ see your doctor regularly, but especially if there is any sign of loss of blood-sugar control.

Insulin

In 1889 the cause of diabetes was traced to a disorder of the pancreas gland. Two Canadian doctors, Frederick Banting and Charles Best identified insulin as the key substance lacking in diabetics in 1921. Insulin was first tried in a human on 11 January 1922 when an extract of animal pancreas was injected. Until then, diabetes was a grave disease for which there was no cure and death was inevitable within a year or so.

Insulin is broken down by the digestive system and is therefore not effective when taken by mouth. In replacing the body's insulin, an external source of insulin must be given every day by injection. Insulin is injected under the skin (*subcutaneously*) routinely unless there is an emergency, such as coma when it is injected into a vein or muscle. External sources of insulin are mainly prepared *biosynthetically* – by genetic engineering using a particular type of bacterium (*Escherichia coli*) – or semi-synthetically using an enzyme to alter pork insulin. Other sources include insulin extracted from cattle pancreases.

When injected into humans, all external sources of insulin produce a response from the immune system. Even genetically engineered human insulin is not free of this effect, because it is mixed with additives and preservatives which may contribute to the immune response. Overwhelming allergy to insulin preparations is uncommon and if there are problems you may need to change to another type of insulin preparation, for example from pork to beef.

One drawback of insulin treatment is the daily round of injections. Researchers have looked for many years for alternative ways to give insulin, for example by suppository or by tablets with special coatings to avoid the enzyme which destroys it in the digestive system. No other route into the body has been satisfactory. However, a nasal spray is now being tested on British volunteers. The spray appears to match more closely the way insulin is released naturally in the body and, if it proves to be effective, should certainly be more acceptable to diabetics, especially children. The spray is not available yet and it will be at least 1995 before the results of tests are known.

INSULIN PREPARATIONS

When insulin injections are manufactured they can be mixed with other substances (for example a zinc salt) which prolong the action of insulin in the body. There are three main types of insulin preparation.

Short-acting insulins, such as **soluble insulin**, act rapidly in the body but their effect lasts up to about eight hours with peak action between two and four hours. A short-acting insulin may be used before a meal to deal with the increase in blood sugar after eating.

Intermediate-acting insulins, such as **isophane insulin injection** and **insulin zinc suspension**, do not begin to act until one or two hours after injection but continue to work for up to 16 hours with a peak effect between four and ten hours. They can be used at bedtime.

Long-acting insulins, such as **protamine zinc insulin**, have slower onset of action but last for longer periods, up to about 35 hours.

How long different insulin preparations work in the body varies from person to person. The insulin requirement for each diabetic has to be carefully assessed and this includes the type of insulin or mix of insulins, the dosage and how often injections must be given. Many people can manage with just two injections a day of a mixture of short- and longer-acting insulins but more complex regimens are increasingly popular because they can improve blood-glucose control. Additional doses of short-acting insulin can be given before meals.

Injections

Insulin can be injected into the upper arms, thighs, buttocks or abdomen. It is a good idea to rotate the site of injection.

Repeatedly injecting into the same site may disturb the fatty tissue under the skin and lead to swelling or pitting. During the first few weeks of insulin treatment some people have allergic reactions at the site of injection, but this is not usually troublesome and soon clears up. Easy-to-carry pen injector devices (brand names Autopen; B-D Pen; NovoPen II; Penject; Pur-In Pen) with cartridges of soluble insulin which meter the dose needed are now very popular. Insulin can also be injected continuously throughout 24 hours by a battery-operated portable infusion pump strapped to the body. This may improve the quality of life for some diabetics, but you need to be well motivated and responsible for monitoring your own blood-sugar levels. An infusion pump is expensive and not generally available in the NHS and is not much used in Britain.

Hypoglycaemia

When you start insulin treatment your doctor or the specialist nurse will usually want you to experience the early warning effects of hypoglycaemia so that you can recognise the signs and know what action to take. Sometimes it may be helpful for a relative or friend to be taught to recognise these symptoms too in case of emergencies. If your type of insulin is changed for some reason, you may find that your awareness and warning signs of hypoglycaemia alter. It is usually necessary to adjust the dose and to monitor your progress carefully in the first few days after starting a new type of insulin.

If you feel a 'hypo' coming on you will need to take some carbohydrate or in a real emergency three or four lumps of sugar with a little water. Repeat this in 10–15 minutes if necessary. Your doctor may suggest that you or a relative carries an emergency supply of **glucagon**, a drug that increases blood-sugar by mobilising a stored source of sugar in the liver. Glucagon can be used to treat acute hypoglycaemic symptoms in an emergency.

Driving and diabetes

If you are a car driver you will need to be particularly careful to avoid a 'hypo' while driving. Loss of warning of hypoglycaemia is quite common especially if you are dependent on insulin. You should try to check your blood-sugar level before you drive and every two hours on long journeys. Always carry a snack and a drink in the car so that you can stop and replenish your blood-sugar levels. If necessary share the driving with someone else, especially on longer drives. You should not drive if you have lost awareness of hypoglycaemic symptoms. You must inform the DVLC (Driver and Vehicle Licencing Centre) and your insurance company that you have diabetes.

INSULIN

Short-acting
SOLUBLE INSULIN
Animal source: NEUTRAL INSULIN; HYPURIN NEUTRAL; VELOSULIN
Human source: HUMAN ACTRAPID; HUMAN VELOSULIN; HUMULIN S; PUR-IN NEUTRAL

Intermediate and long-acting
INSULIN ZINC SUSPENSION
Animal source: INSULIN ZINC SUSPENSION LENTE; HYPURIN LENTE; LENTARD MC
Human source: HUMAN MONOTARD; HUMULIN LENTE
AMORPHOUS INSULIN ZINC SUSPENSION
Animal source: SEMITARD MC
CRYSTALLINE INSULIN ZINC SUSPENSION
Human source: HUMAN ULTRATARD; HUMULIN ZN
ISOPHANE INSULIN
Animal source: ISOPHANE INSULIN; HYPURIN ISOPHANE; INSULATARD
Human source: HUMAN INSULATARD; HUMAN PROTAPHANE; HUMULIN I; PUR-IN ISOPHANE

Biphasic
Biphasic insulins are ready-mixed combinations of short- and a longer-acting insulin in various ratios.
BIPHASIC INSULIN
Animal source: RAPITARD MC
BIPHASIC ISOPHANE INSULIN
Animal source: INITARD 50/50; MIXTARD 30/70
Human source: HUMAN ACTRAPHANE 30/70; HUMAN INITARD 50/50; HUMAN MIXTARD 30/70; HUMULIN M1–M4 (differing proportions); PENMIX 30/70; PUR-IN MIX

Rarely used
PROTAMINE ZINC INSULIN
Animal source: HYPURIN PROTAMINE ZINC

Insulin is a hormone, a complex protein made in the pancreas gland. It controls blood-sugar levels and transports glucose from the bloodstream into the body's cells. Insulin is essential for health and is given to replace the body's source or to supplement it in diabetes mellitus. It is broken down by the digestive system and therefore to be given by injection every day. The correct dose and type of insulin have to be found for each diabetic person. Dosage may have to be adjusted according to diet, exercise and health. Too much insulin causes low blood-sugar (hypoglycaemia). Too little insulin allows too much sugar to remain in the bloodstream (hyperglycaemia) resulting in the production of waste acids and symptoms of ketoacidosis.

Before you use this medicine

Tell your doctor if you are:
☐ pregnant or planning to become pregnant – good control of diabetes is essential before conception and throughout pregnancy ☐ breast-feeding – a small amount of insulin passes through into milk, but is not harmful ☐ taking any other medicines, including vitamins and those bought over the counter.

Tell your doctor if you have or have had:
☐ kidney, liver or thyroid disease ☐ recent illness, such as severe infection ☐ allergy to insulin.

How to use this medicine

Before using insulin, roll the vial slowly between the palms of your hands. Inject insulin under the skin according to the treatment plan worked out with the doctor. Test your levels of blood-sugar regularly.

Until you know how you react to insulin, do not drive. Avoid driving or operating machinery if you have warning signs of a 'hypo'. Always carry glucose sweets or a snack when driving. Avoid alcohol – it increases the blood-sugar lowering effect of insulin and upsets control of diabetes.

Do not stop taking insulin suddenly or change to another type or brand of insulin or syringe without checking with your doctor. Make sure you see your doctor or specialist nurse regularly to check progress, but especially when you first start insulin treatment. If you have to have surgery, including dental work, tell the doctor or dentist that you take insulin. Agree a plan with your doctor for missed doses, because action depends on the dose and type of insulin.

Storage Store unused insulin supplies in the refrigerator at 2–8°C, but do not freeze. If insulin has been frozen do not use it. Check use-by dates and do not use if out of date or the liquid looks lumpy, grainy or discoloured. Make sure you know what the appearance of your insulin injection should be so that you can tell if the solution has deteriorated.

Cartridges in use or carried as spare for a portable injection device may be kept at room temperature, but not exposed to excessive sunlight or heat. **A cartridge in use must not be kept in a refrigerator.**

Over 65 No special requirements.

Interactions with other medicines

Many drugs interfere with the effects of insulin. Do not take other medicines including those sold over the counter such as aspirin without checking first with your doctor or pharmacist.
Monoamine-oxidase inhibitors (antidepressants) increase the risk of low blood-sugar.
Beta blockers (heart and blood pressure drugs) may mask warning signs of and delay recovery from low blood-sugar.
Corticosteroids, **oral contraceptives** and **diuretics** may increase insulin requirements.

Unwanted effects

Likely Irritation or rash at injection site, weakness and sweating.
Unlikely Swelling or dimpling at injection site, rash.

Allergy to insulin is rare. The dose and how often insulin is given to control blood-sugar are very important. You need to take action if blood-sugar levels are too low or too high.
Signs of low blood-sugar Faintness, hunger, sweating, weakness, trembling, blurred vision, confusion, headache. These symptoms mean take extra sugar immediately. Loss of consciousness or seizures need emergency action and medical help.
Signs of high blood-sugar Drowsiness, dry flushed skin, loss of appetite, abnormal thirst, increased urination, breath smells of fruit. You need additional short-acting insulin, contact your doctor or specialist nurse.

Medicines for type 2 diabetes

Drug treatment is started only when diet has failed to control blood-sugar. If your doctor considers that a medicine is necessary it will be to augment the effect of your diet, not replace it. A **sulphonylurea**-type drug encourages the pancreas to produce more insulin while **metformin** reduces glucose production by the liver. They can only be used when the body is still making some insulin.

Most sulphonylureas are similar in effect, but they differ in how long they act in the body. **Tolbutamide** is short-acting, whereas **glibenclamide** works for over 24 hours and **chlorpropamide** acts for even longer. If these longer-acting antidiabetics cause low blood-sugar, the hypoglycaemia will be prolonged and may be hazardous. You should avoid these drugs if you are an older person or have poor liver function. Furthermore chlorpropamide interacts with alcohol and for some people causes uncomfortable flushing. People taking a sulphonylurea medicine have been found to gain weight whereas metformin helps those who are already overweight. The sulphonylureas can cause hypoglycaemia, particularly in older people. **Tolazamide**, **glibenclamide** and **chlorpropamide** are best avoided if you have poor kidney function.

Tolbutamide, the oldest sulphonylurea in use, has a good safety record and is least likely to cause prolonged low levels of blood-sugar. However, the tablets are large and some people find them difficult to swallow, although you can break one in half.

Metformin is used when strict dieting and treatment with a sulphonylurea have not controlled diabetes. It can be used on its own or with a sulphonylurea. Unwanted effects include loss of appetite, feeling or being sick and diarrhoea (usually transient). These effects can be lessened by taking metformin tablets with or after meals. With high doses unwanted effects can be troublesome. Metformin should not be used if you have kidney or liver disease. Alcohol increases the risk of a severe adverse effect (*lactic acidosis* – a medical emergency).

If your blood-sugar level is controlled on a low dose of an antidiabetic medicine, ask your doctor whether you can try a test period without the drug. Do not do this until you have discussed a plan of action with the doctor.

Guar gum is a natural vegetable fibre presented in granule form, which can be taken mixed with liquid before a meal to reduce the blood-sugar level. However, it causes bloating, indigestion, diarrhoea and flatulence which limit its usefulness.

Your doctor may need to give you insulin temporarily in times of stress or illness and during surgery because an antidiabetic medicine may be insufficient.

TOLBUTAMIDE

TOLBUTAMIDE – Tablets
RASTINON – Tablets

Tolbutamide is an oral antidiabetic drug. It lowers high blood-sugar levels in non insulin-dependent diabetics, but is used only after dietary measures have failed to control blood-sugar. Tolbutamide must be used with a suitable diet. Like all sulphonylurea medicines, it encourages the production of insulin in the pancreas. It acts for a relatively short time in the body and rarely causes low blood-sugar levels.

Before you use this medicine

Tell your doctor if you are:
☐ breast-feeding (tolbutamide is not recommended) ☐ taking any other medicines, including vitamins and those bought over the counter.

Tell your doctor if you have or have had:
☐ allergy to sulphonamides ☐ liver or kidney disease ☐ porphyria ☐ adrenal or thyroid disease ☐ diabetic ketoacidosis.

Do not use if you are:
☐ pregnant – tolbutamide may be harmful; diabetes is usually controlled with insulin during pregnancy ☐ an insulin-dependent diabetic.

How to use this medicine

Take the tablets, either as a single dose with or immediately after the first main meal of the day or twice daily in the morning and evening.

Until you know how you react to tolbutamide, do not drive. Avoid driving or operating machinery if you have warning signs of a 'hypo'. Always carry glucose sweets or a snack when driving. Avoid alcohol – it may upset control of diabetes.

Do not stop taking tolbutamide suddenly without checking with your doctor. Your condition may worsen. If you miss a dose, take it as soon as you remember. If your next dose is due within two hours, take it and skip the next dose. Do not take double the dose. If you have to have surgery, including dental work, tell the doctor or dentist that you take tolbutamide.

Over 65 Low blood-sugar is more likely. You may need less than the standard adult dose. Tolbutamide may be used by people with mild to moderate kidney impairment in a reduced dose.

Interactions with other medicines

Various drugs interfere with the effect of tolbutamide. Do not take other medicines including those sold over the counter without checking first with your doctor or pharmacist.

Blood-sugar lowering effects increased by
Beta blockers
Antidepressants – monoamine-oxidase inhibitor
Anti-infectives – co-trimoxazole, trimethoprim, sulphonamides, chloramphenicol
Antifungals – miconazole, fluconazole
Medicines for rheumatism and gout – azapropazone, phenylbutazone, sulphinpyrazone
Blood-sugar may rise with
Corticosteroids; **rifampicin**; **oral contraceptives**; **thiazide diuretics**.

Unwanted effects

Likely Headache, mild digestive system upsets.
Unlikely Dizziness, confusion, weakness, skin rash.

Serious unwanted effects are rare – occasionally blood disorders, itching, jaundice occur. If unwanted effects are troublesome contact your doctor. You need to take action if blood-sugar levels drop.

Signs of low blood-sugar Faintness, hunger, sweating, weakness, trembling, blurred vision, confusion, headache. These symptoms mean take extra sugar immediately. Loss of consciousness or seizures need emergency action and medical help.

Similar preparations

CHLORPROPAMIDE – Tablets

DAONIL – Tablets
GLIBENCLAMIDE

DIABINESE – Tablets
CHLORPROPAMIDE

DIAMICRON – Tablets
GLICLAZIDE

EUGLUCON – Tablets
GLIBENCLAMIDE

GLIBENCLAMIDE – Tablets

GLIBENESE – Tablets
GLIPIZIDE

GLUCOPHAGE – Tablets
METFORMIN

GLURENORM – Tablets
GLIQUIDONE

METFORMIN – Tablets

MINODIAB – Tablets
GLIPIZIDE

SEMI-DAONIL – Tablets
GLIBENCLAMIDE

TOLANASE – Tablets
TOLAZAMIDE

Thyroid disorders

The thyroid gland in the neck produces several hormones that regulate the body's metabolism. **Calcitonin** is essential for a normal calcium balance. Two other hormones, **thyroxine** and **triiodothyronine**, act on all the body's cells to control the rate at which food is converted into energy. To make the hormones the gland needs trace amounts of iodine, a mineral which is usually in plentiful supply in our diet. Different illnesses occur depending on whether too much or too little of the thyroid hormones are produced. Low levels of thyroid hormones cause *hypothyroidism*; if the gland becomes overactive and produces high levels of hormones *hyperthyroidism* occurs.

Goitre is enlargement of the thyroid gland which may be due to abnormal growth of thyroid tissue or can be the body's response to disruption in the production of thyroid hormone.

● *UNDERACTIVE THYROID* ● *(HYPOTHYROIDISM)*

A low level of thyroid hormones produces different illnesses depending on the person's age. If a baby is born with low levels of the hormones, it does not develop normally and will be stunted and mentally handicapped. The condition (*cretinism*) is rare and regular injections of a thyroid preparation usually establish normal development. The thyroid levels of babies are checked routinely after birth. Hypothyroidism in children delays growth and puberty.

For older people it is not certain how the disorder occurs but it may be caused by the body's own immune system attacking the thyroid gland. The illness comes on slowly and is hard to recognise in its early stages, but a blood test can confirm abnormal thyroid function. Hypothyroidism is quite common, occurs more often in women than men and usually after the age of 45. Signs include tiredness, slowing of mental processes, weight increase, slower heart rate, drying and coarsening of the skin, hair loss and puffy face and eyelids. Sensitivity to cold is increased and women who are still menstruating may find that periods are heavier and prolonged or stop prematurely.

● *OVERACTIVE THYROID* ● *(HYPERTHYROIDISM)*

When the thyroid gland is overactive it produces symptoms not unlike acute anxiety and it may be difficult to tell the two conditions apart. Signs of hyperthyroidism (also called *thyrotoxicosis*) include nervousness, tiredness, sweating, trembling, rapid pulse and irregular heart rhythms. In more severe cases, weight loss and increased sensitivity to heat may occur. Women who are still menstruating may find that their periods are heavier, or sometimes lighter and scantier. Sometimes the gland may swell to produce a goitre. Thyrotoxicosis can cause an abnormal bulging of the eyes known as *exophthalmos*. Hyperthyroidism occurs more commonly in women than men and usually in young people. The condition may be more difficult to detect in older people. Blood tests are used to confirm the diagnosis and to measure hormone levels.

● *Exophthalmos*

Bulging eyes associated with hyperthyroidism can be uncomfortable, unsightly and even painful. It can be distressing because a person's physical appearance is altered. It occurs most commonly in women aged 20–45, and in smokers. Eye muscles become swollen and there is a build-up of fat and fluid behind the eyes, pushing the eyes outwards and leading to double vision. In rare, severe cases sight can be threatened by pressure on the optic nerve. This needs treatment with high doses of steroids or other immunosuppressive drugs, or surgery to make more room for the eyes and the swollen muscles. Drug or surgical treatment does not affect the eye disease consistently. Once high levels of thyroid have been controlled, eye problems remain stable in the majority of people (eight out of ten), but may get worse or improve.

Your doctor will aim to preserve vision and to relieve the condition with conservative measures. Raising the head of the bed at night may prevent worsening of the fluid behind the eye. To protect the cornea at night, the eyelids can be taped and a protective patch applied. Simple eye ointment may help to prevent drying out at night, while **methylcellulose** eye drops can lessen the gritty sensation in the eyes during the day. Tinted glasses can reduce the unpleasant sensation from bright lights, protect the cornea from wind and dust and will help cosmetically. Prismatic lenses in glasses will help double vision.

Medicines for thyroid disorders

● *HYPOTHYROIDISM* ●

Treatment consists of replacing the body's thyroid hormone with an external source, usually **thyroxine** tablets containing tiny quantities equal to those the body would make normally. You will need to take tablets for the rest of your life, but this should not be difficult once a suitable dose has been established. Thyroxine must be started at a low dose and gradually increased at two- to four-week intervals. Older people and those with heart disease need a smaller dose and your doctor will supervise you closely until the maintenance dose has been reached. You will need to have regular blood tests during the early stages of treatment to measure the hormone levels. At the start of thyroxine treatment your heart may beat more rapidly and if you have heart disease may cause anginal pain and muscle cramps. Too large a dose may cause symptoms of *hyper*thyroidism, such as restlessness, sweating, flushing, headache and diarrhoea.

Liothyronine has a similar action to thyroxine. Its effects develop more rapidly but it does not act for as long. Liothyronine is sometimes used by injection for treating severe hypothyroid conditions. **Dried thyroid** or **extract of thyroid** contains variable amounts of thyroxine and liothyronine and is not recommended.

THYROXINE

THYROXINE – Tablets
ELTROXIN – Tablets

Thyroxine is a thyroid hormone used for replacing the body's source when the normal working of the thyroid gland is disrupted. It is used for treating an underactive gland (hypothyroidism). Thyroxine also helps to relieve swelling in certain types of goitre when the thyroid gland is enlarged. It may also be used during treatment for thyroid cancer.

Before you use this medicine

Tell your doctor if you are:
□ pregnant or breast-feeding □ taking any other medicines, including vitamins and those bought over the counter.

Tell your doctor if you have or have had:
□ heart problems □ high blood pressure □ overactive thyroid □ sensitivity to thyroxine □ adrenal insufficiency.

How to use this medicine

Take the tablet once a day, preferably before breakfast. If you are older or have heart disease you may take a tablet on alternate days. See your doctor at least once a year for a regular check-up and blood tests to assess thyroid function.

Do not stop taking thyroxine without talking to your doctor. Thyroxine is replacing the body's hormone and tablets must be taken regularly or symptoms will recur. If you miss a dose take it as soon as you remember. Do not take double the dose in one day.

Over 65 You will need less than the usual adult dose.

Interactions with other medicines

Thyroxine interacts with a number of drugs. Do not take other medicines including those sold over the counter without checking first with your doctor or pharmacist.

Oral anticoagulants such as warfarin Increased risk of bleeding with thyroxine.

Unwanted effects

Unlikely Anginal pain, irregular heartbeat, palpitation, muscle cramps, diarrhoea, vomiting, agitation, restlessness, sleeplessness, sweating, weight loss.

Unwanted effects are unlikely but may occur at the start of treatment when your doctor is determining the dosage. If you experience these symptoms contact your doctor.

Similar preparations

TERTROXIN – Tablets
LIOTHYRONINE

TRIIODOTHYRONINE – Injection

• *HYPERTHYROIDISM* •

There are several possibilities for treating an overactive thyroid gland:

☐ treatment with an antithyroid medicine that interferes with the production of thyroid hormones

☐ radioactive iodine to destroy thyroid tissue and lessen the amount of hormones produced
☐ surgery to remove part of the gland – this may be necessary if drug treatment has failed to improve the condition or if the gland is swollen (goitre) and pressing against the wind-pipe.

Drug treatment usually lasts for a period of 18 months. **Carbimazole** is commonly used in Britain, but for someone who has a sensitivity reaction to it **propylthiouracil** may be needed. Treatment starts with a high dose for about four to eight weeks until hormone production is controlled. The dose is then gradually reduced and tailored to each person. About half the people taking an antithyroid medicine improve and the disease may burn out (remit) during treatment. Others may need further treatment sometimes with alternative measures. Over-treatment may result in *hypo*thyroidism, which must then be treated with **thyroxine**. Sometimes a combination of a daily dose of carbimazole plus thyroxine may be used in a 'blocking-replacement' strategy, but this is not suitable treatment during pregnancy.

A beta blocker such as **propranolol** may be used to control symptoms at the start of treatment. It may also be used with an antithyroid drug or as part of the treatment with radioactive iodine.

CARBIMAZOLE

NEO-MERCAZOLE – Tablets

Carbimazole is an antithyroid drug which reduces thyroid hormone levels when the gland is overactive. Prolonged treatment lasts for about 18 months, during which time the disease may burn out. Carbimazole may be used in preparation for surgery (thyroidectomy) or before and after radioactive iodine treatment. Unwanted effects usually occur in the first eight weeks but improve as treatment continues. The most serious but rare adverse effect is bone-marrow depression which may lead to a blood disorder. Your doctor will ask you to report any fever, sore throat or mouth ulcers immediately.

Before you use this medicine

Tell your doctor if you are:
☐ pregnant – carbimazole may be used under very close super-

vision, although hyperthyroidism often remits during pregnancy ☐ breast-feeding – the baby must be carefully monitored ☐ taking any other medicines, including vitamins and those bought over the counter.

Tell your doctor if you have or have had:
☐ liver or kidney disorders ☐ sensitivity to carbimazole.

How to use this medicine

Take the tablets every day as directed by your doctor. At first you may take the dose two or three times a day, but once overactivity is controlled, after four to eight weeks, you may be able to take one dose a day.

Do not stop taking carbimazole suddenly as symptoms may recur. Treatment is usually continued for at least six months but may be up to two years. If you miss a dose take it as soon as you remember, but skip it if it is almost time for your next dose.

Over 65 No special requirements.

Unwanted effects

Likely Feeling sick, headache, dizziness, joint pains, mild stomach upsets, skin rashes and itching.
Unlikely Hair loss, fever, sore throat, mouth ulcers, jaundice.

The most likely effects are common at the start of treatment but usually fade as treatment continues. Skin rashes and itching respond to antihistamine treatment by mouth and carbimazole treatment can be continued. Occasionally your doctor may prescribe **propylthiouracil** in place of carbimazole. **If you have a sore throat or mouth ulcers, stop taking carbimazole and contact your doctor immediately as this may indicate a serious effect on blood cells.**

Similar preparations

PROPYLTHIOURACIL – Tablets

Adrenal disorders

There are two adrenal glands, each one lying above the top of a kidney. Each adrenal gland has a centre, the *medulla*, which secretes **adrenaline** and **noradrenaline**, and an outer layer, the *adrenal cortex*. The medulla and cortex behave as independent glands. The release of adrenaline and noradrenaline from the medulla is controlled by nerves. These body chemicals are especially active during a wide variety of stress conditions, such as anger, fear, cold, low blood-sugar and low blood pressure. Hormone production in the adrenal cortex, like the thyroid and the sex glands, is mainly regulated by the pituitary gland in the brain. Over 30 hormones are produced in the cortex to regulate the body's mineral salts and water balance and its response to stress and injury. There are three main groups:

□ *mineralocorticoids*, such as **aldosterone**, which regulates the mineral salts in the body, acting mainly on sodium to affect the water balance within the body and in turn influence blood volume
□ *glucocorticoids*, such as **hydrocortisone** (also known as **cortisol**), which regulates chemical conversion (metabolism) of sugar, proteins and fats
□ *sex hormones* (**androgens**, **oestrogens** and **progesterone**); the sex glands (*gonads*) are more important sites for making these hormones.

The hormones are grouped according to their main effects but some activities overlap. For example, **hydrocortisone** has mostly *glucocorticoid* activity but also some weak *mineralocorticoid* effects.

The blood level of hydrocortisone varies during the day, with higher levels in the morning and lower levels at night. This is called diurnal variation and can be important in scheduling treatment.

Disorders of the adrenal glands are relatively rare but both underactivity and overactivity can occur. The body's own immune system may be responsible for the destruction or underactivity of the gland and a tumour of the gland can cause overactivity or underactivity.

• *UNDERACTIVE ADRENAL GLANDS – ADDISON'S DISEASE* •

This is a general underfunctioning of the adrenal glands which is usually fatal if untreated. Symptoms include a fall in blood pressure, muscle weakness and patchy darkening (pigmentation) of the skin. Both glucocorticoid and mineralocorticoid hormones have to be replaced. **Hydrocortisone** is given to replace the glucocorticoid hormones twice a day, with the higher dose in the morning and a lower dose in the evening to take account of the diurnal variation in body hydrocortisone. **Fludrocortisone** (brand name Florinef) is usually used to replace the mineralocorticoid hormones. There are few unwanted effects from hydrocortisone because it is taken to replace the body's natural supply. If the glands have to be surgically removed (*adrenalectomy*), hydrocortisone must be replaced.

● *OVERACTIVE ADRENAL GLANDS* ●

If the level of the body's corticoid hormones greatly increases and diurnal variation is abolished, the resulting condition is called *Cushing's syndrome*. If the disorder is due to overactivity in the part of the pituitary that produces the **adrenocorticotrophic hormone** (ACTH) – the hormone responsible for controlling body levels of adrenal hormones – the condition is known as *Cushing's disease*. Extra ACTH prompts the adrenal glands to make more corticoid hormones, which results in many changes to body function. Treatment is usually by surgical means or irradiation.

Corticosteroids

Once the corticoid hormones were identified and extracted from adrenal glands, scientists were able to modify the steroid molecule to make synthetic **corticosteroids**. The term **corticosteroid** is used to describe the hormones produced by the cortex of the adrenal gland and also the man-made or synthetic drugs derived from these natural hormones. Some people refer to corticosteroid preparations as 'steroids' but this may lead to confusion with **anabolic steroids**, which are synthetic derivatives of male sex hormones with limited medical usefulness; their use as body builders and tonics is quite unjustified.

Although corticosteroids are used for replacing the body's hormones in rare disorders, they are used mainly for their anti-inflammatory properties in a wide variety of conditions. Corticosteroids are used for treating disorders where the body's immune system appears to be faulty resulting in inflammation, blood disorders, allergy or rheumatic conditions. These include asthma, rheumatoid arthritis, inflammatory conditions of the bowel, skin and eyes, systemic lupus erythematosus (an arthritic condition) and life-threatening disorders such as acute leukaemia.

Each preparation varies in the balance between its *glucocorticoid*

HOW YOU CAN HELP YOURSELF

☐ If you use a corticosteroid routinely, you should see your doctor regularly for checks.
☐ If you take a corticosteroid by mouth for longer than a period of one month, or you take one regularly, you should carry a 'steroid' warning card. If you have one treatment course of one month duration you should carry a steroid card for two years. Your doctor or pharmacist can give you a card.
☐ Note details of the name of the corticosteroid, the dosage and length of treatment time.
☐ Always have a reserve supply of your medicine. You must not stop taking a corticosteroid suddenly.
☐ If you have an illness such as diarrhoea, vomiting, a temperature or fever, continue taking your corticosteroid. Contact your doctor as you may need a higher dose during these sorts of illnesses.
☐ Always tell a new doctor, your dentist or any other person involved in your health care that you take a corticosteroid or that you have taken one.

and *mineralocorticoid* effects. Glucocorticoid effects are anti-inflammatory, an effect most prized for controlling a number of serious and life-threatening conditions. Research focuses on trying to separate the anti-inflammatory and anti-allergy effects of corticosteroids from their disruptive effects on body metabolism. The corticosteroids vary in their anti-inflammatory effect; for example, **betamethasone** is very potent, but **hydrocortisone** and **cortisone** are weaker. Drugs with strong mineralocorticoid activity such as **fludrocortisone** are not used for their anti-inflammatory effect, because salt and water balance will always be disrupted.

● *Using corticosteroids*

Corticosteroids were much misused and overused when they were first introduced in the 1950s. The long-term consequences of taking cortisone by mouth for a few years, for instance to relieve painful and swollen joints in rheumatoid arthritis, did not become visible until people's backbones and hip bones began to crumble. A corticosteroid has to be taken in a much higher dose than the body's source in order to produce its anti-inflammatory effect. The beneficial anti-inflammatory effect is then also accompanied by the risk of adverse effects. Your doctor must weigh up whether the benefits justify the adverse effects. A corticosteroid can be life-saving.

Whenever possible a corticosteroid should be used locally – for example in enemas or eye drops, by inhalation or by direct injection into a swollen joint – rather than taken by mouth when the risk of adverse effects is greater. An inhaled corticosteroid for controlling asthma symptoms is extremely valuable. It causes few unwanted effects by this route and tiny doses are used compared with those taken by mouth. Many people with nasal symptoms during the hay fever season can expect good relief from a local corticosteroid preparation without unwanted effects (see page 181).

A corticosteroid should always be used at the lowest possible dose for the shortest length of time, particularly in children, because long-term use may affect growth. When you take a corticosteroid by mouth it is always best to take it as a single dose in the morning. This causes less *adrenal suppression* (see page 326).

PREDNISOLONE

PREDNISOLONE – Tablets
DELTACORTRIL ENTERIC – Enteric-coated tablets
DELTASTAB – Tablets, injection
MINIMS PREDNISOLONE – Single-use eye drops
PRECORTISYL – Tablets, high-dose (Forte) tablets
PREDENEMA – Enema
PREDFOAM – Rectal foam
PRED FORTE – Eye drops
PREDNESOL – Tablets
PREDSOL – Enema, suppositories, ear/eye drops
SINTISONE – Tablets
With antibiotic
PREDSOL-N – Ear/eye drops (*not recommended* for eye)
PREDNISOLONE + NEOMYCIN

Prednisolone is a corticosteroid used for suppressing inflammatory and allergic disorders. Like other corticosteroids, it blocks the action of *prostaglandins*, body chemicals that are involved in the inflammatory process. It also dampens the immune system temporarily by reducing the activity of certain white blood cells. Short courses of oral treatment at low doses rarely cause serious adverse effects. Prednisolone is used locally in the eye to reduce inflammation and in joints to relieve pain and swelling, and in some cases to reduce deformity, caused by arthritis. A small amount of corticosteroid may be injected locally to help conditions such as tennis or golfer's elbow or tendinitis.

Before you use this medicine

Tell your doctor if you are:
☐ pregnant or breast-feeding ☐ taking any other medicines, including vitamins and those bought over the counter.

Tell your doctor if you have or have had:
☐ tuberculosis ☐ peptic ulcer ☐ diabetes ☐ heart disease ☐ high blood pressure ☐ glaucoma ☐ any infection ☐ depression ☐ kidney or liver disease ☐ osteoporosis ☐ seizures (epilepsy).

How to use this medicine

Tablets Take the dose according to the doctor's directions. Do not take more than the dose prescribed for you.
Eye drops These are used only after visual acuity tests and checks to see that there is no infection. Your doctor should review treatment every few days. Contact your doctor if symptoms do not improve after five to seven days or the condition worsens. A corticosteroid with an antibiotic such as neomycin is rarely needed.

During prolonged courses of treatment by mouth or injection, eat food low in salt (sodium) and rich in potassium and protein. Avoid alcohol when you take prednisolone by mouth as this may increase the likelihood of developing an ulcer.

Do not stop taking prednisolone suddenly; your doctor will give you a schedule for reducing the dose gradually. Carry a steroid warning card with you if you take prednisolone by mouth for longer than a month.

If you miss a dose take it as soon as you remember. If your next dose is due within 6 hours, take the missed dose and skip the next one. If you need to have surgery, tell your doctor or dentist that you take a corticosteroid.

Over 65 Older people are more susceptible to the adverse effects of corticosteroids, which should only be used if absolutely necessary.

Interactions with other medicines

Various drugs interfere with the effect of prednisolone. Do not take other medicines including those sold over the counter without checking first with your doctor or pharmacist. Interactions do not generally apply to corticosteroids used locally – on the skin, inhaled or injected into a joint.

Rifampicin (used against tuberculosis) and **anti-epileptics**, such as **phenytoin**, reduce the effect of prednisolone.

Unwanted effects

Likely Indigestion.
Unlikely Increased appetite, acne, muscle weakness, nervousness or restlessness, headache, dizziness, sleeplessness, increased body or facial hair, mood changes.

Serious unwanted effects occur only when prednisolone is taken by mouth in high doses or by injection and for long periods of time. See below.

Similar preparations

BETAMETHASONE:
BETNELAN; BETNESOL
CORTISONE:
CORTISTAB; CORTISYL
DEXAMETHASONE:
DECADRON
HYDROCORTISONE:
HYDROCORTISTAB; HYDROCORTONE; EFCORTELAN SOLUBLE; SOLU-CORTEF
METHYLPREDNISOLONE:
MEDRONE; SOLU-MEDRONE; DEPO-MEDRONE
PREDNISONE:
DECORTISYL
TRIAMCINOLONE:
KENALOG; LEDERCORT

SERIOUS UNWANTED EFFECTS

☐ Increased breakdown of protein resulting in muscle wasting and weakness: protein is also removed from skin which becomes thin and marked with purple stripes – also a delay in wound healing
☐ Increased use of carbohydrate to produce heat and energy resulting in diabetes mellitus
☐ Extra sodium is retained in the body resulting in additional water retention; this extra fluid (oedema) causes a rise in blood pressure
☐ Upset in fat breakdown leading to deposits of fat in the face (the characteristic 'moon face'), on the shoulders ('buffalo hump') and on the abdomen
☐ Lessening of the response to inflammation which may mask signs of infection
☐ Reduced ability to fight infection because of a fall in the number of white blood cells

□ Upset calcium balance resulting in the bones thinning and crumbling; extra calcium is removed from the body via the kidneys with an increased risk of kidney stones
□ Increased hair growth on the face, chest and abdomen
□ Acne
□ Absence of periods in women who are menstruating
□ Indigestion and possible peptic ulcer
□ Mood changes and mental disturbances, such as a heightened sense of well-being (euphoria) and depression
□ Reduction in the complex hormonal and nervous response to stress.

● *Adrenal suppression*

In taking an external source of a corticosteroid for more than a few weeks, the adrenal glands respond by not producing the body's usual amount of adrenal hormones. If you stop taking the external source suddenly, the body and the adrenal glands are unprepared, resulting in signs of acute (sudden) adrenal insufficiency. With long-term corticosteroid treatment the adrenal glands shut down because there is an external supply. Long-term treatment must be stopped gradually with the daily dose gently reduced. This may take weeks or even months depending on the dosage and how long you have been treated with a corticosteroid. Too rapid a reduction in dose can lead to collapse and even death. The adrenal glands usually recover, but may function less well.

In times of stress or illness, infection or surgery, or any increased demand on the body's reserves an additional dose of corticosteroid may be needed. For a person with proper functioning adrenal glands, extra hormones are produced to help the body cope with stress or illness. If you take a corticosteroid by mouth, the body cannot respond in the normal way, so the dose must be increased to compensate during the stressful period and then gradually decreased afterwards.

Sex hormone deficiencies

Hormones play a major part in the development and maintenance of the reproductive organs. The sex hormones are mainly produced by the sex glands (*gonads*): the *ovaries* in women and the *testes* in men. The female sex hormones are **oestrogen** and **progesterone**. The male sex hormones are called **androgens**, of which **testosterone** is the most important. The male sex hormones are produced at a constant rate whereas the female hormone production varies over a 28-day cycle. The male and female sex hormones are controlled by the *gonadotrophic hormones* produced by the pituitary gland.

● *FEMALE SEX HORMONES* ●

Women's reproductive organs consist of the two ovaries, the Fallopian or uterine tubes, the womb or uterus, vagina and vulva. The uterus is behind the bladder and in front of the rectum and is connected to the outside by the vagina. The inner lining of the womb is called the *endometrium*. When a girl is born, she has around a million egg-forming cells or follicles in each ovary. As she develops, many follicles die off, leaving around 300,000 at the age of eleven. At the start of menstruation one or possibly two follicles start to ripen every month under the influence of the gonadotrophic hormones. The follicles produce oestrogen, which causes the development of female characteristics: breasts, pubic hair, hair under the arms and widening of the pelvis. Oestrogen and progesterone and synthetic derivatives are used medically to replace body hormones when they are deficient, to prevent conception, to regulate periods and to treat certain cancers.

● *Ovulation*

Female sex hormones are produced in differing quantities over a 28-day cycle which prepares the body for fertilisation. The *follicle-stimulating hormone* (FSH) produced by the pituitary gland causes the egg cell within a follicle to ripen and stimulates oestrogen production. Under the combined influence of FSH, increased levels of oestrogen and the release of a second pituitary hormone – the *luteinising hormone* (LH) – the egg matures and *ovulation* (release of the egg) occurs. The egg is released from the follicle into the ovary and from there it passes into the Fallopian tube. Ovulation occurs in the middle of the menstrual cycle, around day 14, and sometimes causes abdominal pain. The egg travels along the Fallopian tube to the womb.

Under the influence of LH, the empty follicle produces the hormone progesterone. This circulates in blood and stops further ovulation during the cycle. The combined effect of oestrogen and progesterone during the second half of the cycle makes the lining of the womb thicken and prepare for pregnancy. If the egg is not fertilised and pregnancy does not occur, the empty follicle dies and the levels of oestrogen and progesterone fall, triggering menstruation: the egg and the thickened lining of the womb are shed with blood. The first day of blood loss is designated as day one of the cycle.

Hormone deficiency

In young women the delicate balance of sex hormones can be upset at two places in the body – the pituitary gland and the ovaries. In either case the disruption in hormonal production means that there are no monthly periods and sexual development is halted. Tests can show the type of deficiency and your doctor can then prescribe the appropriate preparations to supplement either the gonadotrophins or oestrogen and progesterone. Other causes of periods stopping between puberty and the menopause include excessive loss of weight, as in the slimmer's disease *anorexia nervosa*, hard physical training, thyroid disorders and medicines which increase levels of **prolactin**, the pituitary hormone which controls the production of breast-milk.

The menopause

As a woman grows older the egg-forming cells or follicles decrease until there are approximately 8,000 left around the age of 44. Only a few of these follicles will ripen to produce eggs and fertility gradually declines with age. As the ovaries slowly stop working, less oestrogen and progesterone are produced. At around 50 years the egg supply stops and with it monthly periods. The age at which women's periods begin and when they stop varies but it is rare for periods to continue beyond the age of 55. Each woman's levels of hormones are unique, so your body will have its own way of reacting to the hormonal change which happen around the time of the menopause.

The menopause happens broadly in three stages:

Premenopause when you may experience irregular and more or less frequent periods, mood changes and hot flushes.

Perimenopause when periods become irregular. The date of the last period is known as the menopause. Because irregular periods make it difficult to determine this date you can only be certain your periods have stopped when you haven't had one for at least six months to a year. If periods stop before you are 50 you should allow two years to pass before you can say the menopause has occurred. Even if you have irregular periods, conception can still occur, so you will still need to use contraception until you are sure you are no longer having periods. Post-menopausal symptoms begin at this time, although two out of ten women do not have problems.

Postmenopause Hormonal changes affect the body in a number of noticeable ways. You may experience hot flushes with sweating, especially at night, and palpitations, which may interrupt sleep and lead to fatigue; vaginal and urethral dryness; mood changes; *osteoporosis* (thinning of the bones).

The main symptoms occur around the menopause but the falling level of sex hormones affects the body in many subtle ways. One effect is that up to the menopause a woman is protected against heart disease by oestrogen, but after the menopause the risk of cardiovascular disease such as heart attack or stroke increases.

● *Osteoporosis*

Both men and women start to lose bone gradually from their mid-thirties onwards, but women are more at risk of developing osteoporosis. Bone is lost quite rapidly in the first few years after the menopause and the process continues gradually as you grow older. It results in increased risk of bone fracture, particularly of hip joints, and curvature of the spine as load-bearing bones are crushed. Osteoporosis is more likely to be serious if you have two or more of the following risk factors:
☐ you are thin, of lean build or have small bones
☐ you are white or Asian
☐ you have had an early menopause
☐ you have a high daily alcohol intake
☐ you are having or have recently had oral corticosteroid treatment
☐ you have certain illnesses, including myeloma (a tumour of bone-marrow cells), rheumatoid arthritis, chronic liver disease and glandular disorders such as thyrotoxicosis and Cushing's disease.

Hormone replacement therapy

The menopause is a natural occurrence for every woman. Menopausal symptoms are not life-threatening but if you have distressing symptoms which disrupt your life you may wish to take an external supply of hormones to replace the body's oestrogen and progesterone. This is called hormone replacement therapy (HRT). Low doses of an oestrogen are given with 10–13 days of a *progestogen* (a synthetic equivalent of progesterone) to protect the womb from changes in the endometrial lining brought about by the oestrogen, which could possibly lead to cancer. A progestogen opposes the effects of oestrogen on the womb. If you have already had your womb removed (see 'Surgical menopause', page 332) you do not need to take a progestogen.

HRT can be very beneficial and can help if you have hot flushes, vaginal dryness and urinary problems or are at a high risk of osteoporosis. If you have vaginal symptoms only, these may

HOW YOU CAN HELP YOURSELF

Hot flushes and sweating

☐ Wear several layers of light clothing so that you can peel off or put on a layer as your body temperature changes. Wear cotton because it allows the skin to breathe and air to circulate and use cotton sheets.

☐ Lie on a large towel in bed so that you do not have to change the sheets every time you break out in a sweat.

☐ Have a tepid shower when you feel unbearably hot.

☐ Avoid tea, coffee, alcohol and spicy foods as these aggravate flushes.

☐ If you take any medicines, ask your doctor whether they could give you flushes.

Vaginal and urethral dryness The lining of the vagina becomes thin and dry. Secretions lessen and intercourse may be painful, sometimes with bleeding. There may be infection and discharge. Similar changes can occur in the bladder and the urethra, leading to cystitis (see page 283). You may have stress incontinence – leaking urine when you cough, laugh or sneeze.

☐ Use a lubricant before intercourse.

☐ Regular love making, masturbation and pelvic floor muscle exercises all help to stimulate secretions and keep the vagina moist.

☐ If you have severe symptoms see your doctor. A local oestrogen cream or hormone replacement treatment can help.

☐ Talk about sexual difficulties with your partner or try a counselling service.

☐ For stress incontinence, tone up your pelvic floor muscles: when you pass urine, pull up and back on the muscles in mid-flow to stop urine flow for a few seconds; relax, release the muscle and allow urine to flow and empty the bladder completely. When you have learnt the action you can practise these exercises at any time.

Mood changes The late forties are often the most stressful time in your life, not just because of the menopause but because there may be family, job and social changes as well.

☐ Find time to relax and be peaceful on your own away from children and other worries.

☐ Join a yoga or relaxation class. Yoga can help you to tone muscles as well as relax.

☐ Share your worries with your partner, friend or neighbour.

Thinning of the bones

☐ Regular exercise such as half an hour's daily walking,

jogging or dancing can reduce bone loss. Exercise from childhood onwards is extremely important to build strong healthy bones. Routine exercise is also valuable in helping with weight loss and for getting rid of tension.

☐ Make sure there is enough calcium in your diet. The recommended daily amount is 800mg per day; one pint of milk contains about 700mg of calcium.

☐ If you have had an early menopause or have your ovaries removed, ask your doctor about hormone replacement therapy and calcium supplementation. **Etidronate** (brand name Didronel PMO) is used to increase bone density when fractures of the spine have occurred; it is taken for two weeks, followed by 11 weeks of calcium treatment.

See your doctor once a year to have your blood pressure checked as it tends to go up at the time of the menopause. You should check your breasts every month, but your doctor should also examine them once a year and you may want to consider a breast X-ray (*mammography*). You should have a cervical smear every three years.

You should see your doctor if you have:

☐ irregular bleeding between periods

☐ bleeding after more than six months without a period

☐ severe abdominal pain

☐ a dragging feeling or heaviness in the pelvis; this may mean the organs in the abdomen are beginning to drop (prolapse) because of slack muscles, a common condition which can be surgically treated

☐ frequent urination or inability to hold urine

☐ severe vaginal infection or itchiness of the vulva.

respond to a short course of an oestrogen cream used locally for a few weeks. Hot flushes, vaginal symptoms and night sweats which disrupt sleep can be helped by systemic treatment. HRT also helps to prevent osteoporosis. However, if you already have thin bones HRT cannot reverse this bone loss, but it can prevent further decline in bone density. The risk of cardiovascular disease increases sharply after the menopause due to declining levels of oestrogen, but HRT protects against heart attacks and stroke.

While many of the advantages and disadvantages of HRT are known, the relative risks and benefits of the various HRT preparations have still to be completely established. There is an increased risk of endometrial cancer if you take oestrogen on its own and have not had a hysterectomy, but taking a progestogen for 10–13 days in the month counteracts this. After some years of HRT use there may possibly be increased risk of breast cancer.

HRT is not an elixir of youth, although it is heavily promoted as the pill that will keep women young, sexually active and free from emotional problems. Research shows that reduced oestrogen levels in the body are not responsible for psychiatric problems and replacing the oestrogen is unlikely to cure these problems. Vaginal dryness is helped by oestrogen treatment but general loss of sexual interest has more to do with relationship and other strains on life. The years leading up to the menopause are generally the most stressful in women's lives and problems need to be disentangled from the effects of the menopause.

• *How long should you take HRT?*

Doctors do not agree about the duration of treatment and you will need to discuss this before starting HRT. Menopausal symptoms fade after some time but this varies from woman to woman. If you are taking HRT to relieve menopausal symptoms you could try a course for 6–12 months and then stop gradually and see if troublesome symptoms return. You can always restart if symptoms recur. If you feel comfortable taking HRT and do not experience unwanted effects, you can carry on for many years as long as you visit your doctor for regular checks. If you do not have a womb, ten years' treatment is usual. If you are at risk of developing osteoporosis you may also need treatment for some years, but staying fit and active is also important.

SURGICAL MENOPAUSE

If you are under 50 and have not reached the menopause, but have a gynaecological problem such as cancer of the womb, fibroids or heavy bleeding, you may have the womb surgically removed (hysterectomy). Although your periods stop when you have a hysterectomy, you will go through the menopause later providing your ovaries have not been removed. The ovaries are important organs as they produce oestrogen and progesterone throughout your life from puberty onwards, although after the menopause levels are much reduced. Unless one or both ovaries are diseased, you should not have them removed. If they have to be removed you may experience an immediate and often severe menopause. Your doctor will then recommend hormone replacement therapy.

• *OESTROGEN REPLACEMENT PREPARATIONS* •

Natural oestrogens (**oestradiol**, **oestriol**, or **oestrone**) are generally used because they are believed to cause less nausea and have a lower risk of thrombosis than synthetic alternatives. They can be taken by mouth, given as an injection or an implant, applied to the skin in a patch or used locally as a cream in the vagina.

Tablets are commonly used, especially if you have to take progesterone or the synthetic equivalent (a progestogen) to oppose the effects of oestrogen. Some preparations of oestrogen with a progestogen are taken continuously whereas others (cyclical preparations) are taken for only 21 days followed by a seven-day break. Combined HRT does not provide effective contraception, but nor should it be taken at the same time as an oral contraceptive. Another method of contraception should be chosen if it is needed. Discuss this with your doctor.

Implants are long-acting oestrogen preparations which are inserted under the skin, where they gradually release the hormone over a period of months. They may be used after hysterectomy, when you do not have to take a progestogen. If you have a womb you will have to remember to take a progestogen for 10–13 days of the cycle. Oestrogen is broken down in the liver so not all a dose by mouth is effective in the body. Using an implant can overcome this problem but sometimes oestrogen levels become too high and the effects cannot be stopped quickly.

A skin patch containing oestrogen (brand name Estraderm TTS) releases the drug slowly through the skin (transdermally). This method also avoids oestrogen passing through the liver. A plaster is applied every three to four days to a clean, dry hairless area of unbroken skin below the waist where there is little rubbing from clothes. The plaster should not be applied on or near the breasts. It can be kept on when bathing or showering. Redness, itching and rash sometimes occur but fade when the plaster is removed, so a different site should be used each time it is changed. Estracombi is a patch system providing oestrogen plus two weeks of progestogen per month, so that if you have a womb you will not have to remember to take progestogen tablets as well for 10–13 days of the cycle.

Local oestrogen cream pessaries can be used for vaginal problems, but oestrogen passes into the bloodstream from the vagina in variable amounts. A cream should be used for a short time, say two to three weeks. Long-term use is not recommended, particularly if you have a womb, as you will be absorbing oestrogen unopposed by a progestogen. If symptoms return when you stop using the cream, your doctor may suggest trying another form of HRT. Preparations include **dienoestrol** (brand name Ortho Dienoestrol), **oestriol** (Ortho-Gynest; Ovestin), **conjugated oestrogens** (Premarin), **oestradiol** vaginal tablets (Vagifem) and **stilboestrol** (Tampovagan Stilboestrol and Lactic Acid), which is not recommended.

• *PROGESTERONE REPLACEMENT PREPARATIONS* •

A progestogen (a synthetic equivalent of progesterone) should always be used if you have a womb as it modifies some of oestrogen's effects. Oestrogen replacement on its own stimulates growth of the lining of the womb, which may lead to cancerous changes. A progestogen given for 10–13 days out of 28 abolishes oestrogen's effect on the womb lining. When a progestogen is added, the endometrium may be shed as a 'period'. If you still have irregular periods, a combined preparation will help to make the cycle regular. Progestogens may work against some of the beneficial effects of oestrogen, aggravating menopausal symptoms.

CONJUGATED OESTROGENS

PREMARIN – Tablets, vaginal cream
OESTROGEN

PREMPAK-C – Tablets
OESTROGEN + NORGESTREL

You have to pay double the prescription charge because the pack contains two different medicines.

Conjugated oestrogens are a mixture of natural oestrogens used in low doses for replacing the body's own oestrogen supply as it dwindles at the menopause. They relieve the uncomfortable symptoms of hot flushes, night sweats and vaginal and bladder problems. Hormone replacement therapy also helps to prevent osteoporosis. Premarin is an oestrogen-only product and can be used if you do not have a womb – when a progestogen is not needed. If you have a womb you will need to take the cyclical preparation Prempak-C, which contains oestrogen and the progestogen **norgestrel**. The vaginal cream can be used for short periods to relieve vaginal and bladder symptoms of dryness and pain, but with long-term treatment you will also need to take a progestogen by mouth.

Before you use this medicine

Tell your doctor if you are:
☐ pregnant – do not take HRT during pregnancy ☐ breast-feeding – high doses suppress milk flow ☐ taking any other medicines, including vitamins and those bought over the counter.

Tell your doctor if you have or have had:
☐ high blood pressure or heart disease ☐ liver or kidney disease ☐ diabetes ☐ epilepsy or migraine ☐ asthma.

Do not take if you have or have had:
☐ oestrogen-dependent cancer or breast cancer ☐ abnormal vaginal bleeding ☐ severe liver disease ☐ abnormal blood clots in your veins (deep vein thrombosis) ☐ endometriosis ☐ porphyria ☐ sickle-cell anaemia ☐ herpes during pregnancy ☐ deterioration of the hearing problem otosclerosis.

How to use this medicine

Before you start HRT you should have a complete physical and gynaecological check. Once you have started treatment see your doctor regularly every 6–12 months. You should contact your doctor if you have any unusual breakthrough bleeding.
Tablets Take one tablet daily. Premarin is taken for three weeks followed by one week off. With Prempak-C the oestrogen tablet is taken continuously and norgestrel is taken during days 17–28.
Vaginal cream Apply locally or insert the applicator with the measured dose into the vagina. Intravaginal treatment should be started on the fifth day of bleeding if you are still having periods or otherwise as your doctor directs. Treatment should be continued for three weeks followed by one week off. For long-term treatment you must take a progestogen by mouth.

Do not stop taking this medicine suddenly as symptoms may return. Ask your doctor to give you a schedule to reduce the dose gradually. If you miss a dose take it as soon as you remember. It is very important to remember to take the progestogen tablets. If you have surgery you may need to stop taking HRT a few weeks before the operation.

Over 65 The lowest possible dose should be used, but there are no special requirements.

Interactions with other medicines

The low doses used in HRT are unlikely to cause significant problems. Check with your doctor or pharmacist.

Unwanted effects

Likely Feeling sick, bloating, weight gain, swollen ankles, breast tenderness or swelling, intolerance to wearing contact lenses, changes in hair growth.
Unlikely Breakthrough bleeding, vaginal candidiasis, reduced sex drive, headaches, depression, irritability, pains in chest, groin, leg or calf, sudden loss of co-ordination, weakness or numbness in arm or leg, shortness of breath, breast lumps or discharge, yellowing of the eyes or skin, skin rash.

Effects such as feeling sick and breast tenderness usually wear off after a few weeks' treatment. If not, contact your doctor. If you have breakthrough bleeding, depression or generally feel unwell during treatment see your doctor.

Similar preparations

Oestrogen-only
CLIMAVAL – Tablets
HARMOGEN – Tablets
HORMONIN – Tablets
OVESTIN – Tablets
PROGYNOVA – Tablets

Oestrogen + progestogen
MENOPHASE – Tablets (13 days of progestogen)
NUVELLE – Tablets (10 days of progestogen)
TRISEQUENS – Tablets (10 days of progestogen)

Tibolone (Livial) is a new hormonal steroid treatment for relieving menopausal symptoms such as hot flushes and sweating. It is not yet recommended for preventing bone-thinning after the menopause. It suppresses levels of gonadotrophic hormones produced in the pituitary and can be given about one year after periods have stopped. Tibolone does not stimulate the womb lining, so you do not have to take a progestogen to protect against disordered endometrial growth and there is no monthly bleeding. If you do experience any vaginal bleeding, discuss this with your doctor. The cautions and unwanted effects appear to be similar to those of oestrogens. Experience with this new product is limited and it is not clear how long treatment should continue or whether symptoms return on stopping the drug.

● *MALE SEX HORMONES* ●

The testes make the male sex hormones (*androgens*) under the influence of a gonadotrophic hormone produced by the pituitary gland. This occurs at puberty when the main androgen, **testosterone**, brings about sexual changes. Testosterone has *androgenic* effects which cause the voice box to enlarge and the voice to deepen, hair to grow in various parts of the body and the growth of the reproductive organs. The testes produce sperm, the male reproductive cells, at puberty and for the rest of the man's life. Testosterone also has *anabolic* effects, which cause bone and body growth and muscle development.

Sexual difficulties are rarely due to testosterone deficiency and hormone replacement therapy for men is rarely needed. Testosterone replacement therapy is given when the body is not making its own or levels are too low. This may be due to lack of development or underdevelopment of the testes or a failure of the pituitary gland to produce a gonadotrophin to stimulate testosterone production in the testes. If puberty is delayed in a boy, a course of testosterone may be considered. However, testosterone can eventually stunt growth because it closes off the growing ends of the long bones. Hormonal treatment may therefore be given after growth is completed and always with specialist advice.

In men with low levels of testosterone, replacement therapy may help to overcome impotence and loss of sex drive, but not infertility. Men with low gonadotrophin levels may have gonadotrophin treatment and this helps fertility. Testosterone replacement is usually given by long-lasting intramuscular depot injection every three to four weeks because testosterone is broken down in the liver when it is taken by mouth. However, some preparations of testosterone can be effective when taken by mouth.

Additional male sex hormones will not boost testosterone levels if they are normal nor will they help impotence caused by psychological problems.

Women are sometimes treated with male hormones for certain types of cancer of the breast. Testosterone has been used in some hormone replacement preparations, but there is little scientific evidence to support its use and it is not recommended. Male hormones given to women in large and continued doses can cause masculine features to develop.

REPRODUCTIVE AND URINARY SYSTEMS

Period problems Contraception Bladder disorders

The reproductive systems of both men and women are described briefly in Chapter 6.

The urinary system removes liquid waste from the body. As blood passes through the kidneys, waste products and water are filtered out and then discharged from the body at intervals. In both men and women the urinary system consists of two kidneys, each with a muscular tube, the *ureter*, running to the bladder. The bladder is a muscular storage tank for urine and can hold up to about a pint of fluid until it is convenient to empty it through the tube that leads to the outside, the *urethra*. A tight ring of sphincter muscles at the bladder outlet keep a constant pressure on the urethra to prevent urine escaping.

Infection of the reproductive organs may be sexually transmitted but is not always so, particularly in women. In men infection of the urinary system is uncommon because it is harder for bacteria and other organisms to gain access to the bladder and kidneys through the long urethra. A woman's urethra is shorter and the opening nearer to the vaginal and rectal openings provides easier access for infecting organisms. Bladder infections are common (see 'Cystitis', page 283). See Chapter 5 for medicines active against invading micro-organisms.

Period problems

Period problems include heavy blood loss (*menorrhagia*), painful periods (*dysmenorrhoea*) and premenstrual syndrome – physical symptoms and mood changes that occur before a period. *Endometriosis* (see page 340) is a less common problem, but can cause painful periods. The menstrual cycle is usually 28 days although this can vary from woman to woman and anything from 21–35 days is considered normal. Hormones produced by the pituitary gland and the ovaries control and regulate the reproductive cycle and bleeding when the egg has not been fertilised.

HEAVY PERIODS – MENORRHAGIA

Continued excessive blood loss during periods can be exhausting and interfere with daily living. It is one of the commonest causes of iron deficiency anaemia in women. You may be used to the occasional heavy period but if this pattern continues you should see your doctor. The reason for heavy bleeding should be investigated and your doctor may ask you to keep a record of bleeding over a number of weeks noting each day whether it is heavy, moderate or light and whether you have pain. Excessive blood loss is most commonly the result of abnormal bleeding from the womb, but there may be an underlying gynaecological reason such as endometriosis, pelvic inflammatory disease (PID), a uterine or ovarian growth or the intra-uterine contraceptive device (IUD). Hormonal imbalance such as a thyroid disorder can cause excessive bleeding and so can abnormalities of the blood clotting mechanism.

Your doctor may suggest a minor operation, a *dilatation and curettage* (D&C), a procedure which involves scraping away the lining of the womb (*endometrium*) to allow it to re-grow. The newest treatment for heavy periods is to remove the endometrium using a laser (*laser ablation*). Removal of the womb (*hysterectomy*) is the final solution to heavy bleeding. However, there are a number of drug treatments and you may prefer to try a medicine before accepting a surgical procedure.

The combined oral contraceptive can reduce blood loss but is not suitable for every woman, for example if you have or have had heart disease or blood clotting problems or if you smoke and are over the age of 35 years. A non-steroidal anti-inflammatory drug (NSAID) blocks prostaglandins and reduces bleeding as well as pain. You take the NSAID just before or as soon as menstruation starts and for as many days as bleeding is troublesome. You may be able to shorten the course and/or reduce the dose in subsequent periods. **Tranexamic acid** (brand name Cyklokapron) is a medicine which reduces blood loss by acting on the blood clotting mechanism. It is only taken during heavy bleeding and for a maximum of three menstrual cycles. **Ethamsylate** (brand name Dicynene) works in a similar way.

Progestogen (one type of female sex hormone) taken for part of the cycle is also used for treating heavy bleeding although there is little evidence that it reduces blood loss. If you can take the combined oral contraceptive and you need contraception it is a good choice for controlling heavy bleeding. **Danazol**, a drug that appears to block pituitary hormone is used but has many unwanted effects. It is mainly used for treating endometriosis.

● *PAINFUL PERIODS – DYSMENORRHOEA* ●

Painful periods can happen at any age during your reproductive life, but they are quite common during puberty when you start periods (primary dysmenorrhoea). At this stage the hormones may be unbalanced and may trigger high levels of prostaglandins in the womb which cause pain and cramps. Period pains that begin when you are older (secondary dysmenorrhoea) may be caused by abnormal conditions of the womb or ovaries, such as infection, fibroids or endometriosis. You should see your doctor if period pains continue, so that any underlying problem can be investigated and treated.

Pain can be relieved with aspirin or paracetamol. The combined oral contraceptive stops ovulation and is effective in relieving painful periods. A progestogen on its own is also used.

● *PREMENSTRUAL SYNDROME* ●

Symptoms of premenstrual syndrome (also known as premenstrual tension) may occur for up to ten days before a period. They may vary from cycle to cycle. Psychological changes such as feelings of tension, irritability and depression and physical signs such as headache, bloating, and breast tenderness are common. There may be fluid retention and other symptoms such as itching, backache and muscle and joint pains. Attacks of certain conditions, for example asthma, migraine, epilepsy and rhinitis are more frequent than at other times. Once you have had your period the symptoms disappear. The symptoms appear to be triggered by the hormonal changes during the menstrual cycle, but particularly by a low level of progesterone.

Your doctor may ask you to keep a record of your menstrual cycle, the timing and nature of symptoms, how long they last and when your period begins. Treatment is not very satisfactory but the combined oral contraceptive sometimes seems to help. **Progestogens** have been used although there is little evidence of their value. **Pyridoxine** (vitamin B_6) and evening primrose oil have also been tried, but again there is little sound evidence to support their use in the premenstrual syndrome.

● *ENDOMETRIOSIS* ●

Occasionally small pieces of the lining of the womb, the endometrium, grow in other parts of the pelvic cavity outside the womb. Most commonly growths occur on the ovary, on the surface of the womb, bladder or bowel. Every month these pieces of tissue swell and bleed causing pain. Some blood is absorbed,

HOW YOU CAN HELP YOURSELF

☐ For painful or heavy periods you may need to rest in bed with a hot water bottle
☐ Take an analgesic regularly for pain relief
☐ Try to avoid stressful activities just before and during your period
☐ Note the dates of your periods and any unusual bleeding or symptoms
☐ Do not ignore menstrual problems; if they continue for a few cycles see your doctor
☐ You may like to contact one of a number of self-help groups for information and/or support – for example, the Endometriosis Society. See 'Useful addresses'.

but some may remain to form cysts on the ovaries or tissues may become sandwiched together with scar tissue to form adhesions. You may have severe pain just before or during the first few days of your period. Intercourse may be painful. Endometriosis can sometimes lead to infertility. The abnormal tissue can be removed surgically; hysterectomy or removal of one or both ovaries may be necessary. Drug treatment can sometimes avoid the need for surgery, particularly in mild cases.

The condition may respond to treatment with a progestogen given throughout the menstrual cycle; otherwise a six-month course of **danazol** (brand name Danol) is often effective. Danazol lowers the oestrogen and progesterone hormone levels during the cycle by blocking the *gonadotrophin* hormones. Ovulation stops in many women who take danazol but a low dose may not have this effect. You must make sure that you use effective non-hormonal contraception while you are on a course of danazol because it can cause masculine features to develop in a female foetus. You should not take danazol if you are pregnant. Danazol commonly causes weight gain, acne and a decreased interest in sex but these unwanted effects disappear once you stop treatment. Other unwanted effects include headache, nausea, dizziness, muscle cramps, lassitude, voice changes and extra hair growth.

Gestrinone (brand name Dimetriose) is similar to danazol, but needs to be taken only twice a week because it acts in the body for several days. The twice-weekly dosage may be preferred by some women, but if you forget more than one dose, treatment is interrupted until the next cycle. As with danazol, you must not become pregnant while taking gestrinone.

MEFENAMIC ACID

MEFENAMIC ACID – Capsules, tablets
PONSTAN – Capsules, tablets, soluble tablets, liquid

Mefenamic acid is a non-steroidal anti-inflammatory drug (NSAID) which relieves pain and swelling in arthritis and is used as an analgesic for relieving pain and for reducing fever in children. It is also used for relieving painful periods (primary dysmenorrhoea) and for treating excessive bleeding (menorrhagia). It acts by blocking the activity of *prostaglandins*, body chemicals involved in the transmission of pain. Like all NSAIDs mefenamic acid may cause gastrointestinal upsets and should not be given to anyone with a peptic ulcer.

Before you use this medicine

Tell your doctor if you are:
☐ pregnant or breast-feeding ☐ taking any other medicines, including vitamins and those bought over the counter.

Tell your doctor if you have or have had:
☐ liver or kidney disease ☐ high blood pressure.

Do not use if you have or have had:
☐ allergy to aspirin or other NSAIDs ☐ severe kidney disease ☐ peptic ulcer or digestive disorders including inflammatory bowel disease.

How to use this medicine

Take one tablet or capsule three times a day after food. Soluble tablets should be dissolved in half a tumblerful of water before taking. Children can be given the liquid for lowering a raised temperature but treatment should not be for longer than seven days, except for those with juvenile arthritis.

Mefenamic acid may occasionally cause drowsiness or dizziness. If affected do not drive or operate machinery. Avoid alcohol as it may increase the risk of stomach bleeding.

Over 65 You may need less than the adult dose. Use with caution if you are dehydrated or have kidney disease.

Interactions with other medicines

NSAIDs interact with a number of different medicines. Always check with your doctor or pharmacist.
Lithium Possibility of increased blood levels and risk of toxicity.

Unwanted effects

Likely Heartburn or indigestion, feeling sick, diarrhoea.
Unlikely Drowsiness, dizziness, constipation, abdominal pain or cramps, skin rash, wheezing or breathlessness.

If you develop severe diarrhoea or a skin rash while taking mefenamic acid, stop taking it and contact your doctor. You should not take mefenamic acid ever again. Contact your doctor immediately if you have bloody or black, tarry stools or vomit blood. In rare cases mefenamic acid may cause numbness or tingling arms or legs, if this happens contact your doctor.

Similar preparations

See other NSAIDs in Chapter 8

Contraception

Contraception is the prevention of conception and pregnancy. There are several different methods: hormonal contraception, barrier methods such as the condom (sheath) or diaphragm, intrauterine devices (IUD), and, more permanently, sterilisation.

HORMONAL CONTRACEPTION

In 1961 the UK Family Planning Association introduced the combined oral contraceptive, the 'pill', into its clinics and a new era of birth control began. The pill remains a popular and convenient method for preventing pregnancy and around three million British women, particularly those who have not yet had children, choose oral contraception. There are two main types of oral contraceptives: oestrogen and progestogen combined in one tablet (the combined oral contraceptive) and the progestogen-only type.

HOW YOU CAN HELP YOURSELF

☐ Plan your contraception: discuss the matter with your doctor or visit a family planning clinic.
☐ Find out what the various methods are and discuss the benefits and risks.
☐ Give up smoking, particularly if you take the combined pill, as this will lessen the rare but serious risks of blood clots and other cardiovascular problems.
☐ If you take an oral contraceptive, visit your doctor regularly for blood pressure measurements and checks on your breast and reproductive organs.
☐ Use a condom to protect against HIV and other sexually transmitted diseases.

Oral contraceptives

The combined oral contraceptive containing an oestrogen and a progestogen is a most effective form of contraception and the most popular type of pill. The doses of both oestrogen and progestogen are now much lower than in the preparations available when the pill was first introduced. Lower doses have lessened unwanted effects without reducing contraceptive efficacy. **Ethinyloestradiol**, an oestrogen commonly used in the pill, is present in quantities varying from 20 micrograms in low-dose preparations to 50 micrograms. **Mestranol**, another synthetic oestrogen is converted to ethinyloestradiol in the body and is used in several preparations. The progestogens **norethisterone**, **levonorgestrel** and **ethynodiol** are used in various brands of the combined pill. Newer progestogens (**desogestrel**, **gestodene** and **norgestimate**) may have a more favourable effect on body metabolism and are effective at lower doses than the older progestogens. You should use a preparation with the lowest oestrogen and progestogen content to give good cycle control and the fewest unwanted effects.

When an external source of oestrogen and progestogen is taken the body's hormonal control of ovulation is disrupted. The delicate balance and control between the sex hormones produced by the ovaries and the pituitary gland hormones, *follicle-stimulating hormone* (FSH) and *luteinising-hormone* (LH), produces the normal menstrual cycle and ovulation (see page 327). The hormones in the combined pill add to the body's supplies of oestrogen and progesterone so that the hormone levels are similar to those of pregnancy. In other words, the combined pill produces a state of 'pseudo-pregnancy'. The oestrogen content of the pill prevents the egg cell from ripening in the ovary by stopping FSH production, while the progestogen component acts on the cervix – the entrance to the womb – to form a sticky, mucous plug to prevent sperm entering. Progestogen also blocks LH production.

The combined pill can be started on day 1 of your period and is usually taken once a day for 21 days. You will then have seven days without the pill or may have seven inactive (placebo) tablets (in every day 'ED' formulations) to take before starting the next packet of pills. Bleeding usually occurs during this pill-free week. You will not need additional contraception unless you started the course on the fifth day of your period, when ovulation may not be stopped during the first cycle and you should use additional contraception. If you miss a pill, especially at the beginning or end of the packet, you are less well protected and may need to take additional contraceptive measures (see 'If you miss a pill', page 347).

The phased combined oral contraceptive is designed to provide a low total hormone dose and to mimic more closely the body's hormone patterns. There are two or three phases and each provides a different proportion of oestrogen and progestogen. Different phases are indicated by different coloured tablets and you have to take care to start with the correct tablets for day 1.

The progestogen-only pill can be taken if you are unable to take oestrogen in the combined pill, for instance if you smoke, have high blood pressure or heart disease or have diabetes. The progestogen-only pill can provide good and effective contraception if you are approaching the menopause. Its main drawbacks are that periods may disappear or become heavy and irregular with breakthrough bleeding and you have to be conscientious in taking the pill at the same time each day (or within three hours) – see 'If you miss a pill'.

● *Injections*

Medroxyprogesterone (brand name Depo-Provera) is a long-acting progestogen given by injection. Its effect lasts three months and it may be useful as an interim measure, for example before your partner's vasectomy becomes effective. It is as effective as the combined pill, reversible and can be used without an upper age limit in smokers and if you cannot tolerate oestrogen. Irregular periods can happen and transient infertility may occur after stopping treatment. **Norethisterone enanthate** (brand name Noristerat) is another long-acting progestogen given as an injection which is effective for eight weeks. Future developments with progestogen compounds include the vaginal ring and pellets for insertion under the skin. These ways of giving progestogen may reduce unwanted effects and will avoid daily pill-taking.

Should you take the pill?

Taking any medicine carries some risks as well as bringing benefits. When you take the pill you should understand that you are taking a medicine that will modify your body's hormonal system even though you are not unwell. Discuss with your doctor the pros and cons of taking oral contraception and of other contraceptive methods. It is important to find an effective contraceptive method that you and your partner are happy and relaxed with. Oral contraception is not suitable for every woman and your doctor will need to check carefully that you do not have a condition that prevents you from using this form of contraception.

The combined pill is very effective as long as you take the pill regularly. It is convenient and does not get in the way of lovemaking. If you are a healthy, non-smoker and have no risk factors such as heart disease, you may take the pill up to the age of 45. Period problems such as painful or heavy bleeding are helped by taking the combined pill. Premenstrual tension may be reduced and you are less likely to have other gynaecological disorders, for example cancer of the lining of the womb and of the ovary, ovarian cysts, tubal pregnancy (ectopic pregnancy), infections of the womb and Fallopian tubes (pelvic inflammatory disease), anaemia because of heavy periods and non-cancerous diseases of the breast (benign breast disease).

However, oestrogen increases the risk of abnormal blood clots forming, particularly in the deep veins of the legs or pelvis. The clot may break off and travel to the heart, lungs or the blood vessels in the brain to cause conditions such as heart attack, angina or stroke and possibly death. Lower doses of oestrogen in the pill (below 50 micrograms) have reduced this risk considerably. There is also a risk of high blood pressure, jaundice, cancer of the liver and gallstones. There is still a debate about whether you are at greater risk of developing breast cancer by the age of 35 if you started the pill when you were young. For women who start the pill after the age of 25 the risk does not increase for however long you take it up to the age of 45. The combined oral contraceptive protects against ovarian and endometrial cancer and any cancer-promoting effects have to be balanced against these well established facts.

If you smoke you should stop taking the combined pill at the age of 35 because the risks of heart disease become too high. Other factors that increase risks are heart disease or a family history of heart disease or circulatory disorders, varicose veins, being overweight, diabetes mellitus, long-term treatment with other medicines and prolonged immobilisation due to illness or accident.

The progestogen-only pill avoids some of the risks of the combined pill and the effects of oestrogen. It is reasonably reliable and if you take it at the same time each day its effectiveness is improved. It is convenient and does not get in the way of lovemaking. It can be used while breast-feeding and allows a rapid return to fertility when stopped. The risks are irregular periods, heart or circulatory disease, ectopic pregnancy and ovarian cysts.

IF YOU MISS A PILL

● *Combined and phased pills*

It is important to bear in mind that the critical time for loss of protection is when a pill is forgotten at the *beginning* or *end* of a cycle. The following advice is now recommended by family planning organisations:

'If you forget a pill, take it as soon as you remember, and the next one at your normal time. If you are 12 or more hours late with any pill (especially the first or last in the packet) the pill may not work. As soon as you remember, continue normal pill taking. However, you will not be protected for the next seven days and must either not have sex or use another method such as the sheath.

If these seven days run beyond the end of your packet, start the next packet at once when you have finished the present one – do not have a gap between packets. This will mean you may not have a period until the end of two packets but this does you no harm. Nor does it matter if you see some bleeding on tablet-taking days. If you are using every day (ED) pills, miss out the seven inactive pills. If you are not sure which these are, ask your doctor.'

● *Progestogen-only pills*

The following advice is now recommended by family planning organisations:

'If you forget a pill, take it as soon as you remember and carry on with the next pill at the right time. If the pill was more than three hours overdue you are not protected. Continue normal pill-taking but you must also use another method, such as the sheath, for the next 48 hours.

If you have vomiting or very severe diarrhoea the pill may not work. Continue to take it, but you may not be protected from the first day of vomiting or diarrhoea. Use another method, such as the sheath, for any intercourse during the stomach upset and for the next 48 hours.'

The morning-after pill

If you have unprotected intercourse but had not planned to, you can prevent an unintended pregnancy by taking hormone tablets within 72 hours. Your doctor can prescribe four high-dose oestrogen and progestogen pills, two of which must be taken within 72 hours of the first episode of unprotected intercourse and the second two pills exactly 12 hours later. The tablets (Schering PC4), each containing **ethinyloestradiol** 50 micrograms and **levonorgestrel** 250 micrograms, probably prevent the implantation of a fertilised egg or stop ovulation depending at what stage of the menstrual cycle they are taken. The high doses of oestrogen and progestogen in this pill can make you feel sick or vomit but these symptoms are short-lived and rarely serious. If you are sick after taking the first tablets, the doctor will have to give you a further course of tablets, perhaps with an anti-emetic to stop you being sick again.

This method cannot be used in established pregnancies, nor for intercourse which has taken place more than 72 hours earlier. It will not protect you against future intercourse later in the cycle. These high-dose tablets are effective but there is a failure rate of about two to four per cent if you have unprotected intercourse in mid-cycle, when ovulation occurs. Although no cases have been reported, there is a theoretical risk of abnormalities in the developing baby if the course of tablets fails. You will need to see your doctor again three to four weeks after the course of tablets to make sure you are not pregnant. Your next period should come as normal, but you should not worry if it is up to a week later than the expected time as this is common after high-dose hormonal treatment.

An alternative to the morning-after pill, which is usually for emergency treatment, is the insertion of an intrauterine device (IUD). This is effective if the device is inserted within five days of unprotected intercourse.

ETHINYLOESTRADIOL

Combination preparations *(see also page 354)*
ETHINYLOESTRADIOL 20 MICROGRAMS:
MERCILON[1]

ETHINYLOESTRADIOL 30 MICROGRAMS:
CONOVA 30; EUGYNON 30; FEMODENE[1]; FEMODENE ED[1]; LOESTRIN 30; MARVELON[1]; MICROGYNON 30; MINULET[1]; OVRAN 30; OVRANETTE.

ETHINYLOESTRADIOL 35 MICROGRAMS:
BREVINOR; ▼CILEST[1]; NEOCON 1/35; NORIMIN; OVYSMEN

ETHINYLOESTRADIOL 50 MICROGRAMS:
OVRAN; SCHERING PC4 (emergency contraception)

Poor choice (less effective cycle control)
LOESTRIN 20
ETHINYLOESTRADIOL 20 MICROGRAMS

Phased preparations
BINOVUM; LOGYNON; LOGYNON ED; SYNPHASE; TRIADENE[1]; TRI-MINULET[1]; TRINORDIOL; TRINOVUM; TRINOVUM ED

For severe acne
DIANETTE – Tablets
ETHINYLOESTRADIOL 35 MICROGRAMS + CYPROTERONE 2MG

1 Contains newer progestogen

Ethinyloestradiol is a synthetic female sex hormone. It is used mainly in combination with a progestogen in the combined oral contraceptive to prevent pregnancy. If taken regularly, which is essential for low-dose preparations, the combined oral contraceptive offers very effective contraception. In high doses oestrogen is used with a progestogen for emergency contraception in the morning-after pill.

Ethinyloestradiol is also used in lower doses to supplement the body's oestrogen levels and to relieve menopausal symptoms. It can be taken without a progestogen if you have had a hysterectomy. When oestradiol is combined with cyproterone it is effective treatment for severe acne which has not responded to antibacterial therapy. It is also an effective oral contraceptive. Ethinyloestradiol is a potent oestrogen and is sometimes used in the treatment of breast cancer.

Before you use this medicine

Tell your doctor if you are:
□ pregnant – the pill should not be taken as there may be a small risk of malformation in the baby □ breast-feeding – oestrogen + progestogen does not usually affect established milk flow, but suppression may occur if it is not established; a progestogen-only contraceptive is preferable □ taking any other medicines, including vitamins and those bought over the counter.

Tell your doctor if you have or have had:
☐ diabetes ☐ heart disease or high blood pressure ☐ kidney disease ☐ migraine ☐ epilepsy or seizures ☐ depression ☐ asthma ☐ varicose veins ☐ sickle-cell anaemia.

Do not take if you have or have had:
☐ blood clots ☐ recurrent jaundice – acute and chronic liver disease ☐ porphyria ☐ high levels of blood fats (hyperlipidaemia) ☐ breast or endometrial cancer ☐ oestrogen-dependent tumours ☐ severe migraine ☐ unexplained vaginal bleeding ☐ itching of whole body during pregnancy (herpes gestationis) ☐ certain types of jaundice (Dubin-Johnson or Rotor syndromes) ☐ deterioration of the ear problem otosclerosis during pregnancy.

How to use this medicine

Take the pill marked day 1 or number 1 or the correct day of the week on the first day of your period. Take one pill daily, if possible at the same time each day until you finish the 21 pills in the pack. For every day (ED) preparations you take 28 pills. If you start the pill on the first day of bleeding, you will be protected from the first day and do not need additional contraceptive measures. If you start your course of pills on the fifth day of bleeding, you will need to take additional precautions for seven days.

After you have taken the course of 21 pills, you have a pill-free week during which time bleeding may occur. You will probably have less bleeding and it may be a different shade of red. Sometimes bleeding occurs while you are taking the pills – this is called breakthrough bleeding. Do not stop taking the pills but mention this to your doctor or nurse when you go for a check up. For ED preparations you start a new pack as soon as you have finished the course of 28 pills.

If you change from one combined pill to another, if possible take the first pill of your new pack on the day immediately after finishing your old pack. Bleeding will be delayed until you have finished the new course, although you may get some irregular bleeding in the meantime. You will not need additional contraception.

For other uses of ethinyloestradiol take the tablet as directed.

If you have to have surgery you may need to stop taking ethinyloestradiol four weeks before major surgery or any surgery to the legs. You can usually start taking the pill two weeks after the operation. If you have to lie in bed for some time because of an accident or a long illness then it is best to stop taking the pill until you are active again.

Do not stop taking the pill unless you have decided that you want to have a baby. You should wait until you have had two periods after stopping the pill before you try to get pregnant. Ask your doctor about other contraceptive precautions to cover this time. If you become pregnant straight away, this should not be harmful. If you are taking ethinyloestradiol for other reasons, your doctor will give you a schedule to reduce the dose gradually.

If you miss a dose, take it as soon as you remember – see 'If you miss a pill', page 347.

Over 65 There are similar oestrogens in hormone replacement preparations.

Interactions with other medicines

Ethinyloestradiol interacts with a number of medicines. Do not take other medicines without checking with your doctor or pharmacist. If you are taking long-term medication (for example, for epilepsy) you may need to take a higher-dose pill. These are the most important interactions:

Antibacterials: rifampicin reduces the effectiveness of the pill. Other broad-spectrum antibiotics, such as **ampicillin** and **tetracycline** may do this although the risk is small. You may need to use additional contraceptive measures such as the condom while you are on a course of antibiotics.

Anticoagulants Blood thinning effect reduced by ethinyloestradiol.

Antiepileptics: carbamazepine, **phenobarbitone**, **phenytoin** and **primidone** reduce the effectiveness of the pill.

Antifungals: griseofulvin reduces effectiveness of the pill.

Cyclosporin, used to suppress immune responses, has blood levels increased by the pill.

Unwanted effects

Likely Feeling or being sick, headache, breast tenderness, changes in weight.

Unlikely Pains in the legs, groin or chest, changes in sexual desire, depression, skin changes, decreased tolerance to wearing contact lenses.

Unwanted effects are usually mild and fade as you continue treatment. However, there are a number of rare adverse effects and if you have any of the following symptoms, you must contact your doctor immediately:

☐ A sudden sharp or severe pain in the chest ☐ sudden shortness of breath or painful breathing ☐ unexplained cough ☐ painful or inflamed veins in the legs ☐ a crushing type of chest pain or simply heaviness in the chest ☐ the very first attack of migraine ☐ worsening of existing migraine □ sudden and unusually severe headache □ dizziness or fainting, quite different from anything you have had before □ change in normal vision or speech □ sudden partial or complete loss of vision □ weakness or numbness in one arm or leg □ swelling in the limbs.

Similar preparations

Combination preparations
MESTRANOL 50 MICROGRAMS:
NORINYL-1; ORTHO-NOVIN 1/50

LEVONORGESTREL

Progestogen-only preparations
LEVONORGESTREL
MICROVAL; NEOGEST; NORGESTON

Combination preparations
EUGYNON 30; MICROGYNON 30; OVRAN 30; OVRANETTE; OVRAN

Phased preparations
LOGYNON; LOGYNON ED; TRINORDIOL

Emergency contraception
SCHERING PC4

Levonorgestrel is a synthetic version of the female sex hormone progesterone. It is a single ingredient of the progestogen-only pill or it is used with an oestrogen such as ethinyloestradiol in the combined pill. Levonorgestrel acts on the cervix, the entrance to the womb, to form a sticky, mucous plug making it difficult for sperm to enter. Levonorgestrel also interferes with luteinising hormone (LH) production. The progestogen-only pill may cause periods to disappear or become irregular. Breakthrough bleeding is sometimes a problem, although this often settles with long-term use. It is suitable for smokers of any age, older women and those who have unwanted effects with oestrogens.

Some progestogens similar to levonorgestrel are used in the treatment of cancers, including breast cancer.

Before you use this medicine

Tell your doctor if you are:
☐ pregnant – the pill should not be taken; there may be a small risk of malformation in the baby ☐ breast-feeding – low doses of progestogen may pass through into the milk but are not harmful. You can take a progestogen-only pill from day 21 after your baby is born and this will protect you immediately. If you start after this time, you may need additional protection during the first 48 hours of pill-taking ☐ taking any other medicines, including vitamins and those bought over the counter.

Tell your doctor if you have or have had:
☐ diabetes ☐ high blood pressure or heart or circulatory disease ☐ tubal pregnancy (ectopic pregnancy) ☐ ovarian cysts ☐ malabsorption syndromes ☐ migraine or migraine triggered by the combined pill.

Do not take if you have or have had:
☐ blood clots ☐ unexplained vaginal bleeding ☐ severe arterial disease ☐ liver disease ☐ itching of whole body during pregnancy or unexplained jaundice ☐ certain types of jaundice (Dubin-Johnson or Rotor syndromes).

How to use this medicine

Take the pill marked with the correct day of the week on the first day of your period. Take one pill daily, at the same time each day, preferably in the early evening. Accurate pill-taking will improve reliability. You will be protected from the first day and do not need additional contraceptive measures. Continue taking a pill every day until you finish all the pills in the pack.

When you have finished the first pack, start your next pack the next day. Take a pill from the pack for the appropriate day of the week. Progestogen-only pills are taken without a break.

If you change from the combined pill to progestogen-only, start taking the new pill the day after completing the combined pill course so that there is no break in pill-taking.

Do not stop taking the pill unless you have decided that you want to have a baby. You should wait until you have had two periods after stopping the pill before you try to become pregnant. Ask your doctor about other contraceptive precautions to cover this time. If you become pregnant straight away, this should not be harmful. If you are taking levonorgestrel for another reason, your doctor will give you a schedule to reduce the dose gradually.

If you miss a dose, take it as soon as you remember and take the next one at the normal time – see 'If you miss a pill', page 347.

Over 65 There are similar progestogens in hormone replacement preparations.

Interactions with other medicines

Levonorgestrel may interact with other medicines or the effectiveness of the pill may be reduced – see also interactions for **ethinyloestradiol**. Do not take other medicines without checking with your doctor or pharmacist.

Unwanted effects

Likely Absent or irregular periods or changes in menstrual pattern, changes in weight, breast tenderness, swollen feet and ankles.
Unlikely Feeling or being sick, headache, depression.

The most common unwanted effect of the progestogen-only pill is irregular periods (spotting between periods or absence of periods).

Similar preparations

Progestogen-only preparations

FEMULEN
ETHYNODIOL

MICRONOR
NORETHISTERONE

NORIDAY
NORETHISTERONE

Combined with ethinyloestradiol

▼CILEST
NORGESTIMATE

CONOVA 30
ETHYNODIOL

FEMODENE/FEMODENE ED
GESTODENE

MARVELON
DESOGESTREL

MERCILON
DESOGESTREL

MINULET
GESTODENE

Injections

DEPO-PROVERA
MEDROXYPROGESTERONE ACETATE

NORISTERAT
NORETHISTERONE

• *OTHER METHODS OF CONTRACEPTION* •

Barrier methods are popular now because they can protect against sexually transmitted diseases and prevent the spread of human immunodeficiency virus (HIV). The sheath or condom is very effective if used properly. Condoms are readily available and free from the risks of hormonal contraception. However, the failure rate can be high if the condom is not applied properly to the penis and before genital contact occurs. Training in how to use the condom is available at family planning clinics.

Diaphragms and caps placed over the cervix prevent the sperm reaching the womb. The diaphragm can be inserted several hours before intercourse but must be left in place for at least six hours afterwards. The diaphragm or cap needs to be fitted for each woman and requires a little training and practice before regular use as a contraceptive.

Diaphragms and condoms are usually used with spermicides – chemicals which kill sperm cells – for additional protection. Spermicides do not give adequate protection when used alone. The effectiveness of condoms and diaphragms can be reduced if you use them with an oil-based lubricant or ointment, for example if you are using a local treatment for a candidal infection or use an oestrogen cream for menopausal symptoms. Oil-based vaginal and rectal preparations, including pessaries, ointments, creams, gels and suppositories can damage latex rubber so that not only is contraceptive efficacy reduced but there is less protection from sexually transmitted diseases. Check with your doctor or pharmacist whether local vaginal or rectal treatment or the lubricant that you use is compatible with the condom or diaphragm.

An intrauterine device (IUD) or coil is a small solid device placed in the womb to prevent pregnancy. Most devices are now made of copper wound onto the stem of a plastic carrier; some have silver cores. New developments including a hormone-releasing device may improve the IUD's popularity. The IUD is suitable for older women who have had children and it can now be left in place for five years before replacement with a new one. Any device fitted after the age of 40 may be safely left in place until the menopause.

The IUD is not ideal for younger women who have not had children and who may have a number of sexual partners. Its use has been associated with pelvic inflammatory disease (PID) and infertility.

The device is usually fitted at the end of menstruation. It may cause pain and spotting between periods and heavier or prolonged bleeding for a few months but this usually lessens with time. If you find these unwanted effects unacceptable the device can be removed. An IUD should not be used if you are pregnant, have severe anaemia, very heavy periods, a history of tubal (*ectopic*) pregnancy, malignant tumours in the genital organs, pelvic inflammatory disease or you are having treatment which suppresses the immune system. A copper-carrying device is not suitable if you are allergic to copper.

Sterilisation of either the man or woman is popular with couples and has replaced the contraceptive pill as the most widely used method of birth control when the woman is over 30 or the family is considered complete. It is very effective contraception and difficult to reverse. The surgical procedure for either the male operation (vasectomy) or the female operation on the Fallopian tubes is straightforward, but the decision to go ahead with the method needs careful thought and discussion with your doctor.

Bladder disorders

Bladder disorders include inflammation in the bladder (*cystitis*: see page 283) and the urethra (*urethritis*), loss of control in passing urine (*urinary incontinence*) and difficulty emptying the bladder (*urinary retention*). Infections in the bladder are usually caused by bacteria and are therefore treated with appropriate antibacterial drugs or preparations that change the acidity of urine. Signs of cystitis include the urge to keep passing urine although there is hardly anything to pass and it is painful to do so. Urethritis is inflammation or infection of the urethra, the tube that takes urine from the bladder to the outside. Urethritis is common in women after the menopause when changes to the reproductive organs may also affect the bladder and cause inflammation, frequent urination, difficult or painful urination and incontinence. Hormone replacement therapy (see Chapter 6) can help.

● *LOSS OF BLADDER CONTROL* ●

The sphincter muscles around the outlet of the bladder keep a constant pressure on the urethra and prevent urine escaping. As the volume of fluid increases in the bladder, stretch receptors in the bladder wall transmit this information to activate the nerves controlling the bladder. When the bladder is full, the nerves controlling urination signal the bladder muscles to contract. The sphincter muscles are then consciously relaxed to allow urine to flow out.

Urinary incontinence is the involuntary passing of urine. You find that you have no control over whether urine is passed, even if you try to stop it, or you may lose the nerve sensations that tell you the bladder is full or that urine is being passed. Whatever the cause it can be a distressing and embarrassing problem. Urinary incontinence is a common complaint; research shows that five to ten per cent of adults in Britain have a problem and that half of them need to use an appliance or incontinence pads. Women are seven to eight times more likely to be affected than men and more than half of all women have experienced some loss of urinary control.

TYPES OF INCONTINENCE

☐ **Stress incontinence** A small amount of urine leaks from your bladder as a result of even slight exertion – laughing, sneezing, coughing, jogging or lifting a heavy object – anything which exerts pressure on the abdomen to override the bladder's closure mechanism. Stress incontinence is nothing to do with psychological stress. Its main cause is the stretching and weakening of pelvic muscles which support the contents of the abdomen. This is common after childbirth and can get worse if nothing is done about it.
☐ **Dribble incontinence** Urine escapes gradually in drips or a thin trickle. This can be caused by severe constipation; by an over-stretched bladder; or, in men, an enlarged prostate gland (which partially obstructs the urethral opening and prevents the bladder being completely emptied).
☐ **Urge incontinence** The desire to pass water is so great that you cannot delay long enough to reach the toilet. This may be due to an infection – cystitis, for example – or some other irritation that makes the bladder contract involuntarily. Alternatively, you may not be able to reach the toilet in time because of an illness such as arthritis or medicines which slow your reactions or increase the volume of urine.
☐ **Nocturnal enuresis** Bedwetting in children who have bladder control during the day.
☐ **Double incontinence** Loss of control over both bowel and bladder emptying.

Management

Sometimes the onset of incontinence is gradual, for example in older people, but for others it can be sudden. The condition is worrying whether you lose small amounts of urine or a stream. You should see your doctor as soon as you realise you have a problem. Your doctor will ask you the following questions and it would be helpful to think about the answers and to jot them down beforehand:

☐ **Onset** When did the problem first start? was it sudden or gradual?

HOW YOU CAN HELP YOURSELF

☐ Know that incontinence is a common problem which can be investigated, treated or managed.
☐ Seek help and advice from your doctor, who may also be able to arrange for a continence adviser to visit you.
☐ A number of organisations can provide services and advice, including Age Concern, Disabled Living Foundation, Incontinence Advisory Service, National Action on Incontinence, and the Enuresis Resource and Information Centre. See 'Useful addresses'.
☐ If you are a relative or carer of someone who is incontinent find out as much as you can so that you can be understanding and reassuring.
☐ Take practical measures, such as having a commode or bedpan in every room and wearing clothing that is easily undone. Ask the Clothing Advisory Service for advice (see 'Useful addresses').
☐ Do not cut down on the amount you drink as your body needs a certain amount of fluid each day. Take your fluids earlier in the day and avoid drinks late in the evening so that sleep is not disturbed.
☐ Take care to empty your bladder completely each time; bending forward at the waist may help.
☐ Keep a note of when and how often you or the person you care for has incontinence.
☐ Exercise pelvic floor muscles (see Box). These exercises should be routine for women after childbirth and are particularly helpful for stress incontinence.
☐ Make sure you know where there are toilet facilities when you are away from home.

☐ **Volume** Is the loss a constant dribble or an occasional flood?
☐ **Frequency** How often does it happen? once a day, several times a day, or constantly?
☐ **Timing** Does it tend to happen more at night or during the day?

Your doctor will want to find out the cause of incontinence as it can be a symptom of some underlying condition. The aim is to treat the condition which should then cure or improve the incontinence. If there is an infection then a course of antibiotics should help. Surgery may be necessary to correct a prolapse of the womb or to remove an enlarged prostate gland.

Sometimes there is no underlying cause; the bladder muscles simply contract resulting in urinary frequency, urgency and

EXERCISES FOR PELVIC FLOOR MUSCLES

☐ In a comfortable position tighten the muscles around your back passage as if you were controlling an attack of diarrhoea. Do this several times until you are sure you have identified the correct muscles.
☐ Once you are familiar with the muscles gently pull them up, tightening them slowly to a count of four and then slowly relaxing them.

There is no need to set aside a special time or place for these exercises: they can be done sitting, standing, or even whilst walking.
☐ When you pass urine, deliberately stop and start the flow by contracting the same muscles. Do this several times each time you pass urine – but make sure you always empty your bladder properly.

sometimes incontinence. Treatment with an *antimuscarinic* medicine may be helpful for urinary frequency and incontinence as it can lessen bladder muscle contractions and increase bladder capacity. Medicines used include **propantheline** (brand name Pro-Banthine), **flavoxate** (Urispas), **oxybutynin** (Ditropan) or a tricyclic antidepressant.

OXYBUTYNIN

▼CYSTRIN – Tablets
▼DITROPAN – Tablets

Oxybutynin is an antimuscarinic drug which relaxes the bladder muscles, allowing the bladder to hold more urine. It reduces the frequency of passing urine and is used for urinary incontinence, urgency and frequency in the unstable bladder. Oxybutynin may be used, with other drug measures, for treating bedwetting in children usually aged over seven years.

Before you use this medicine

Tell your doctor if you are:
☐ pregnant or breast-feeding ☐ taking any other medicines, including vitamins and those bought over the counter.

Tell your doctor if you have or have had:
☐ thyroid disease ☐ heart disease ☐ kidney or liver disease ☐ irregular heart rhythms ☐ enlargement of the prostate gland.

Do not use if you have:
☐ obstruction of the bowel ☐ bladder outflow obstruction ☐ severe ulcerative colitis or toxic megacolon ☐ myasthenia gravis ☐ glaucoma.

How to use this medicine

Take one tablet two or three times a day. Occasionally your doctor may increase the dose to one tablet four times a day.

Do not drive or do other activities that require alertness until you know how you react to oxybutynin. Small amounts of alcohol should not be a problem.

If you miss a dose, take it as soon as you remember, but skip it if it is almost time for your next dose. Do not take double the dose.

Over 65 Usually take less than the standard adult dose.

Interactions with other medicines

Oxybutynin causes atropine-like unwanted effects such as dry mouth, visual disturbances and constipation. Many other medicines have these effects and if two or three of these drugs are used together, unwanted effects are increased; in older people confusion is likely. Do not take other medicines without checking with your doctor or pharmacist.

Unwanted effects

Likely Dry mouth, constipation, blurred vision, feeling sick, abdominal discomfort, facial flushing, difficulty in passing urine.
Unlikely Headache, urinary retention, dizziness, drowsiness, dry skin, diarrhoea, irregular heart rhythms.

The most common unwanted effect is dry mouth which can make you drink more and so aggravate urinary symptoms. Sucking a sweet or chewing gum will encourage saliva flow to keep the mouth comfortable.

Similar preparations

PRO-BANTHINE – Tablets
PROPANTHELINE

URISPAS – Tablets
FLAVOXATE

Not all cases of incontinence can be adequately controlled and it may be necessary to use a special appliance or pads. There is a wide variety of appliances, portable urinals, collection bags for day and night use, and drainage tubes which your doctor can prescribe. The exact type of appliance depends on individual needs in different situations. For example bulky absorbent pads may be good at night, but something less obtrusive will be more appropriate during the day. There are also specially designed pants and discreet pads which can help you lead an unrestricted life. Incontinence pads are provided by hospitals and community health services free of charge to NHS patients.

Skin care is very important and the area should be kept clean and dry as far as possible to prevent sores. A barrier cream (see page 415) may help after washing and drying.

Self-catheterisation is a technique that you may be able to learn and operate yourself. A catheter is a drainage tube that is inserted into the bladder to allow the urine to run out and be collected in a bag. Catheterisation is usually performed by a nurse or some other qualified person but some people with incontinence can be taught to do this for themselves. If you have incontinence or other urinary difficulties where the bladder contains a significant residual volume of urine then you may be a suitable candidate for self-catheterisation. You will need to catheterise yourself at least four times a day to prevent the bladder overfilling. The technique is not difficult, neither is it painful nor dangerous, but you will need to be taught by a doctor or continence adviser or nurse. You will also need to know how to look after the catheter and who to contact for advice at any time.

The advantages of self-catheterisation are that you can become 'dry', you can do without bulky external drainage appliances and you no longer need to remain within reach of a toilet. There should be no more smells of stale urine or embarrassing moments. Furthermore by establishing effective urinary drainage you will protect your kidneys from the effects of back pressure and urinary infection. Serious adverse effects are infrequent, especially in women. Bleeding sometimes occurs, but does not usually signify a serious problem, although you should always mention this to the nurse or doctor.

Bedwetting – nocturnal enuresis

Children usually do without nappies and gain control of their bladder function during the day by the age of two or three. Control over bladder function at night may come later, perhaps not until five or six years. Bedwetting occurs on most nights in about 15 per cent of five-year-olds and persists in as many as five per cent by the age of ten. Over 100,000 teenagers suffer from bedwetting; the Enuresis Resource and Information Centre publishes a guide especially for this age group. If there is no underlying cause, such as a urinary tract infection, bladder training with or without the use of an enuresis alarm can be tried. An alarm system consists of a pad or mat which is placed under the child at night so that when urine is passed it completes an electric circuit, causing an alarm to sound and wake the child. After several weeks' use, the child becomes conditioned and wakes before passing urine or loses the urge to do so at night. There are also alarms that the child can wear with the detector placed in underpants and the alarm clipped to the clothing. Alarms are successful in about 65 per cent of children without any underlying cause of incontinence.

There are various alarm systems and only those conforming to Department of Health specifications or the British Standard should be used. None is available on NHS prescription but your doctor may be able to arrange one free on loan through the district services.

Drug treatment of bedwetting is not recommended for children under seven years and is generally only used when other measures have failed. Tricyclic antidepressant medicines such as **amitriptyline** (see page 210) or **imipramine** are effective, but behaviour disturbances and relapse are common after treatment stops. Unwanted effects include dry mouth, blurred vision, constipation, confusion and drowsiness; the drugs are toxic in overdosage. **Desmopressin** (brand name Desmospray) is also used; the relapse rate is high but unwanted effects fewer and mild compared with the tricyclic antidepressants. **Oxybutynin**, a new antimuscarinic drug may be used in children over five, but experience with it is limited; unwanted effects are similar to those of the tricyclic antidepressants.

● *INABILITY TO EMPTY THE BLADDER* ●

Urinary retention usually occurs because the bladder muscles fail to contract sufficiently to push out all the urine. Urinary retention is a less common condition than incontinence, but causes include an enlarged prostate gland or tumour, or loss of nerve control over bladder function. Acute (sudden and severe) retention is painful and is treated by catheterisation. Your doctor will look for an underlying cause and surgery may be needed. Chronic (long-term) retention may be treated with a medicine to increase the strength of bladder muscle contraction. Drugs used include those that enhance the activity of the nerves to the bladder, such as **carbachol**, **bethanechol** (brand name Myotonine) and **distig-**

mine (Ubretid). The alpha blockers **indoramin** (brand name Baratol) and **prazosin** (Hypovase – see also page 127) relax the sphincter muscles and increase urine flow when enlargement of the prostate gland obstructs bladder function.

8

MUSCLES AND JOINTS

Osteoarthritis Rheumatoid arthritis Gout Strains and sprains

The skeleton is the frame which encloses and protects the body's vital organs and to which muscles are attached. Over 200 bones make up the skeleton, allowing great variety of movement. The spaces between the ends of bones are joints, which are supported by strong *ligaments* and moved by the contraction of *muscles*. Muscles are connected to the skeleton at fixed points by *tendons*.

Covering the end of a bone and attached to it is a layer of tough tissue or *cartilage* which protects the bone. The greatest mobility occurs in *synovial joints* such as the knee or shoulder. In these joints the space between the adjoining ends of bones is enclosed by a strong membrane. This membrane produces *synovial fluid*, which lubricates the inside of the joint, permitting smooth movement and cushioning the bones as the joint bends, straightens or rotates.

Muscles, tendons and ligaments are tough tissues built to take the stresses and strains of body movements. However, they are subject to wear and tear with age or if used too much or too violently, for example during sporting activities. Joints also take a great deal of strain and as you grow older the cartilage protecting the end of the bone can break down causing pain and swelling. Disease can also affect joints to produce pain and inflammation.

Osteoarthritis

Osteoarthritis causes the cartilage covering the end of the bone to become thin and rough. The bone thickens and bony outgrowths or 'spurs' grow around the joint. The joint may become inflamed and weakened; in severe cases it becomes deformed. Osteoarthritis comes with age and does not normally start before the age of 50. The cause is not fully understood, but as you get older you are more likely to get osteoarthritis, particularly in the weight-bearing joints – the lower back, hips and knees. Age does not necessarily bring osteoarthritis, but it is more likely to develop if the joint has been used a great deal or has been damaged before, for example at work or playing sport, or if it was malformed at birth.

Symptoms include pain, stiffness, swelling and tenderness in the affected joint. Often the condition progresses as the cartilage is worn away and eventually bone grates on bone; there is increasing pain and disability. Pain and stiffness are usually worse at the end of the day or after exercise. The severity of osteoarthritis varies considerably from person to person and mild forms may cause only a slight loss of cartilage with no symptoms.

HOW YOU CAN HELP YOURSELF

☐ Lose weight if you are overweight. Extra weight means an additional load on the weight-bearing joints and more wear and tear.
☐ Rest, particularly if you have osteoarthritis in a weight-bearing joint, before the pain becomes unbearable.
☐ Exercise. Ask your doctor what exercise you can do and how much. Gentle exercise will help to prevent the muscles around the joint from becoming stiff and weak. Swimming is useful because the water allows you to take weight off the joints while exercising the muscles, but some exercise, such as walking on rough ground, may aggravate osteoarthritis in a knee or hip.
☐ Avoid sitting or standing in one position for long periods of time as this will make you stiff. Learn to reorganise postures and activities which seem to aggravate pain or stiffness and try to avoid them.
☐ Local heat may help an arthritic knee, for example. Use a hot water bottle or infra-red radiant lamp.
☐ Massaging the joint helps the circulation and may give comfort. Your doctor may be able to refer you to a physiotherapist who can advise on keeping joints mobile. Physiotherapy teaches you the best way to move and use your body; it is better to see a physiotherapist in the early stages of arthritic disease rather than later.
☐ Find out about suitable aids and possible adaptations to your home to help you live and move about more easily. Local social services departments can sometimes help, but they may want a letter from your doctor.

Medicines for osteoarthritis

Arthritis treatments control and ease symptoms and maintain joint function rather than cure the disease. A simple analgesic such as paracetamol or aspirin can be used for relieving pain and should be tried first. For more severe pain, swelling and stiffness your doctor may prescribe a non-steroidal anti-inflammatory drug (NSAID).

An NSAID has two separate actions. In a single dose it has similar pain-relieving activity (analgesia) to that of paracetamol and can therefore be used to ease mild or intermittent pain. Additionally, if taken regularly it reduces the underlying inflammation which may be making the joint swollen, hot and very painful; paracetamol does not do this. This combination of analgesic and anti-inflammatory effects makes NSAIDs particularly useful for treating the continuous pain associated with arthritis.

Aspirin, the original NSAID, has to be taken in much higher doses and for longer periods than you would take for a headache to relieve painful arthritic conditions. It should only be taken in these higher doses on the recommendation of a doctor. When taken in regular high dosage aspirin has about the same anti-inflammatory effect as other NSAIDs, but at these doses aspirin is likely to cause unwanted effects such as stomach irritation, gastric bleeding, nausea and ringing in the ears (tinnitus). Stomach upsets can be reduced by taking aspirin after meals or in one of the many other formulations such as dispersible, buffered or enteric-coated preparations. Tinnitus, deafness and dizziness are signs of mild overdosage and will be lessened by reducing the dose.

Benorylate, an aspirin–paracetamol compound, can be taken twice a day and is slightly kinder to the stomach than aspirin alone. *Salicylate* compounds (brand names Disalcid; Trilisate) are similar to other aspirin preparations. Aspirin has been widely used in higher dosages for its anti-inflammatory effect but other NSAIDs are better tolerated and more convenient to take.

NSAIDs are known as 'non-steroidal' drugs to distinguish them from corticosteroids which are powerful steroidal drugs with dramatic anti-inflammatory properties (see page 321). Although effective in arthritic conditions, corticosteroids by mouth are reserved for use only after other treatments have proved unsuccessful. However, a corticosteroid injected directly into a swollen and painful joint may produce very effective short-term pain relief usually without adverse effects.

NSAIDs do not alter the progress of arthritic conditions but reduce inflammation and therefore pain by blocking *prostaglandin* production. Prostaglandins are body chemicals involved in the process of inflammation and the transmission of pain, in the body's immune response and in tissue damage. NSAIDs are therefore used to treat a variety of conditions involving prostaglandin activity, for example headaches, pain following surgery, period pains, backache and soft tissue injury (muscles, tendons and ligaments), strains and sprains.

All NSAIDs have similar anti-inflammatory activity, but there is considerable variation in how individuals respond to any one

NSAID. Your doctor may need to try several different NSAIDs before you find one that suits you. Most NSAIDs are rapidly absorbed and start to relieve symptoms during the first day of treatment but a sustained effect may not be seen for a week or more. However, you should not expect pain-relief 24 hours a day nor to take on activities that were previously restricted. Your doctor will want to give each treatment a fair trial, so three weeks may be needed to assess anti-inflammatory activity. NSAIDs are usually taken by mouth as tablets or capsules, but some are now produced in cream or gel form for applying to the skin to treat strains, sprains and bruising.

You should never take two NSAID preparations at the same time. This includes taking ibuprofen bought over the counter for pain relief at the same time as a prescribed NSAID.

The main differences between the NSAIDs are in the severity and frequency of unwanted effects, such as stomach upsets and diarrhoea. Occasionally bleeding and ulceration occur in the stomach or duodenum. Other unwanted effects include ankle swelling, headache, dizziness, vertigo and tinnitus. NSAIDs can cause hypersensitivity reactions such as asthma and skin rashes and should not be used if you are allergic to aspirin or have asthma.

NSAIDS AND ALLERGIC DISORDERS

NSAIDs may cause hypersensitivity reactions. If you develop skin rashes and wheezing after taking aspirin, you may also be allergic to any of the prescribed NSAIDs or ibuprofen bought over the counter. Similarly, if you have asthma and your condition worsens while taking an NSAID, stop taking the medicine and seek medical help immediately. An NSAID applied to the skin can also trigger allergic reactions or asthma because some of the drug is absorbed into the body.

NSAIDs should be used with caution by older people and particularly by anyone who has poor kidney, liver or heart function. Many older people have some degree of kidney impairment, so an NSAID should always be used at the lowest possible dose for the shortest time to achieve an effect. If you are over 65 your doctor should avoid prescribing an NSAID for a long period if at all possible. If long-term treatment is necessary you should not have repeat prescriptions without regular check-ups. Your doctor should check your kidney function periodically if you are taking an NSAID for any length of time. You should not take an NSAID if you are pregnant.

Sometimes an NSAID can cause fluid to be retained in the body; one of the signs is ankle swelling. If you have heart failure this will aggravate the problem further and your doctor would not usually prescribe an NSAID under these circumstances. Fluid retention can also increase blood pressure and, if this is already raised, could possibly lead to a heart attack or stroke.

If you have an active peptic ulcer, you should not take NSAIDs because they upset the stomach and may aggravate an ulcer, causing serious bleeding. If you have had a peptic ulcer, you should normally avoid NSAIDs, but some people with serious rheumatic diseases may need one to relieve swelling, stiffness and pain. Your doctor may then decide to prescribe an H_2-receptor blocking drug, such as **ranitidine** (brand name Zantac) or **misoprostol** (Cytotec), to prevent further injury to the stomach lining. See page 73.

IBUPROFEN

On prescription

IBUPROFEN – Tablets

BRUFEN – Tablets, liquid, soluble granules, modified-release tablets

FENBID – Modified-release capsules

JUNIFEN – Children's liquid

CODAFEN CONTINUS — Modified release tablets
IBUPROFEN + CODEINE

From a pharmacy/on prescription

Creams and gels:

IBUGEL; IBULEVE; PROFLEX

Tablets and capsules for symptoms such as rheumatic and muscular pain, backache, migraine and headache include:
INOVEN; NUROFEN; MIGRAFEN; RELCOFEN (See also page 241).

Ibuprofen is a non-steroidal anti-inflammatory drug for relieving the swelling and pain of rheumatoid arthritis (including juvenile arthritis), ankylosing spondylitis (stiffening of the spine), osteoarthritis and other arthritic conditions. Ibuprofen blocks prostaglandin production, reduces inflammation and eases pain. It has fewer unwanted effects than other NSAIDs but its anti-inflammatory effect is weaker. High doses are needed for treating rheumatoid arthritis, which may result in more serious unwanted effects, and it is not suitable for inflammatory conditions such as acute gout. It reduces fever and is used as an analgesic in lower doses. Ibuprofen can be bought over the counter for pain relief in muscular and rheumatic conditions, dental pain, period pains and headache.

Before you use this medicine

Tell your doctor if you are:
☐ pregnant – do not use, especially during the last three months ☐ breast-feeding ☐ taking any other medicines, including vitamins and those bought over the counter.

Tell your doctor if you have or have had:
☐ heart disease or high blood pressure ☐ kidney or liver disease.

Do not use if you have or have had:
☐ allergy to aspirin ☐ severe kidney disease ☐ heart failure ☐ peptic ulcer or oesophagitis ☐ asthma or nasal polyps.

How to use this medicine

Take the tablets in divided doses with food or after meals. Sustained-release preparations may be taken once or twice daily. Granules should be dispersed in water before taking. Children with rheumatoid arthritis usually take the liquid (not Junifen, which is only for reducing fever). The cream is applied to an injured area three or four times daily.

Avoid alcohol as it irritates the stomach lining and increases the risk of stomach upsets. If you miss a dose, take it as soon as you remember. If your next dose is due within two hours take one dose and then skip the next.

Over 65 You may need less than the standard adult dose, especially if you have poor kidney function. If you are on long-term treatment, ask your doctor if you should have a kidney test periodically.

Interactions with other medicines

Do not take other medicines without checking with your doctor or pharmacist.

Oral anticoagulants, such as warfarin increase the risk of gastrointestinal bleeding or peptic ulcers.

Lithium Greater risk of lithium toxicity because blood levels are increased.

Unwanted effects

Likely Indigestion, heartburn, feeling or being sick, diarrhoea. **Unlikely** Skin rashes, wheezing, breathlessness, dizziness, light-headedness, headache, hearing disturbances, ankle swelling and fluid retention, unusual bleeding or bruising.

Contact your doctor if you develop any of the unlikely unwanted effects or if you have bloody or black, tarry stools, stomach pain or cramps, or you vomit blood or material that looks like coffee grounds.

Similar preparations

ALRHEUMAT – Capsules
KETOPROFEN

CLINORIL – Tablets
SULINDAC

DICLOFENAC – Tablets

DIFLUNISAL – Tablets

DOLOBID – Tablets
DIFLUNISAL

▼EMFLEX – Capsules
ACEMETACIN

FELDENE – Capsules, soluble tablets, suppositories, gel
PIROXICAM

FENOPRON – Tablets
FENOPROFEN

FLEXIN – Modified-release tablets
INDOMETHACIN

FROBEN – Modified-release capsules, tablets, suppositories
FLURBIPROFEN

INDOCID – Capsules, modified-release capsules, liquid, suppositories
INDOMETHACIN

INDOMETHACIN – Capsules, suppositories

KETOPROFEN – Capsules

LEDERFEN – Capsules, tablets, soluble tablets
FENBUFEN

LODINE – Capsules, tablets
ETODOLAC

MEFENAMIC ACID – Capsules, tablets

MOBIFLEX – Tablets
TENOXICAM

NAPROSYN – Tablets, liquid, granules, suppositories
NAPROXEN

NAPROXEN – Tablets

NYCOPREN – Tablets
NAPROXEN

ORUDIS – Capsules, suppositories
KETOPROFEN

ORUVAIL – Modified-release capsules, injection, gel
KETOPROFEN

PIROXICAM – Capsules

PONSTAN – Capsules, soluble tablets, children's liquid
MEFENAMIC ACID

RELIFEX – Tablets, liquid
NABUMETONE

RHEUMACIN LA – Modified-release capsules
INDOMETHACIN

RHEUMOX – Capsules, tablets
AZAPROPAZONE

SLO-INDO – Modified-release tablets
INDOMETHACIN

SURGAM – Tablets
TIAPROFENIC ACID

TIAPROFENIC ACID – Tablets

TOLECTIN – Capsules
TOLMETIN

VOLTAROL – Tablets, modified-release tablets, soluble tablets, injection, suppositories, gel
DICLOFENAC

Phenylbutazone, one of the early NSAIDs, is a potent anti-inflammatory drug but may cause occasional serious adverse effects. Its use is now limited to hospital treatment of ankylosing spondylitis, a rheumatic condition affecting the spine, when other treatments have not succeeded.

Rheumatoid arthritis

Rheumatoid arthritis is a disease of the whole body, not just the joints. It is an *autoimmune* disease – the body's defence mechanism, which normally protects you from infection, attacks your own tissue, including the joints. White blood cells normally recognise and attack foreign matter such as bacteria and make antibodies to fight off infection. In rheumatoid arthritis the body's immune system fails to recognise the body's own cells and turns its attack on the cells of the *synovial membrane*, causing swelling, heat and pain in the joint. If this process continues for many months or years, the protective cartilage lining the bones becomes eroded, damaging the joint irreversibly. All the body's joints can be affected but it is usually those of the hands, knees and feet that are involved. The joints are often affected symmetrically – both hands or both feet.

A swollen and painful joint becomes stiff and difficult to move and the symptoms are usually worse in the morning. Other symptoms include fever, weight loss, tiredness and anaemia. In severe cases rheumatoid arthritis involves the eyes, blood vessels, skin, heart or lungs, but this is rare. Rheumatoid arthritis is more common in women than men and can occur at any age, but usually between 20 and 60. The disease has dramatic ups and downs and can clear up completely. About 30 per cent of sufferers recover within a year or so from the first attack; 65 per cent continue to have symptoms sporadically throughout life and five per cent become severely disabled.

GETTING HELP

Your doctor Explain your symptoms clearly to your doctor so that together you can reach a better understanding of your problem and its treatment. See your doctor early in an attack so that treatment can be tailored to your needs. Find out what you can take for additional pain relief.

Rheumatoid arthritis is a disease involving the whole body which needs a total management plan involving other experts, such as eye specialists, surgeons, physiotherapists, social workers and teachers. Ask your general practitioner whether you should see a rheumatologist to discuss a strategy for managing the disease.

Self-help groups A number of organisations (for example, Arthritis Care) provide information and advice about many aspects of arthritic diseases. Join a local branch for support from fellow sufferers.

Social services Find out if you are eligible for any allowances or benefits from the DSS. The Disability Rights Handbook, published by The Disability Alliance, is a good source of information. Your local council may be able to help with a care assistant, meals on wheels and home aids or modifications.

The cause of rheumatoid arthritis is unclear although there is a great deal of research to find reasons as to why the body should attack its own tissues. There may be a hereditary element and a particular gene found in 70 per cent of rheumatoid arthritics is present in only 25 per cent of the population. It is likely that some external trigger such as a virus or bacterium sets off the inflammatory process. Most recent research points to a particular bacterium and trials are in progress to see if antibacterial treatment during the active form of the disease may help.

• *OTHER DISEASES AFFECTING THE JOINTS* •

Doctors often test blood for a molecule called *rheumatoid factor* to diagnose rheumatoid arthritis. It may also be present in rare forms of arthritis where, as in rheumatoid arthritis, an active inflammation (rather than one arising from wear and tear, as in osteoarthritis) attacks the tissues. *Ankylosing spondylitis* means 'a joining up of inflamed vertebrae' and mainly affects the spine and pelvic joints, causing severe stiffening. It may be hereditary and is most common in young men. In severe cases the spine becomes fixed in a bent position, but current treatment can often prevent such disability. *Systemic lupus erythematosus* is a rare immunological

HOW YOU CAN HELP YOURSELF

Rest and exercise Splints can be helpful, especially at night, to rest the affected joints and prevent deformity. They are best fitted by a skilled physiotherapist. Physiotherapy can help mobility and improve muscle strength. Exercising in water or swimming is beneficial; ask the physiotherapist what other exercises you can do regularly as part of the daily management of the disease.
Lose weight This will reduce the load on the weight-bearing joints. Special diets are not necessary, although some people claim that avoiding certain foods helps them. Always eat a balanced diet with plenty of fresh fruit and vegetables and seek advice if you are not sure about your diet. Short-term studies have shown that fish oils (for example, cod liver oil) can sometimes help inflammation and stiffness.
Local treatment of a painful joint can be soothing: for example, apply heat with a hot water bottle or infra red lamp or cold with a cold compress made out of a plastic bag full of ice cubes. Gentle massage may also sooth.
Save effort Find out about suitable aids and possible adaptations to your home to help you live and move about more easily. Make sure the pharmacist supplies your medicines in containers you can open.

disorder which causes widespread damage; it mainly affects young women with symptoms including skin rashes, joint pains and tiredness. Other types of rheumatoid-like arthritis include *psoriatic arthritis* and *Reiter's disease*. A form of arthritis that affects children called *juvenile rheumatoid arthritis* (Still's disease) usually disappears before adulthood but may damage the joints permanently.

Medicines for rheumatoid arthritis

Your doctor will aim to control pain, and if possible the disease process, maintain the function of joints and prevent disability and permanent deformity. There are several approaches to treatment and no one method may be completely successful.

A simple analgesic such as paracetamol may relieve pain, while one of the NSAID group (see 'Osteoarthritis') can help inflammation and stiffness, although it may take time to find a suitable preparation. You will need to take the NSAID regularly whether you are in pain or not because it will help to reduce and control inflammation on a long-term basis. Suppositories used at night may help morning stiffness. However, neither paracetamol nor NSAIDs slow down or stop the disease itself. If symptoms are severe and not controlled by an NSAID after some months of treatment, you may be given a medicine aimed at modifying the arthritis. These *antirheumatic* medicines affect the disease process. Rheumatoid arthritis may improve spontaneously or after a number of years 'burn out' (remit) but this is unpredictable. The disease-modifying drugs can help this process by allowing eroded cartilage to heal or at least stopping further erosion. However, they act slowly and it may take six months before there is a response. They are not prescribed before anti-inflammatory drugs are tried because they can cause serious adverse effects and need careful monitoring.

• *DISEASE-MODIFYING DRUGS* •

These medicines are used in serious arthritic diseases and may improve active inflammatory joint disease and also other symptoms of rheumatoid arthritis. All these medicines produce adverse effects, but with regular blood, kidney or liver tests and careful monitoring for toxicity, they can be very effective treatments. Your doctor will tell you which signs are important to report. These include bruising, sore throat, rash or itching and a change in vision.

Gold compounds (brand names Myocrisin; Ridaura) may be given by mouth or injection, although the injection has been in use for many years and is the standard against which newer drugs are compared. Unwanted effects include diarrhoea, skin rash and adverse effects on the kidneys and blood cells. Treatment has to be stopped if serious unwanted effects occur. Gold by mouth is easy to take but slightly less effective than gold injections and often causes diarrhoea. Both forms require monthly testing of blood and urine.

Penicillamine (brand names Distamine; Pendramine) has a similar action to gold. Unwanted effects occur frequently and include disturbance of taste, nausea, loss of appetite, mouth ulcers and skin rashes. These effects fade when treatment is stopped. Like gold, penicillamine also affects kidney function and blood cells so that periodic testing is needed.

Sulphasalazine (brand name Salazopyrin) is an effective anti-inflammatory drug for rheumatoid arthritis and is also used for treating ulcerative colitis. Unwanted effects include rashes and gastrointestinal upsets. It can also affect blood cells, usually in the first three to six months of treatment, so blood and liver function tests are necessary.

Chloroquine and **hydroxychloroquine** (brand names Nivaquine; Plaquenil) are probably less effective in rheumatoid arthritis. Long-term use is limited by their effect on the eyes. Corneal deposits are common, but rarely cause problems. However, very occasionally these drugs affect the retina and this can lead to blindness. You should have your eyes examined before starting treatment and then every three to six months. Eye damage is very rare on the daily doses used and if continuous treatment does not exceed two years. These drugs cause fewer unwanted effects than the others in this group. Chloroquine is also used for preventing and treating malaria.

Immunosuppressive drugs – **azathioprine**, **methotrexate** or **cyclophosphamide** – are effective but are reserved for severe and disabling symptoms because of adverse effects, particularly on blood. Regular blood tests are essential.

GOLD COMPOUNDS

MYOCRISIN – Injection
SODIUM AUROTHIOMALATE

Sodium aurothiomalate is a gold compound used for treating severe symptoms of rheumatoid arthritis in adults and children. It slows the progression of joint disease but cannot repair existing damage. Like the other drugs that affect rheumatic disease, gold is not usually prescribed until the NSAIDs and other measures have been tried. Sodium aurothiomalate is given by intramuscular injections over a period of some months until a total, cumulative dose of one gram has been injected. There is no immediate benefit from gold treatment and it may take four to six months before you notice any improvement. An NSAID is usually given for pain relief during this time. If there is little improvement by the time the cumulative dose reaches one gram, treatment is usually stopped. If you respond by this stage, injections are continued, but less often, and treatment may last for five years. Gold treatment has to be carefully monitored because of adverse effects. Treatment has to be stopped in up to a third of all cases.

Before you use this medicine

Tell your doctor if you are:
☐ pregnant – avoid gold injections ☐ breast-feeding ☐ taking any other medicines, including vitamins and those bought over the counter.

Tell your doctor if you have or have had:
☐ kidney or liver impairment ☐ skin rash – urticaria or eczema ☐ colitis (inflammation of the intestines) ☐ heart or high blood pressure problems ☐ drugs that cause blood disorders ☐ annual chest X-ray.

Do not use if you have or have had:
☐ severe kidney or liver disease ☐ blood disorders or bone marrow problems ☐ exfoliative dermatitis – peeling skin ☐ systemic lupus erythematosus ☐ necrotising enterocolitis – a severe intestinal condition ☐ fibrous lung disease – pulmonary fibrosis ☐ porphyria ☐ reactions to previous gold treatment.

How to use this medicine

Sodium aurothiomalate must be given by deep *intramuscular* injection – usually into the buttocks – and the area gently massaged. After a small test dose, an injection is given once a week, reducing to a dose every two to four weeks.

Before starting treatment and again before each injection, the doctor or nurse will test your urine, look at the skin and take a blood sample to be tested. Other tests for kidney and liver function may be needed periodically. If you miss a dose treatment can be continued without a problem.

Record your injections and the amount of gold you have and the results of tests on a medicines worksheet or a special card given to you by the rheumatologist.

Over 65 No special precautions but care will be needed in monitoring adverse effects.

Unwanted effects

Likely Dizziness or faintness, flushing or redness of face, feeling or being sick, abdominal cramps or pain, loss of appetite, joint pain.

Sodium aurothiomalate sometimes causes rashes or blood disorders or affects kidney function. Contact your doctor immediately if you have any of the following:
☐ skin rash or itching ☐ metallic taste in mouth ☐ sore throat or fever ☐ sore mouth or tongue ☐ mouth ulcers ☐ bleeding gums ☐ ankle swelling ☐ unusual bleeding or bruising ☐ diarrhoea or stomach pains ☐ bloody or cloudy urine ☐ coughing or shortness of breath ☐ numbness or tingling of the hands or feet ☐ yellow eyes or skin.

Some adverse effects can occur after you have stopped gold treatment. Always check with your doctor if you are concerned.

Similar preparations

RIDAURA – Tablets
AURANOFIN

● *CORTICOSTEROIDS* ●

A corticosteroid may be used in severe, possibly life-threatening situations. High doses have to be used to control the condition and then the corticosteroid is gradually reduced to the lowest possible maintenance dose or stopped completely. Sometimes the condition recurs as the dose is lowered and this makes it difficult to stop corticosteroid treatment. If you have to continue taking the corticosteroid you may become physically dependent on a lifelong maintenance dose. Adverse effects are likely if you continue treatment for more than a few months although low doses may avoid some serious unwanted effects. These include diabetes, muscle wasting in the limbs, a moon-shaped face and weight gain to the torso. You will need to carry a steroid warning card (see page 322). To avoid extended use, high doses of the corticosteroid **methylprednisolone** are given by injection for three days to control the active inflammatory disease while longer-term and slower-acting non-steroidal treatment is started.

A corticosteroid used at a joint can bring relief without the adverse effects of a long-term systemic corticosteroid because the drug reaches the affected part direct and acts within a confined area. A corticosteroid injected into a joint can relieve pain, increase mobility and reduce deformity. This technique is generally used for joints such as knees, shoulders and fingers. Infected joints should not be injected as this will reduce immune defences around the joint and could lead to severe worsening of the infection. After the injection there may be a temporary increase in pain and swelling but this subsides as the corticosteroid starts to reduce inflammation.

● *SURGERY* ●

In some cases, severe joint damage and pain develop despite treatment. In these cases, surgery may be advised, for example joint replacement. Hip replacement is the most common operation; most people are discharged from hospital two to three weeks afterwards. Great improvements have been made recently in knee joint replacements: research continues into replacements for other joints such as elbows, ankles and knuckles.

ALTERNATIVE TREATMENTS

Acupuncture is the alternative therapy which is best documented in treating arthritis. It has been demonstrated to relieve pain, but cannot cure the underlying structure of a damaged joint. One theory is that is stimulates the brain to release endorphins, the body's own painkillers. As the effect is only temporary, treatments will have to be repeated regularly.

Osteopathy can provide relief of back and shoulder pain by manipulation of the spine and joints. However, it can be dangerous to have this treatment if your disease is in an active inflammatory stage, so make sure of your diagnosis before visiting a practitioner.

Herbal remedies a number of herbs have been recommended for the treatment of arthritis. Some people believe that herbs may do some good, and certainly will not do any harm. However, like orthodox medicines herbal remedies can cause adverse effects and their long-term toxic effects are not always known. Herbs commonly recommended are Devil's Claw and Comfrey. Adverse effects have been demonstrated for both of these – Devil's Claw may lead to termination of pregnancy, and Comfrey has been associated with liver disease.

Homoeopathy works on the theory that substances which cause particular symptoms will cure those same symptoms if taken in an extremely small dose. Attempts have been made to assess formally the impact of homoeopathy on arthritis, but the results have been inconclusive. It is possible to get homoeopathic treatment on the NHS from a medically trained doctor.

Other remedies Many other cures and treatments have been proposed over the years, ranging from keeping new potatoes in the pockets to aromatherapy (the external use of essential oils derived from plants). Copper bangles are popular; there is no medical evidence that they do any good, but some people find them helpful. Green-lipped mussel extract, or 'Seatone', is sold as a supplement to relieve arthritic symptoms. Unfortunately the evidence for its usefulness is not convincing.

Surgery can also be performed on structures around the joints: tendons may be repaired or transplanted, synovial membranes may be cut out.

Gout

Gout is a form of arthritis caused by a disorder of the metabolism. *Uric acid*, one of the waste products of normal metabolism, leaves the body via the kidneys in urine. If its concentration becomes too high in blood, uric acid starts to form crystals which are deposited in various parts of the body, most commonly in the joints of the foot (particularly the big toe), ankles, knees and hands. Crystals of uric acid also form lumps under the skin (*tophi*), often visible in the cartilage of the ear, and stones in the kidneys. The deposits of uric acid in the joints can lead to inflammation, causing intense pain which develops over a few hours. The joint quickly becomes red, swollen and extremely tender, so that any sort of pressure on the area is unbearable. Attacks of gout can recur and if untreated, the joints become damaged and eventually deformed.

The amount of uric acid increases in the body if too much is being made or if the kidneys are unable to remove it from the body adequately. The disorder can be inherited and is more common in men. Diet is an important factor and certain foods, for example red meat, sardines, and offal increase the risk of an attack. High alcohol intake is known to trigger attacks. Gout can also occur in kidney failure, in certain blood disorders and as an unwanted effect of some medicines, such as thiazide diuretics.

HOW YOU CAN HELP YOURSELF

☐ Once you have had an attack it may recur. Ask your doctor whether you should have a supply of medicine to relieve an acute attack. **Do not take aspirin** (see below) including any over-the-counter products that may contain aspirin or a salicylate.

☐ Rest the affected joints.

☐ Reduce alcohol intake. Any type of alcoholic drink can precipitate an attack of gout.

☐ Drink plenty of non-alcoholic fluids especially if you are taking a medicine for preventing further attacks of gout.

Medicines for gout

Medicines are used for relieving pain and inflammation in an acute attack of gout and also for the long-term control of the disease to prevent the development of joint and kidney damage. **Aspirin** and **salicylates** must not be used to treat an acute attack of gout nor during long-term control of the condition, as they can raise the uric acid levels and aggravate symptoms.

• *ACUTE ATTACKS* •

NSAIDs are effective in relieving pain and swelling (see page 366). Those used include **indomethacin**, **azapropazone**, **diclofenac**, **ketoprofen**, and **naproxen**. High doses are usually prescribed for a short period to bring the acute symptoms under control. Unwanted effects are unlikely to be a problem because treatment with the NSAID is short.

Colchicine, derived from the seeds of the autumn crocus, is an established treatment for relieving the acute pain and inflammation of gout. It is as effective as indomethacin and can be used if someone cannot tolerate NSAIDs. Unwanted effects include nausea, vomiting and abdominal pain. It is toxic in higher doses, causing profuse diarrhoea, rashes and kidney damage, and these effects limit its usefulness. Colchicine is sometimes used to confirm the diagnosis of gout because it is so specific in relieving symptoms.

• *LONG-TERM CONTROL* •

If you have recurrent attacks of gout, your doctor may suggest that you take one of two types of medicine for controlling the levels of uric acid in your blood. Once you start treatment you will need to continue it indefinitely to control uric acid levels. **Allopurinol** reduces the formation of uric acid while **probenecid** or **sulphinpyrazone** (*uricosuric* drugs) increase its excretion. None of these drugs must be started during an acute attack of gout because they can prolong and exacerbate symptoms. Colchicine or an NSAID may therefore be given to prevent an acute attack of gout at the start of treatment with allopurinol or the uricosuric drugs. The NSAID **azapropazone** may be helpful in controlling chronic symptoms because it increases the excretion of uric acid in addition to relieving pain and inflammation in acute attacks.

ALLOPURINOL

ALLOPURINOL – Tablets
ZYLORIC – Tablets

Allopurinol is used in the long-term control of gout to prevent recurrent attacks. It lowers blood levels of uric acid by inhibiting the activity of an enzyme involved in the production of uric acid. It will not relieve a gout attack and may even precipitate one at the beginning of treatment. However, keep taking it through an attack of gout in addition to other medicines prescribed to relieve the attack. Allopurinol gradually controls uric acid levels, so attacks of gout stop. It also stops uric acid stones forming in the kidneys and can be used if you have a kidney disorder.

Before you use this medicine

Tell your doctor if you are:
☐ pregnant or breast-feeding ☐ taking any other medicines, including vitamins and those bought over the counter.

Tell your doctor if you have or have had:
☐ a previous reaction to allopurinol ☐ poor kidney or liver function.

How to use this medicine

Take a tablet once a day or higher doses divided up to three times a day with food. Drink about two litres of non-alcoholic fluids a day. Do not drive or do other activities that require alertness until you know how you react to allopurinol. Avoid alcohol: it increases the blood levels of uric acid.

Do not stop taking this medicine without talking to your doctor. Symptoms of gout may return. If you miss a dose, take it as soon as you remember. Do not take double the dose.

Over 65 You need the lowest effective dose.

Interactions with other medicines

Anticancer drugs (**azathioprine**, **cyclophosphamide** and **mercaptopurine**) The effects are enhanced by allopurinol because it blocks their breakdown in the body.
Anticoagulants Blood-thinning effects of **warfarin** and **nicoumalone** are increased.

Unwanted effects

Likely Diarrhoea, feeling or being sick, stomach pains.
Unlikely Skin rashes, itching, red, thick or scaly skin, malaise, headache, vertigo, drowsiness, metallic taste in mouth, numbness

or tingling of hands and feet, sore throat or fever, yellow eyes or skin, hair loss.

Allopurinol is usually well tolerated. Contact your doctor if you develop a skin rash especially if you have fever. The drug usually has to be stopped but your doctor may start it again cautiously if the rash was mild and fades.

Similar preparations

Uricosuric drugs to increase uric acid excretion from the body

ANTURAN – Tablets
SULPHINPYRAZONE

BENEMID – Tablets
PROBENECID

Strains and sprains

Injuries to soft tissues such as muscles, tendons and ligaments are common. They can occur through vigorous exercise or through repetitive use of a particular part of the body, for example strain on the wrist during typing or piano playing.

Muscles ache after unaccustomed exercise and in many sports, muscles, tendons, ligaments and also bones are under great stress. Physical fitness and training parts of the body to withstand stress increases suppleness and strength and helps to prevent injury. However, accidents happen – muscles, tendons or ligaments can be torn or pulled, resulting in pain for a few days, but sometimes more permanent damage. Taking overenthusiastic exercise without building up to a suitable level of fitness may lead to injury or inflammation.

After a few days of rest most sudden injuries begin to improve and you can start gentle exercise and massage to strengthen the injured part. If the injury does not improve, see your doctor or a physiotherapist. Some injuries may need surgery. Repetitive strain injuries, such as tennis elbow, can recur and become long-term problems. They can be enormously frustrating because they prevent you from enjoying pastimes. Even with specialist treatment from a rheumatologist or physiotherapist they can remain painful.

HOW YOU CAN HELP YOURSELF

Use the **RICE** principle
Rest the injured area. This helps to stop bleeding, both internal and external and prevents further damage.
Ice, crushed in a sock or polythene bag or a frozen ice pack applied to the injured area can help to contain swelling. Avoid too much cold as it can burn skin. Cooling sprays are of little value.
Compression with firm bandaging, such as a crepe bandage, helps to stop internal bleeding. Avoid bandaging so tightly that you reduce the circulation to the area.
Elevation – keep the damaged limb or area raised to allow excess fluid to drain away and reduce swelling. In some areas Sports Injury Clinics offer a specialised service, often including physiotherapy, for injuries less than two or three days old. Some encourage self-referral, but a doctor's letter is usually required for chronic sports injuries.

Medicines for strains and sprains

• *ANALGESICS* •

To relieve pain a simple analgesic such as paracetamol or aspirin can be used. Aspirin reduces swelling, but paracetamol has no anti-inflammatory activity. See page 234. Compound analgesics rarely have any advantage over a simple analgesic. An NSAID could be used to reduce swelling, tenderness and pain, but unwanted effects may occur (see page 366). However, pain-relief brings the temptation to use the injured part without allowing nature to take its course during periods of enforced rest. This often leads to the injury being repeated, causing long-term symptoms.

• *CORTICOSTEROIDS* •

A local corticosteroid or NSAID injection (see page 377) may help injuries such as tennis or golfer's elbow – inflammation of the tendons and joint between the muscles or the forearm and the bone just above the elbow. However, the improvement following an injection does not reduce the necessity for a careful resumption of activity if a renewed injury is to be avoided. In *tendinitis*, a painful and inflamed tendon, the corticosteroid is injected into the sheath surrounding the tendon. With injuries that have not responded to local corticosteroid treatment, surgery may be necessary.

• *LOCAL 'RUBS' AND LINIMENTS* •

Pain, whether it is on the surface of the skin or deep within the body, can be relieved by any method which causes irritation of the skin. This is known as counter-irritation and can be most comforting in injuries of the muscles, tendons and joints. Rubefacients are counter-irritants which produce inflammation, opening up the blood vessels to cause redness and warmth. When applying a rubefacient, massage and rubbing are the beneficial actions rather than the medicine itself. Therefore a product that costs more, either because of some claimed property or when expensively packaged – in an aerosol for example – has no advantage over a cheaper brand in a tube or bottle. Most rubefacients contain a salicylate such as **methyl salicylate** with menthol for a distinctive smell. When applying a rubefacient you must be careful to avoid contact with eyes, lips and other mucous membranes and inflamed or broken skin. Rubefacients are not generally suitable for children. Liniments are very harmful if accidentally swallowed; keep them well out of reach of children.

NSAIDs applied to the skin seem to be a logical way of trying to get some of the benefits of systemic NSAIDs without the unwanted effects. However, the topical preparations seem to have a brief effect only and are of uncertain value. There are established and cheaper ways of dealing with soft tissue injuries (see the RICE principle) and for relieving pain (see above).

9

EYES, EARS, MOUTH AND THROAT

Eyes

Conjunctivitis Blepharitis Glaucoma
Dry eye Contact lens problems

The eye, the organ of sight, is a sphere about 2·5cm (1 inch) in diameter, well protected above by the brow and behind by a pad of fat. Six muscles work in pairs to control the movement of each eyeball. Covering most of the eye is a tough whitish coat, the *sclera*. The *cornea* at the front forms a clear protective covering for the coloured iris and pupil and a further outer layer, the *conjunctiva*, covers the cornea and the white of the eye. The *iris* is a muscular ring which controls the inner hole, the *pupil*, through which light passes into the *lens* and then reaches the *retina*, the sensitive lining at the back of the eye, which converts light into nerve impulses. The *optic nerve* leading from the retina carries these signals to the brain, where they are interpreted as sight. The size of the pupil is regulated by the muscles of the iris. In dim light the pupil opens wide to let in as much light as possible, whereas in strong light it narrows to pinpoint size to protect the retina from damage. Many medicines which act on the nervous system affect eyesight; for example, atropine-like drugs cause blurred vision. Tears are the eye's own cleansing and antibacterial system. Each time you blink tears wash across the cornea and conjunctiva, keeping the eye surfaces moist and clean. Tears are made in glands above the eyelid and with each blink liquid is squeezed from the gland. *Tear ducts* at the corner of the eye collect tears into a *tear sac* which then drains into the nose.

The space behind the lens is filled with a jelly-like substance called *vitreous humour* which helps to keep the eye's shape within the socket. The front part of the eye, behind the cornea and in front of the iris is filled with a watery liquid called *aqueous humour*.

Conjunctivitis

Inflammation of the conjunctiva is a common eye condition which can be caused by bacterial or viral infection or may be a symptom of allergy, especially in hay fever sufferers. More rarely conjunctivitis develops from other causes, for example chemical irritation from eye cosmetics or an underlying problem such as thyroid disease.

An inflamed conjunctiva is red and swollen. The eye feels as if it has particles or a foreign body in it and there is a sensation of grittiness. There may also be pain although if the conjunctivitis is caused by infection this will ease as tears cleanse the conjunctiva during each day. A bacterial infection produces pus, a sticky discharge which sometimes makes it difficult to open the eyes especially on waking. Viral conjunctivitis, which often occurs in epidemics, produces a watery discharge. You may also have a sore throat with both bacterial and viral conjunctivitis. One or both eyes may be infected and sometimes the eyelids are swollen and drooping. Allergic conjunctivitis causes redness, inflammation, itching which is sometimes severe and watery eyes.

HOW YOU CAN HELP YOURSELF

Eye problems are a nuisance and should never be ignored. It is difficult to distinguish between infection and allergy, so you should always ask your doctor for advice. A 'red eye' has a number of different causes; get prompt treatment especially if sight is affected or if only one eye is involved.

☐ If your eyes are infected, keep a face towel especially for your own use and wash it regularly.

☐ Wash your hands before and after using any eye preparation.

☐ Avoid using eye cosmetics until the infection has cleared up.

☐ Eye drop preparations should never be shared or lent to anyone: when you have finished the course of treatment, return unused amounts to the pharmacy. Never keep opened eye drop preparations for treating another infection.

Medicines for conjunctivitis

A bacterial infection can be treated with an antibacterial preparation applied locally to the eye, either as drops or as ointment – sometimes both are used. The active ingredient is often an antibiotic, commonly **chloramphenicol**, but **neomycin, framycetin**, **gentamicin**, **polymyxin B** and **fusidic acid** are also useful. **Propamidine** (brand name Brolene) drops may sometimes help conjunctivitis and inflammation of the eyelids (*blepharitis*) and are available from a pharmacy. However, great care is needed in treating an eye infection yourself and if the condition does not appear to be clearing up after two days, you should consult your doctor.

The sulphonamide drug **sulphacetamide** (brand name Albucid) is rarely helpful and is no longer recommended. Preparations containing **mercuric oxide** should not be used even for short periods and are not recommended.

WARNING

Some antibiotic preparations contain a corticosteroid (see Chapter 6: Hormones). These preparations must never be used if you have an infection or if you have 'red eye'. 'Red eye' is sometimes caused by *Herpes simplex* virus, which produces an ulcer in the eye. A corticosteroid used locally in the eye may aggravate this condition and possibly lead to serious complications such as loss of vision or even loss of the eye. Furthermore, if a corticosteroid is used for more than a few weeks 'steroid glaucoma' may result in people who have a tendency to develop long-term simple glaucoma.

A combination of an antibacterial and a corticosteroid is rarely needed.

Preparations not recommended include:

BETNESOL-N
BETAMETHASONE + NEOMYCIN

CHLOROMYCETIN HYDROCORTISONE
CHLORAMPHENICOL + HYDROCORTISONE

EUMOVATE-N
CLOBETASONE + NEOMYCIN

FML-NEO
FLUOROMETHALONE + NEOMYCIN

MAXITROL
DEXAMETHASONE + NEOMYCIN + POLYMYXIN B

NEO-CORTEF
HYDROCORTISONE + NEOMYCIN

PREDSOL-N
PREDNISOLONE + NEOMYCIN

SOFRADEX
DEXAMETHASONE + FRAMYCETIN + GRAMICIDIN

VISTA-METHASONE N
BETAMETHASONE + NEOMYCIN

APPLYING MEDICINES TO THE EYE

A medicine can be applied *topically* (direct to the affected area) in eye drops, ointment or lotion. Sometimes a medicine is given byinjection into the conjunctiva for severe infections that have not responded to topical treatment. A plastic device placed in the eye which releases a controlled amount of the drug over a specific period (for example Ocusert) can be used for long-term conditions such as glaucoma.

Eye drops

Just one or two drops of liquid are placed (instilled) in the eye per dose because this is all the eye can hold. Drops should be instilled into the top outer corner of the eye so that they spread over the whole eye before reaching the tear duct. Within 15 seconds the drug is diluted by tears, so it does not have long to act. For this reason eye drops have to be used frequently – at least once every two hours until the infection is controlled and thereafter four times a day.

The drug almost always gets into the body, as it is absorbed into the circulation via the blood vessels in the conjunctiva and it drains down the tear ducts into the nose. If you lightly press a finger against the corner of the eye beside the nose for a few moments after applying the drops you can keep the drug in contact with the conjunctiva for longer. If you have two different eye drop preparations you should leave several minutes between using one type of drops and the other.

When applying eye drops take care not to touch the eye or anything else with the dropper. Eyes can easily become infected through the dropper or an infection can be transferred from one eye to the other. An eye drop preparation is sterile before it is opened, but once opened it can easily become contaminated, so a preservative is included. If you use the preparation carefully – washing hands before applying drops, not touching the eye with the dropper and replacing the dropper in the bottle immediately after use – the drops can be used for up to one month. After this time the risk of contamination is too great.

Preservatives commonly used in eye drops include **benzalkonium chloride**, **thiomersal** and **phenylmercuric nitrate**. They are used in small amounts, but cause allergy in a few people. If your eye condition worsens after you have started treatment, contact your doctor – you may be allergic to one of the ingredients in the preparation.

Single-use eye drops do not contain a preservative. Each container holds a sterile dose, but must be thrown away after its first use because there is nothing in the preparation to prevent contamination once opened.

Eye ointments

Eye ointments contain the medicine in a greasy base. Preparations are sterile until opened and can be used for up to one month providing the usual hygiene measures are observed (see 'How you can help yourself'). Eye ointment is generally easier to apply than drops. The medicine acts for up to 15 minutes and less is absorbed into the body than with drops. Eye ointment does not have to be used as frequently as drops – twice-daily applications are sometimes adequate and an eye ointment is ideal for night-time use.

Eye lotions

Solutions for washing out the eye can be used to soothe the eye or to flush out irritants or foreign bodies. Eye lotions are sterile until they are opened. A soothing lotion for use at home should not be used for longer than one month. In a first aid kit, an eye lotion such as **sodium chloride** should be used for a maximum of 24 hours after opening and not returned to the kit for future use.

CHLORAMPHENICOL

CHLORAMPHENICOL – Eye drops, eye ointment, ear drops
CHLOROMYCETIN – Eye drops, eye ointment, capsules, liquid, injection
KEMICETINE – Injection
MINIMS CHLORAMPHENICOL – Single-use eye drops
SNO PHENICOL – Eye drops

Chloramphenicol is an antibiotic, now mostly used topically for bacterial infections of the eye and ear. It is potentially toxic when taken by mouth or injected, so such treatment is reserved for life-threatening infections against which it is effective, such as typhoid fever and a certain type of meningitis. The following information applies to topical preparations only.

Before you use this medicine

Tell your doctor if you are:
☐ pregnant or breast-feeding ☐ taking any other medicines, including vitamins and those bought over the counter.

Tell your doctor if you have or have had:

☐ sensitivity to any of the ingredients, such as preservatives.

How to use this medicine

Eye drops Instil two drops into the upper outer corner of the eye at least every two hours for the first 24 hours, reducing to four times daily as the infection is controlled. Continue to use the drops for 48 hours after the infection seems to have cleared and the eye appears normal.
Eye ointment Apply a small amount to the eye or within the lower lid three or four times daily. The ointment can be used at night and eye drops used during the day.
Ear drops Apply two or three times daily to the external ear.

If you miss a dose, apply as soon as you remember.

Over 65 No special requirements.

Unwanted effects

Likely with eye drops Short-term stinging or burning; **with ear drops** sensitivity to the ear drop solution: around one person in ten is sensitive to **propylene glycol**.

If your ear condition seems to worsen contact your doctor because you may be sensitive to the solution containing chloramphenicol. Chloramphenicol eye preparations rarely cause problems, but they are not recommended for prolonged use.

Similar preparations

CIDOMYCIN – Eye/ear drops, eye ointment
GENTAMICIN

FUCITHALMIC – Eye drops
FUSIDIC ACID

GARAMYCIN – Eye/ear drops
GENTAMICIN

GENTICIN – Eye drops, eye ointment
GENTAMICIN

NEOMYCIN – Eye drops, eye ointment

NEOSPORIN – Eye drops
POLYMYXIN B + NEOMYCIN + GRAMICIDIN

SOFRAMYCIN – Eye drops
FRAMYCETIN

● *NON-BACTERIAL INFECTIONS* ●

There is no treatment for viral conjunctivitis but this clears of its own accord in two to three weeks. Your doctor may give you an antibiotic to guard against a secondary bacterial infection. Some viral infections, such as herpes simplex, can be treated with specific antiviral eye preparations. Fungal infections affect the cornea rather than the conjunctiva and are not common. Eye symptoms caused by hay fever are usually treated with **sodium cromoglycate** eye drops or ointment (see page 179).

A corticosteroid is usually used under expert supervision, for example to reduce inflammation after an eye operation. A corticosteroid eye preparation should not be used for relieving allergic symptoms.

Blepharitis

Blepharitis is inflammation of the edge of the eyelids, making them sore, red and itchy. There are two types: one is caused by a bacterium (*Staphylococcus*) which produces pus, ulceration and dry dandruff-like scales and the other is an eczematous condition, similar to *seborrhoeic eczema*, with greasy flakes of skin clinging to the eyelashes. Eczematous eyelids can also become infected with bacteria. Infection around an eyelash may cause a stye.

Treatment involves cleaning the eyelids very carefully and then, if there is infection, applying an antibacterial ointment regularly. In the eczematous condition the scalp and eyebrows may also be affected and if these areas are treated with a medicated shampoo, the eyelids often improve. Styes are treated with an antibiotic ointment.

Glaucoma

Aqueous humour is continuously formed within the eye and absorbed back into the veins. Any imbalance between the formation and absorption of this liquid leads to increased pressure within the eye and to a condition known as *glaucoma*. As pressure builds up, the blood vessels to the optic nerve become squashed, reducing the blood flow to the nerve. Eventually the nerve is irreversibly damaged, resulting in permanent loss of sight. Glaucoma is a major cause of blindness but early detection and treatment with medicines or surgery can prevent irreversible damage. It usually occurs in older people.

● *ACUTE GLAUCOMA* ●

Acute glaucoma develops suddenly and is a medical emergency. It occurs when the angle between the iris and the cornea becomes completely closed, preventing aqueous humour from draining away, and pressure from the excess fluid increases rapidly. The eye becomes red and extremely painful; you may have a headache and vomit; vision becomes blurred as the pressure distorts the cornea. You may experience warning symptoms – seeing haloes around lights – and these may occur some weeks or even months before the main attack.

Acute glaucoma needs immediate medical attention in order to prevent permanent loss of sight. Treatment includes lowering the pressure within the eye by reducing the amount of fluid with an intravenous injection of a diuretic followed by surgery. An operation called an *iridectomy* usually solves the problem and long-term treatment with a medicine is rarely needed. The operation involves cutting a tiny hole in the cornea and removing a strip of the iris to allow excess fluid to drain away continuously. There is a risk of the condition occurring in the other eye, so a prophylactic iridectomy is often carried out on that at the same time.

● *CHRONIC SIMPLE GLAUCOMA* ●

This is the most common type of glaucoma, which develops slowly and insidiously. Fluid drains away less efficiently but the production of fluid is unaffected. More aqueous humour remains within the eye and the pressure builds up slowly and painlessly. As the optic nerve is gradually damaged the field of vision is reduced, so that eventually only a small area of central vision remains (tunnel vision) before sight is lost completely. Most people with glaucoma do not have symptoms until they notice some loss of vision, but by this stage the optic nerve is irreversibly damaged. Treatment can prevent further deterioration but cannot restore damage already done. Surgery is often used to relieve chronic glaucoma, including reshaping the eye with a laser.

Medicines for glaucoma

Medical treatment aims to reduce the pressure within the eye (*intra-ocular* pressure) and prevent further reduction in your field of vision. Drug treatment, usually in the form of eye drops, lessens the production of aqueous humour or increases its outflow. A topical beta blocker, such as **timolol**, is generally the first

HOW YOU CAN HELP YOURSELF

☐ If you have a close relative with glaucoma – parent, brother or sister – take particular care to have your eyes checked regularly. Anyone with a family history of glaucoma is entitled to free sight tests.
☐ If you have treatment with eye drops, you will need to use them regularly every day, possibly for life. If you have to use more than one type of eye preparation at the same time of day, allow five to ten minutes between each application.

choice; it reduces the rate of production of aqueous humour within the eye, lessening pressure. A beta blocker is often useful for treating mild glaucoma, but should not be used if you are asthmatic or if you have obstructive airways disease, abnormally slow heartbeat, heart block or heart failure. **Pilocarpine** is an alternative choice (see below). Your doctor may need to add other medicines, depending on how well the intra-ocular pressure remains controlled.

Pilocarpine eye drops increase the outflow of aqueous humour by opening up the drainage channels. However, pilocarpine is a *miotic*: it has the unwanted effect of making the size of the pupil smaller. Pilocarpine also affects 'accommodation', the eye's ability to focus, which results in blurred vision and brow-ache. This is particularly troublesome for younger people and those who are short-sighted. Pilocarpine acts for about three to four hours and drops have to be instilled four times daily, depending on your condition. **Physostigmine** is similar to pilocarpine but has a more powerful action and is usually used in combination with pilocarpine.

Adrenaline eye drops (brand names Epifrin; Eppy; Simplene) increase the outflow of fluid as well as reducing the rate of production of aqueous humour. Adrenaline is a *mydriatic*: it dilates the pupil and must not be used to treat acute glaucoma. It is longer-acting than pilocarpine and only needs to be used once or twice daily. In some people, adrenaline may cause severe stinging and redness in the eye. If you have high blood pressure or heart disease, adrenaline should be used with caution. **Dipivefrine** (brand name Propine) is similar. **Guanethidine** (brand names Ganda; Ismelin) enhances and prolongs the effects of adrenaline. It is sometimes used on its own, but your eyes need checking at least every six months, because it may affect the conjunctiva and cornea if it is used for long periods.

Acetazolamide is a diuretic taken by mouth to relieve chronic simple glaucoma and used as an injection to reduce pressure rapidly in acute glaucoma.

TIMOLOL

TIMOPTOL – Eye drops

Timolol is a beta blocker (see also Chapter 2: Heart and Circulation) used in the eye to reduce the pressure caused by the build up of aqueous humour. It is used for treating eye conditions such as chronic simple glaucoma and ocular hypertension (raised intra-ocular pressure which does not damage the eye). It lowers intra-ocular pressure by reducing the rate of production of aqueous humour. It may be used as supplementary treatment after surgery in either acute or chronic glaucoma. Although timolol is used in the eye, some of it is absorbed into the body so that effects occur throughout the body. Timolol or any other beta blocker for use in the eye should not be used if you have asthma or other breathing difficulties or heart disease.

Before you use this medicine

Tell your doctor if you are:
□ pregnant – discuss with your doctor; the effect of timolol eye drops has not been studied □ breast-feeding □ taking any other medicines, including vitamins and those bought over the counter.

Tell your doctor if you have or have had:
□ diabetes □ circulation problems □ thyroid disorders.

Do not use if you have or have had:
□ asthma □ obstructive airways diseases such as chronic bronchitis or emphysema □ heart block or heart failure □ bradycardia (slow heartbeat).

How to use this medicine

Use one drop twice daily in the affected eye; the dropper bottle automatically measures one drop. See your doctor after four weeks for a check-up. If the intra-ocular pressure stabilises satisfactorily you may be able to switch to once-a-day treatment.

Do not drive or do other activities that require alertness until you know how you react to timolol. The eye drops may cause blurred vision.

Do not stop using timolol suddenly or your condition may worsen. If you miss a dose, apply it as soon as you remember. If you are using timolol twice a day, apply the missed dose as soon as you remember, but skip it if it is nearly time for your next dose. Do not apply double the dose.

If you have to have an operation tell your doctor or dentist that you use timolol drops.

Over 65 No special requirements.

Interactions with other medicines

Although timolol is used in the eye, it may be absorbed into the body and interact with medicines in the same way as taking a beta blocker by mouth (see **atenolol** drug profile, page 117). Do not take other medicines without first checking with your doctor or pharmacist.

Unwanted effects

Likely Blurred vision, dry eyes for short periods, headache.
Unlikely Eye irritation, allergic reaction.

Timolol eye drops are rarely troublesome. Discomfort in the eyes usually fades as treatment continues.

Similar preparations

BETAGAN – Eye drops
LEVOBUNOLOL

BETOPTIC – Eye drops
BETAXOLOL

MINIMS METIPRANOLOL – Single-use eye drops
METIPRANOLOL

TEOPTIC – Eye drops
CARTEOLOL

ACETAZOLAMIDE

DIAMOX – Tablets, modified-release capsules, injection

Acetazolamide is a diuretic used for treating chronic simple glaucoma. It reduces pressure within the eye by decreasing the amount of aqueous humour produced. It is taken by mouth and can be added to other drug treatments, such as beta blocker eye drops, usually as a short-term measure when the intra-ocular pressure needs further reduction. Acetazolamide is also used before surgery in acute glaucoma. Unwanted effects may be troublesome, so acetazolamide is not generally recommended for long-term treatment or for use as a diuretic (see Chapter 2: Heart and Circulation). If you take acetazolamide routinely you may need to have periodic blood tests.

Before you use this medicine

Tell your doctor if you are:
☐ pregnant – avoid acetazolamide ☐ breast-feeding ☐ taking any other medicines, including vitamins and those bought over the counter.

Tell your doctor if you have or have had:
☐ kidney disease or kidney stones ☐ adrenal gland disease (Addison's disease) ☐ diabetes ☐ liver disease ☐ low blood levels of sodium or potassium ☐ sensitivity to sulphonamides.

How to use this medicine

Take one tablet up to four times daily with food. The modified-release capsule can be taken once or twice a day and may be easier to remember if you have to take acetazolamide regularly.

Drink plenty of non-alcoholic fluids while you take acetazolamide to prevent kidney stones. Acetazolamide may reduce the amount of potassium in your body, so eat plenty of potassium-rich foods such as fresh fruit and vegetables (see page 111).

Do not drive or do other activities that require alertness until you know how you react to acetazolamide. Avoid alcohol because it aggravates dehydration caused by acetazolamide.

Do not stop taking this medicine suddenly or your condition may worsen. If you miss a dose, take it as soon as you remember, but skip it if it is almost time for your next dose. Do not take double the dose.

Over 65 You are more likely to experience unwanted effects.

Interactions with other medicines

Lithium Acetazolamide, like other diuretics, may lower sodium levels in the body and increase lithium toxicity.
Other diuretics, especially thiazides enhance the potassium lowering effect. Avoid combinations of diuretics.
Aspirin increases the level of acetazolamide in the body and the risk of unwanted effects.
Heart drugs such as **digoxin** and other blood pressure lowering

medicines may need dosage adjustment if taken at the same time as acetazolamide.

Unwanted effects

Likely Feeling or being sick, stomach upsets, drowsiness, dizziness, lethargy, increased frequency of passing urine, numbness, tingling in hands or feet.
Rare Skin rashes, fever, sore throat, unusual bruising or bleeding, confusion, ringing or buzzing in the ears, temporary deafness.

Acetazolamide is a useful treatment for glaucoma. It is not usually given for long periods, but if it is, you will need blood tests and other tests to check kidney function and the level of salts in the body. Likely unwanted effects generally fade as treatment continues and disappear once treatment is stopped. If you feel unwell while you take acetazolamide, discuss the symptoms with your doctor. If you develop a skin rash or hearing loss, stop taking acetazolamide and contact your doctor.

Similar preparations

DARANIDE – Tablets
DICHLORPHENAMIDE

Dry eye

Dry eye is a common condition, particularly in post-menopausal women and old people, often associated with rheumatoid arthritis. The normal composition of tears may become deficient or less tear fluid may be made. You may have a feeling of grit in the eye or heaviness or drooping of the lids. You may have a headache and difficulty in opening your eyes and there may be mucus. Symptoms usually get worse in hot or smoky environments, and in the evening. Some drugs diminish tear flow.

Treatment involves using a tear substitute and if possible, avoiding situations that make your eyes worse. 'Artificial tear' drops are viscous: they thicken tear film and reduce tear drainage. They are usually used hourly at first to bring symptoms under control and then at least four times a day. A lubricating eye ointment may help further at night. Drops containing **phenylephrine** (brand name Isopto Frin) are not recommended. Many tear substitutes contain a preservative which can cause a local allergic reaction. If this happens you may have to use a single-use preparation without a preservative, such as **hydroxethylcellulose** (Artifical Tears), or **sodium chloride** solution, but these need more frequent application.

One bottle of eye drops used four times daily for both eyes should last four weeks and then be discarded. Your doctor can prescribe these products or you can buy them at a pharmacy, some at less than the prescription charge.

'ARTIFICIAL TEAR' DROPS

Active ingredient	*Product name*	*Preservative*
HYPROMELLOSE	HYPROMELLOSE EYE-DROPS	benzalkonium
	BJ6	chlorhexidine
	ISOPTO ALKALINE	benzalkonium
	ISOPTO PLAIN	benzalkonium
HYPROMELLOSE + DEXTRAN '70'	TEARS NATURALE	benzalkonium
ACETYLCYSTEINE + HYPROMELLOSE	ILUBE	benzalkonium
HYDROXYETHYLCELLULOSE	MINIMS ARTIFICIAL TEARS	none (single-use)
LIQUID PARAFFIN	LACRI-LUBE	lanolin derivatives
POLYVINYL ALCOHOL	HYPOTEARS	benzalkonium + disodium edetate
	LIQUIFILM TEARS	benzalkonium + disodium edetate
	SNO TEARS	benzalkonium + disodium edetate
SODIUM CHLORIDE SOLUTION	MINIMS SODIUM CHLORIDE	none (single-use)

Contact lens problems

Many people wear contact lenses instead of glasses, for cosmetic reasons or because it helps in sporting activities. Contact lenses can also be used for treating certain eye disorders and hiding unsightly eyes. A contact lens is small, paper-thin and usually fits over the cornea. Lenses provide all-round vision and avoid the problems of dusty or steamed-up glasses and frames that slip down your nose. There is a wide range of lenses of different materials and types. The lens material and type influence not only how well you can see and how comfortable the lenses are, but also the complications they may cause. Ideally, the lens material should not interfere with the oxygen supply to the cornea and the eye's lens or with the usual working of the eye, such as tear secretion.

Lens materials are broadly referred to as hard or soft. Hard lenses may be *gas-permeable*, where the material allows oxygen to pass through it, or non gas-permeable, where oxygen cannot pass through. The original hard lens material, *polymethyl methacrylate* (PMMA), is impermeable to oxygen, so it can be supplied only from the layer of tears under the lens. The newer gas-permeable materials allow varying amounts of oxygen through.

Other factors such as how well the material fits over the cornea, how stable it is and how wettable are important. Soft lens materials are of two types – *hydrogels* which contain varying amounts of water (hydrophilic lenses) and are the most used, and *silicone rubber*. Most soft lenses allow oxygen through to the cornea. Soft lenses are easier to fit and, unlike most hard lenses, are readily available from the optician. They are more comfortable in the first few days but thereafter the difference is small. Soft lenses are more fragile and do not last as long as hard lenses.

● *COMPLICATIONS* ●

A contact lens is a foreign body in intimate contact with the eye and can cause complications. Any type of lens can damage the cornea causing problems such as pain, infection, foreign body sensation or discharge. If you get any problems with your lenses you should see an ophthalmologist as soon as possible. Both types of lenses can cause complications and there seems to be little difference between them. Most injuries arise from problems with the lenses themselves, including scratches, deformation and contamination. Research has shown that good lens hygiene is important in reducing the incidence of complications. Looking after your lenses carefully and cleaning them regularly is essential.

Contact lenses are usually inserted daily, but high-water-content soft lenses and some hard lenses allow so much oxygen to get through to the cornea that they can be worn for up to three months. However, these *extended-wear* lenses are much more likely to cause infection with bacteria, fungi or viruses, tissue damage and inflammation. Most opticians would recommend shorter periods of wear for these particular lenses, especially if the lenses are worn just for convenience or cosmetic reasons.

● *LENSES AND MEDICINES* ●

If you need to use eye drops or ointment you should not wear your lenses during the course of treatment, unless your lenses are for a medical purpose or your doctor says you may leave them in. Some medicines can spoil hydrophilic soft lenses and unless eye drops are known to be safe to use with these lenses, you must take them out before starting treatment and not wear them again until treatment has stopped.

The plastic used for many hydrophilic contact lenses interacts with some preservatives used in eye drop preparations. This may cause irritation in the eye. **Benzalkonium chloride** is a common preservative and is unsuitable with all soft lenses. **Thiomersal** does not usually cause problems, **chlorhexidine** is satisfactory for some lenses and **phenylmercuric acetate** or **nitrate** is usually acceptable for short periods.

Some medicines that you take by mouth make it uncomfortable for you to wear contact lenses, for example atropine-like drugs and beta blockers.

Ears

Middle-ear infection   Glue ear
Outer-ear problems   Wax

There are three parts to the ear. The outer ear is the visible part; the middle and inner ear are within the head protected by the skull. The outer ear flap (*pinna*) is mainly made of cartilage. It funnels sound along the ear canal to the eardrum (*tympanic membrane*), which separates the outer ear from the middle and inner. The middle ear contains three tiny bones within an air-filled cavity. The *eustachian tube* runs from the middle ear to the back of the throat, allowing pressure in the middle ear to be the same as the outside air pressure. The inner ear contains the organs of balance (*cochlea*) and of hearing (*labyrinth*).

Middle-ear infection

Middle-ear infection (*otitis media*) is common, especially in young children. Symptoms include pain, fever and temporary deafness. The middle ear can easily become infected if you have a nose or throat infection because bacteria or viruses gain access to it via the eustachian tube. Viral infections have to run their course but are usually less serious than bacterial infections, which can be treated with antibiotics. Unless treated, pus from a bacterial infection may accumulate in the middle ear until the pressure builds up and the ear drum bursts or perforates. Hearing may then be impaired permanently. It is sometimes difficult for your doctor to tell whether your infection is caused by bacteria or a virus. Many middle-ear infections are caused by viruses, but your doctor may give you an antibiotic just in case there is a secondary bacterial infection. If the infection recurs you may need long-term antibiotic treatment, perhaps right through the winter months. Pain can be relieved with an analgesic such as paracetamol.

Local treatment with ear drops applied to the outer ear does not help acute middle-ear problems. **Choline salicylate** (brand name Audax) is a mild analgesic but is of doubtful value when applied to the ear.

Glue ear

Glue ear (*sero-mucinous otitis media*) is the commonest cause of childhood deafness and affects at least one pre-school child in ten. Fluid that forms in the middle ear usually drains away but does not do so if it becomes thick and sticky; the cause of this is unknown. The transmission of sound through the middle ear is affected and hearing is impaired. Although it often follows middle-ear infection, there may be no history of ear problems at all. Poor ventilation of the middle ear via the eustachian tube may contribute as may recurrent tonsillitis and adenoid trouble. A child with a cleft palate or Down's syndrome is particularly likely to have glue ear. Glue ear interferes with the acquisition of normal speech and learning.

Sometimes glue ear improves spontaneously; about a quarter of the children who develop glue ear in their first year improve and half the children who develop it between the ages of one and four do. The condition improves in the summer but relapses again in the winter. Glue ear is less common in children over six and in such cases often resolves of its own accord. However, at whatever age you suspect that your child has a hearing problem you should discuss your concerns with your general practitioner. If glue ear is suspected your doctor should refer you to a specialist because of the risk of permanent damage to middle-ear function and impaired language development.

The aim of treatment is to clear the sticky fluid from the middle ear and to control any infection. An antibiotic may help where there is infection, but there is little evidence that decongestants or antihistamines are helpful, although these preparations are often tried. Decongestants such as **pseudoephedrine** (brand names Sudafed; Dimotane Plus; Galpseud) may cause irritability, sleep disturbance and even hallucinations. Antihistamines cause daytime drowsiness and unsteadiness.

Surgery for glue ear is now common, particularly for children between five and eight. The surgeon is likely to insert *grommets* and/or to remove the *adenoids* if hearing is significantly impaired and does not improve within a few months. Grommets are tiny tubes inserted through the ear drum to allow fluid to drain into the outer ear. After a few months the grommet normally falls out and the ear drum heals. *Myringotomy* is surgical puncture of the ear drum to drain fluid without inserting grommets.

You should discuss the pros and cons of surgery with your doctor; the operation may distress children and involves hospital admission at an age when this can be particularly upsetting. Any general anaesthetic carries some risk and removal of adenoids may occasionally lead to severe blood and fluid loss. The risks from myringotomy and insertion of a grommet are much less. Against these possible problems you will have to weigh up the risk of witholding surgery. Your child may be underperforming at school and behind in social development because of persistent deafness. Very rarely hearing may become permanently impaired.

Grommets that fall out need not be replaced unless symptoms recur. The child may swim, but not dive, because water may get into the middle ear and possibly cause infection. Some doctors recommend using moulded ear plugs and a swimming cap to cover the ears.

Outer-ear problems

The ear canal is lined with very fine skin covered with tiny hairs. Glands in the skin produce an oily fluid which combines with shed cells from the outermost layer of skin to form a covering of wax. The hairs catch dust and dirt which are then trapped in the wax; this is part of the ear's protective mechanisms against invading microbes.

Inflammation of the outer ear canal (*otitis externa*) is an eczema-like skin reaction. If the skin becomes broken, for example from scratching, bacteria or fungi may cause infection. The ear may itch and be quite painful; there may be some discharge and hearing may be impaired temporarily. These symptoms are similar to those of a middle-ear infection and it will be important to see your doctor for correct diagnosis.

● *Applying ear drops*

It may be difficult for you to put ear drops into your own ear so ask someone to help you. Three to four drops should be instilled into the ear canal without the dropper touching the ear. Drops are hard to keep in the ear for any length of time, so you should lie

HOW YOU CAN HELP YOURSELF

☐ The ear has its own self-cleansing mechanism, so avoid using cotton buds to clean out the wax. Wax is continuously produced and moves along the ear canal to the outer ear where it is removed with routine washing.
☐ If the ear becomes itchy, try not to scratch it as this will encourage infection.
☐ If you develop an ear problem see your doctor.
☐ If you have treatment, ask someone to help you apply the ear drops.
☐ Regular swimmers are more likely to get outer ear problems because water breaks down the ear's protective and cleansing mechanisms. Use well-fitting ear plugs or petroleum jelly to protect the ears.

down with the affected ear facing upwards for ten minutes after the solution has been instilled to allow time for the ear drops to take effect. If there is a discharge, this should be gently mopped up before gauze soaked with the drops is placed in the ear.

Medicines for the outer ear

If the ear is itchy and inflamed, but not infected, treatment involves using ear drops that are either astringent – causing the tissue to contract – such as **aluminium acetate**, or anti-inflammatory (a corticosteroid), both of which will help to clean the ear and soothe the inflammation. The outer ear may be full of debris and discharge and this will need gently removing. Drops can then be instilled or, alternatively, a piece of ribbon gauze soaked in the drops can be placed gently into the ear canal. A corticosteroid such as **betamethasone** (brand names Betnesol; Vista-Methasone) or **prednisolone** (Predsol) reduces itching and irritation but should not be used for prolonged periods as it may increase the likelihood of infection. If the ear is infected your doctor may give you ear drops containing an anti-infective drug such as **neomycin** or **framycetin**. The drops can be used for about one week but prolonged use may produce bacteria which become resistant to the drug or allow a fungal infection to develop. **Chloramphenicol** ear drops may be used but they contain **propylene glycol** which causes sensitivity in about one person in ten. Ear drops containing an anti-infective and a cortocosteroid may be used when the skin is infected as well as inflamed and eczematous. Compound anti-infective preparations containing several antibiotics, a corticosteroid, and sometimes an antifungal drug, are not recommended. An acute (sudden and severe) infection, such as a boil, may need treatment with an antibiotic by mouth.

ANTI-INFECTIVE PREPARATIONS

Anti-infective only

ACHROMYCIN
TETRACYCLINE

CANESTEN
CLOTRIMAZOLE

CHLORAMPHENICOL – High risk of sensitivity

CIDOMYCIN
GENTAMICIN

GARAMYCIN
GENTAMICIN

GENTICIN
GENTAMICIN

Anti-infective with corticosteroid

AUDIOCORT
NEOMYCIN + TRIAMCINOLONE

BETNESOL-N
NEOMYCIN + BETAMATHASONE

GENTISONE HC
GENTAMICIN + HYDROCORTISONE

LOCORTEN-VIOFORM
CLIOQUINOL + FLUMETHASONE

NEO-CORTEF
NEOMYCIN + HYDROCORTISONE

OTOMIZE
NEOMYCIN + DEXAMETHASONE

PREDSOL-N
NEOMYCIN + PREDNISOLONE

VISTA-METHASONE N
NEOMYCIN + BETAMETHASONE

Compound preparations: not recommended

OTOSPORIN; SOFRADEX; SOFRAMYCIN; TERRA-CORTRIL; TRI-ADCORTYL OTIC

The Committee on Safety of Medicines has told doctors that the risk of drug-induced deafness with **chlorhexidine**, **framycetin**, **neomycin** and related preparations, or with **polymyxin**, is increased if any of them is used in the outer ear when the ear drum has perforated. If you think your ear drum might be damaged tell your doctor before he prescribes ear drops. Some specialists use these ear drops cautiously for treating severe middle-ear infections when the ear drum is perforated. The infection itself can impair hearing and your doctor will weigh the risks and benefits of using this type of preparation in the middle ear.

Wax

Wax provides a protective layer over the skin of the outer ear. It is a normal bodily secretion and does not need removing unless it is blocking the ear canal and drum and causing deafeness or irritation.

The ear can be unblocked by using wax-softening drops. Sometimes using these drops for a few days may loosen the wax sufficiently to unblock the ear. Alternatively you may need to have the ear syringed with warm water by your doctor or practice nurse. If the wax is hard and impacted in the ear, using a wax-softening preparation before syringing will make the wax come out more easily.

A simple remedy is recommended – such as olive oil, almond oil or sodium bicarbonate ear drops. Any of these is effective and can be bought over the counter for less than the prescription charge. The oil can be warmed before use and you will need someone to help you put the drops into the ear. Lie with the affected ear uppermost for at least five minutes afterwards. A small plug of cotton wool may help to retain some of the fluid after treatment. Oil and wax may seep out, especially during sleep, and pillows can be protected with an old towel. Use the drops twice a day for three to four days.

Some brand name preparations contain solvents that may irritate the skin of the outer ear and should be avoided. Also, these preparations for removing wax are no better than simple oils and are generally more expensive. They include Audinorm; Cerumol; Dioctyl; Exterol; Molcer; Waxsol.

Mouth and throat

Mouth ulcers Thrush Sore throat

The mouth is the starting point of the digestive system. A *mucous membrane*, which secretes a slimy substance, lines the mouth, gums, palate and throat; saliva enters the mouth from glands beneath the tongue and near the ears. Special skin on the tongue contains most of the taste buds. The roof of the mouth consists of a hard (bony) palate and a soft (muscular) palate. At the back lie the *tonsils* and the *pharynx* – when these are inflamed they cause a sore throat (*tonsillitis* or *pharyngitis*). *Laryngitis* is inflammation of the vocal cords, which causes a sore throat along with hoarseness, loss of voice and a cough.

Mouth ulcers

Mouth ulcers are sore, swollen areas where the skin has broken in the mucous membrane in the mouth. At least three quarters of mouth ulcers are *minor aphthous* ulcers, which are not serious, but are painful and recur from time to time. Women have mouth ulcers more frequently than men and they occur most commonly between the ages of 10 and 40. A day or two before the ulcer or ulcers break out part of your mouth may feel sore or burnt; pain and inflammation increase, particularly when you eat. The ulcers, up to five in number, are round or oval-shaped and whitish to yellow in the centre; the surrounding skin is red and swollen. Ulcers occur most commonly on the lips, cheeks and side of the tongue.

Ulceration of the mouth has a number of different causes, including badly fitting dental plates, but the mouth often acts as a barometer of health. Skin disorders often start in the mouth while vitamin deficiency or blood disorders such as iron-deficiency anaemia also cause a sore mouth or ulceration. Disorders of the digestive system such as inflammatory bowel disease (Crohn's disease and ulcerative colitis) and coeliac disease may be linked to mouth ulceration. Other causes include infection, injury, reactions to medicine, and radiotherapy. Aphthous ulcers clear up of their own accord although they may take up to 14 days to heal. However, if you have an ulcer or a sore mouth which persists for more than two weeks, you should see your doctor. The underlying condition will need treating in addition to the ulcers.

Medicines for mouth ulcers

Local treatment aims to soothe the pain of ulcers while natural healing takes place. There are many remedies, including mouthwashes, protective pastes, gels and antiseptic lozenges. All of these may relieve symptoms in some people and you will need to find a preparation that suits you. Local corticosteroids or **tetracycline** are often prescribed for mouth ulcers; other preparations are available from a pharmacy.

● *Mouthwashes*

Mouthwashes are particularly useful when the ulcers are in awkward parts of the mouth and inaccessible. Simple mouthwashes of **sodium chloride** (for a home-made version use a rounded teaspoonful of salt to a pint of water) or **compound thymol**

glycerin are soothing and may relieve the pain of ulceration caused by injury such as biting the inside of your mouth or by ill-fitting dentures. The mouthwash should be made up with warm water and can be used frequently to relieve swelling and pain.

Antiseptic mouthwashes such as **chlorhexidine** (brand names Corsodyl; Eludril) or **povidone-iodine** (Betadine) help to relieve pain and may speed healing of the ulcerated area; they are anti-infective, acting against bacteria and candida. Neither liquid should be diluted before use. Chlorhexidine temporarily stains teeth, dentures and tongue a brown colour, through an interaction with some foods and drinks, such as tea, coffee and red wines. Occasionally the teeth and fillings may have to be scaled and polished to remove the stain completely.

Benzydamine mouthwash or spray (brand name Difflam) can relieve the discomfort of various ulcerative conditions. It reduces the symptoms of radiation-induced mouth inflammation. The mouthwash can be used without dilution but some people find this causes stinging; diluting the liquid with an equal volume of water reduces this. Numbness and tingling of the mouth may occur but are short-lived. The mouthwash is not suitable for children under 12 years, but the spray can be used. **Zinc sulphate** mouthwash is an astringent which some people find helps recurrent aphthous ulcers.

● *Protective pastes*

Carmellose gelatin paste (brand name Orabase) protects the ulcer by forming a barrier over it and in this way it relieves discomfort. A thin layer can be applied when needed, usually after meals. The paste sticks to the ulcer, but it is quite difficult to apply especially to some less accessible parts of the mouth. Carmellose gelatin paste is also made with the corticosteroid **triamcinolone** (brand name Adcortyl in Orabase). The paste sticks to the ulcer and allows the corticosteroid to penetrate the damaged area. A thin layer must be carefully applied, not rubbed in, two to four times a day. In addition to treating aphthous ulcers the paste can be used for sore areas of the mouth caused by dentures, provided these are not infected.

● *Lozenges*

Hydrocortisone lozenges (brand name Corlan) are most effective if they are used just before the ulcer develops. The lozenge is allowed to dissolve slowly in contact with the ulcer four times a day. Prolonged use may allow candida to flourish. A corticosteroid should not be used if the mouth is infected, unless the infection is already being treated.

Compound benzocaine lozenges may relieve soreness in the mouth and painful ulcers. Benzocaine is a local anaesthetic which acts as an analgesic for a short time after it has been applied. **Lignocaine** lozenges or ointment are also used. When a local anaesthetic is used in the mouth care must be taken not to anaesthetise the throat before meals as this might lead to choking. Prolonged use is not recommended because itching and soreness may develop.

● *Gels*

Preparations containing a **salicylate**, an aspirin derivative, have some analgesic action. **Choline salicylate** (brand names Bonjela; Teejel) may provide relief for recurrent aphthous ulcers. It should not be used more frequently than every three hours because excessive application or confinement under a denture irritates the mouth and may cause further ulceration. These non-aspirin salicylate preparations can be used for teething problems in babies from 4 months and young children, although the benefit may come from rubbing the gums or pressure of application rather than the drug. Frequent use can lead to salicylate poisoning (see page 234). **Carbenoxolone** gel (brand name Bioral) may relieve inflammation and be of some help.

Thrush

Thrush is a fungal infection caused by the yeast *Candida albicans* which lives harmlessly on the body until conditions change and allow it to proliferate (see also Chapter 5: Infections). Thrush infection in the mouth is common in babies and frail old people. Some drug treatment encourages candida to grow unchecked, for example broad-spectrum antibiotics. Any drug that dampens the body's immune system, such as an oral corticosteroid or anti-cancer treatment, will allow candida to proliferate. Some of the dose of an inhaled corticosteroid (for preventing asthma) is deposited at the back of the throat and this can lead to candidal overgrowth. Radiotherapy treatment to the head and neck region can also allow candida to flourish. Conditions which interfere with the immune system, including diabetes mellitus, hormone disorders, blood disorders, advanced cancer and AIDS, make you more susceptible to candidal overgrowth.

Oral thrush affects the mucous membrane on the insides of the cheek, the palate and throat, and also the tongue. Creamy white patches (*plaques*) which look like milk curds can be seen on a reddened mucous membrane. In babies oral thrush is often associated with a face rash. Milk curds, with which candida may sometimes be confused, occur only on the insides of the cheeks and can be easily removed from the mucous membrane. They do not cause symptoms.

Denture stomatitis is inflammation of the mucous membrane caused by dentures which then become infected with candida. The mucosa becomes red on the palate directly under the upper denture, but often does not cause symptoms. Candidal infection is usually associated with poor dental hygiene or an ill-fitting denture. *Angular cheilitis* is painful cracking at the angles of the mouth. Folding and fissuring at the sides of the mouth may be due to reduction of facial contour after loss of teeth or wearing down of dentures. Denture stomatitis and angular cheilitis often occur together and any infection should be treated. A sore mouth and angular cheilitis can occur with lack of iron or vitamin B_{12}.

Medicines for oral thrush

Any underlying cause of candidal overgrowth should be considered by your doctor. For example, if an antibiotic or corticosteroid (oral or inhaled) is the probable cause then it may help to reduce the dose or change treatment. With an inhaled corticosteroid, using a spacer or rinsing the mouth with water after inhalation may help. Topical treatment with an antifungal medicine such as **nystatin**, **amphotericin** or **miconazole** is effective in controlling candidal infection. Treatment must be continued for two days after the infection appears to have cleared. Combinations of these drugs are no more effective than either drug alone and amphotericin reduces the effect of miconazole. Intermittent or prolonged treatment may be needed where the underlying cause cannot be cleared up or is unavoidable.

● *Oral suspension*

Nystatin oral suspension (brand names Nystan; Nystatin-Dome) or amphotericin suspension (Fungilin) is swirled around the mouth several times before swallowing, four times a day after food. Nystatin suspension can be mixed with a little flavoured drink or, for a baby, added to a reduced bottle feed. Nystan suspension does not contain sugar, lactose or gluten.

● *Lozenges and pastilles*

Nystatin pastilles (Nystan) or amphotericin lozenges (Fungilin) can be sucked four times a day after meals. They stay in contact with the infected areas for longer; children and older people may find them more acceptable than the suspension.

Oral gel

Miconazole oral gel (Daktarin) is an orange-flavoured, sugar-free gel which is applied to the affected areas four times daily after meals. The gel should be kept in the mouth for as long as possible before swallowing. For babies the gel can be put on the candidal patches using a clean finger. A small tube of gel can be bought from a pharmacy.

Denture stomatitis and angular cheilitis

Denture stomatitis can be treated with an antifungal medicine but also needs improved oral and dental hygiene. Dentures should not be worn at night and should be thoroughly cleaned with a brush at the end of the day. They should be left in diluted **hypochlorite** solution (such as Milton) or water with 1–2ml of nystatin suspension which should be replenished nightly. The denture(s) should be rinsed in water the following morning before use. **Chlorhexidine** solution is less effective against candida but can be used as additional treatment for short periods. The mouthwash should be used 15 minutes before the denture is re-inserted.

Treatment of angular cheilitis sometimes needs to be prolonged: miconazole gel or nystatin cream or ointment is used. New dentures which restore the facial contour and reduce the folding at the corners of the mouth may help.

Sore throat

Discomfort at the back of the mouth and throat is commonly caused by local infection. It may also be due to allergy or drying of the mucosa caused by breathing through the mouth.

A sore throat is most commonly a viral infection which will get better with time; treatment with an antibiotic will not benefit a viral infection. Sometimes a sore throat may be caused by *streptococci* bacteria, which will require a systemic antibiotic, not a local preparation. If the antibiotic **ampicillin** or **amoxycillin** is given for a sore throat caused by glandular fever (a viral infection), a rash often develops, althogh this does not mean you are allergic to the antibiotic.

Many antiseptic lozenges, sprays and gels are available over the counter, but there is little evidence that they are of benefit for a sore throat. Sucking a medicated lozenge, for example, stimulates the flow of saliva, but the same effect can be achieved with a boiled sweet. Antiseptic preparations may sometimes irritate the mouth and cause a sore tongue and lips. Some preparations contain a local anaesthetic such as **benzocaine**; they relieve pain but may cause itching and soreness.

• *Antiseptic gargles*

During gargling the liquid is unlikely to get to the sore part of the throat unless it is swallowed. Even if it is swallowed – and this is not recommended – there is no evidence that a gargle helps. Two soluble aspirin tablets dispersed in half a tumblerful of water can be gargled and then swallowed. However, any benefit is likely to come from the systemic effect of aspirin rather than a local one.

• *Mouthwashes*

Mouthwashes cleanse and freshen the mouth. Simple mouthwashes such as salt or **compound sodium chloride** mouthwash or **compound thymol glycerin** are useful and inexpensive. **Hydrogen peroxide** mouthwash also has a cleansing effect; **sodium perborate** (brand name Bocasan) is similar but must not be used continuously for more than seven days. It should not be taken by children under five or by people with reduced kidney function. **Chlorhexidine** (brand names Corsodyl; Eludril), **hexetidine** (Oraldene), **cetylpyridinium** (Merocet) and **povidone-iodine** (Betadine) are antibacterial, but will not help a sore throat caused by a virus.

10

SKIN CONDITIONS

Eczema Psoriasis Acne
Scabies Lice Sunburn
Cuts, bites and stings
Warts and verrucae

Skin is the body's largest organ. It protects the internal organs from external injury and keeps out harmful organisms such as bacteria. Together with the tissues underneath (*subcutaneous layers*) it acts as a store for water and fat, helping to conserve the body's fluids, although some of the body's waste products leave the body via the sweat glands in skin. Nerve endings in the skin transmit the sensations of touch, pressure, pain and temperature and warn of possible injury. Skin plays an important part in regulating body temperature.

The thin top layer of skin cells is called the *epidermis*; the deeper layer below is known as the *dermis*. The epidermis varies in thickness in different parts of the body. Eyelids have the thinnest skin while on the palms of hands and soles of feet the epidermis is thick, hard and horny. On the outer surface dead cells are continually being rubbed off and replaced by new cells which are always forming in the bottom layer of the epidermis. Skin cells live for about three weeks, gradually moving towards the surface, where they die. The rate of formation of skin cells is highest during sleep and lowest during exercise and stress. Living cells make *keratin* which toughens the skin surface and makes up hair and nails. Some of the cells in the epidermis manufacture *melanin*, a pigment that absorbs some of the ultraviolet rays from the sun and protects against their harmful effects.

When you get hot your body loses water through the *pores* in the skin and this has a cooling effect. Each pore is a tiny opening through which fluid is released from the sweat glands in the dermis. The dermis also contains blood vessels and nerve endings. *Sebaceous glands* in the dermis make a type of oil (*sebum*) which lubricates and protects your skin and hair. The roots of the short hairs which grow from most parts of the skin are contained within channels (*follicles*) in the dermis. Although there are a number of disorders that may occur specifically on the epidermis and the dermis, skin often acts as a barometer of body health. Some skin conditions are outward signs of an underlying disorder. *Dermatitis* is the general term for skin problems when the skin is inflamed.

Eczema

Eczema is a form of dermatitis characterised by itchy, red, scaly skin. Tiny blisters may form which leave a raw surface when scratched. The skin may become infected at this stage, usually with bacteria. If you have eczema for a long time the skin eventually becomes thickened, with the outer layer constantly flaking off as scales.

● *Eczema from external causes*

This is also known as *contact dermatitis* and is a common skin problem.

Irritant contact eczema occurs when the skin's surface is damaged by contact with an irritant substance, for example detergents (washing up liquid, shampoo, washing powders), disinfectants, acids or alkalis. The skin can react immediately or only after repeated contact. The hands are commonly affected, particularly in certain occupations, for example housework, hairdressing and building work.

Allergic contact eczema can occur when the immune system reacts to an external substance which has been touched, eaten or inhaled. There are thousands of substances with the potential to trigger an immune reaction – see Box over the page for some of the common culprits. A rash develops on the skin as white blood cells release substances that open up the blood vessels in the dermis, making the surrounding area hot, red and swollen or inflamed. The reaction can take several days to develop after exposure to the trigger substance. It may develop at the point of contact – for example a nickel-containing bracelet may cause a distinct reaction around the wrist – but not necessarily. You can suddenly become allergic to a substance that has not caused a problem before. Although you can treat the skin rash, the best solution will be to discover what has caused the reaction and, if possible, avoid it on future occasions.

● *Eczema from internal causes*

There may be a family history with these types of skin conditions, but the mechanisms are not well understood.

Atopic eczema is common in babies and children and often starts during the first year of life. In some cases it may be associ-

COMMON CAUSES OF ALLERGIC CONTACT DERMATITIS

☐ Nickel: jewellery (even some silver and gold), zips, coins, stainless steel, arch supports in shoes, door handles
☐ Rubber and associated chemicals: rubber gloves, shoes, insoles, rubber boots, chemicals
☐ Chromium: leather watch straps, wet cement, printing work, shoes, paints
☐ Epoxy resins: glues, insulating materials
☐ Lanolin: moisturisers and cosmetic creams, some medicinal creams and ointments
☐ Preservatives: most cosmetics and prescribed creams
☐ Plants: primula, chrysanthemum, poison ivy
☐ Formaldehyde: crease-resistant clothes.

ated with asthma and/or hay fever and there is often a family history of these conditions. The skin is usually affected on the face in infants, and in the elbow creases and behind the knees in children. The condition improves in many children as they grow older, but occasionally the problem persists into adulthood. In some cases atopic eczema may be linked with allergy to the house dust mite or to foods – for example, cow's milk, eggs or fish.

Seborrhoeic eczema is a flaking and itchy skin condition that affects children and adults. In babies the scalp and forehead are commonly involved and the skin surface appears as a heaped mass of yellowish-brown scaling, sometimes known as 'cradle cap'. Adults have a scaly scalp and severe dandruff and a rash may develop on the face and chest, under the arms and in the groin.

Varicose eczema occurs on the lower legs in association with varicose veins or previous deep vein thrombosis (see page 155). The skin becomes fragile and itchy and minor scratches can lead to a leg ulcer.

Asteatotic dermatitis is usually a result of skin drying out and most commonly affects older people or those suffering from minor malnutrition. The skin on the backs of the hands and fronts of the legs dries out giving an appearance similar to crazy paving with deep fissures. The condition is aggravated by soaps and other irritant substances and by scratching.

Medicines for eczema

Treatment depends on the cause of eczema and if an underlying cause can be found and removed, the condition may clear up

HOW YOU CAN HELP YOURSELF

☐ Avoid ordinary soap, bath additives and other detergents as these can aggravate eczema.
☐ Take showers or short, cool baths. Use a soap substitute, such as emulsifying ointment and a soothing, moisturising preparation on dry skin.
☐ Wear cotton clothes to keep the body cool. Avoid wool or wool mixtures as these can irritate.
☐ Keep bedrooms free of dust to minimise contact with the house dust mite (see also 'Asthma', page 160).
☐ Wear rubber or plastic gloves with cotton linings when cleaning or washing up to protect against the effects of water and detergents. Use a moisturising hand cream afterwards.
☐ Gentle exercise and support stockings or tights can help varicose veins and varicose eczema. These measures may prevent an ulcer forming on the leg.
☐ Contact The National Eczema Society which has branches and local groups providing support and information. See 'Useful addresses'.

without treatment. In cases where an underlying factor cannot be established – for example, atopic eczema – treatment generally involves applying a preparation to the skin. Sometimes an oral preparation may be helpful – for example, an antihistamine to relieve itching.

• *TYPES OF SKIN PREPARATION* •

Small amounts of a drug can be absorbed into the body through the skin (topical treatment) and it is just as important to think of creams and ointments as medicines as those that are taken by mouth or injected. The active ingredient can be applied to the skin in a number of ways, using different 'vehicles'. The vehicle may be a cream, ointment, lotion, paste, dusting-powder, collodion, application or paint. The drug is either dissolved or suspended in it. The vehicle carries the drug but may itself have beneficial effects on the skin, affecting how moist the skin is and how well the drug reaches the lower layer of skin (dermis), and it may well have its own mild anti-inflammatory and soothing effect.

☐ A cream is a fat or oil-in-water preparation. It is less greasy than an ointment, mixes well with skin secretions and is easier to apply. Many creams have an *emollient* effect (see over). A barrier cream contains ingredients such as **dimenthicone**, **zinc** or **titanium** compounds to keep water and irritant substances away from the skin.

☐ An ointment is a greasy preparation often containing soft paraffin, liquid paraffin, wax or lanolin. It does not dissolve in water and lies on the surface, protecting and lubricating the skin. some modern ointment bases also mix with water and wash off readily. Ointments are useful for long-term dry skin conditions.
☐ A gel is a jelly-like base containing the active drug. Skin gels are usually clear so that when they dry they are hardly visible on the skin surface – an advantage for facial treatment.
☐ A lotion is a liquid with the drug dissolved or suspended in it. It is useful for applying a drug to a large or hairy area of the body. A lotion cools by evaporation and soothes inflamed unbroken skin. A shake lotion such as calamine lotion leaves a fine powder on the skin surface as it dries and is useful for encouraging scab formation.
☐ A paste contains various amounts of insoluble powders, such as starch, **zinc oxide** or **titanium dioxide**. It is a thick and stiff preparation which acts as a barrier and protects the skin surface, used for marked thickening and scaling of the skin which occurs in psoriasis or long-term eczema.
☐ A dusting-powder is a mixture of dry powders such as talc and **zinc oxide** which absorbs moisture. It should only be used on unbroken skin.
☐ A collodion is a thick liquid painted on to the skin and left to dry to form a protective film over the area. Collodion may be used to seal a minor cut or wound, or to hold a dissolved drug in contact with the skin for a long period.
☐ An application is a thick liquid for putting on the skin.
☐ A paint is a liquid usually applied with a brush to the skin or mucous surfaces, such as the mouth.

• *SOOTHING PREPARATIONS* •

For dry scaling skin an *emollient* preparation can be used. Emollients, consisting of mixtures of water, fats, waxes and oils, soothe and moisten dry skin. They should be used generously and frequently; treatment should continue even after the condition begins to improve. Use of an emollient is essential for atopic eczema, when the skin is usually very dry. Emollients can be applied as creams, ointments, lotions or added to the bath, but all have a similar function. There is a wide range of preparations from simple formulations to more complex and expensive products. Choice depends on which preparation suits you and your skin.

Aqueous cream is a simple, effective and inexpensive preparation free of ingredients that can cause sensitisation. In general, creams contain more preservatives than ointments. Some preservatives (for example **parabens**) may worsen an existing condition by causing contact allergic dermatitis in addition to the original problem and so may some emollient ingredients (for example **lanolin** – hydrous wool fat). **Camphor**, **menthol** or **phenol** are included in some preparations and may ease itchiness. **Calamine** and **zinc oxide** add a little more to the efficacy of an emollient and are useful in dry eczema. **Zinc** and **titanium** formulations are mildly astringent. **Urea** cream is used for moisturising scaly skin and may be helpful for a baby with eczema or for older people.

● *TAR PREPARATIONS* ●

These are sometimes used for treating chronic eczema and also psoriasis, where there is marked thickening of the skin and scaling. **Coal tar** lessens itching and inflammation and reduces the thickness of scaly lesions. It is also mildly antiseptic. Tar products can irritate the skin and sometimes cause an acne-like rash; they should not be put on broken or very inflamed skin. Thick patches of skin need a stronger concentration of coal tar and pastes are generally used. These pastes cannot be used on the face, but newer preparations such as Carbo-Dome are suitable. A **zinc paste and coal tar** bandage may be used for treating limbs with conditions such as varicose eczema. When large areas of the body are affected coal tar baths may help. **Coal tar and hydrocortisone** cream is mildly potent and may help some eczematous conditions.

Shampoos containing tar extracts are used for seborrhoeic eczema and scaling of the scalp (for example, Alphosyl; Genisol; Ionil T; Polytar). For a baby with cradle cap a little olive or arachis oil can be rubbed gently into the scalp before shampooing with a baby shampoo.

Ichthammol is milder than coal tar and is sometimes used for treating eczema. A **zinc paste and ichthammol** bandage can be used on the limbs.

● *EVENING PRIMROSE OIL* ●

Oil from the seed of the evening primrose is available in capsule form (brand names Epogam; Efamol; Epoc; Naudicelle) and is claimed to relieve symptoms of atopic eczema. You have to take up to 12 capsules a day and it may take two to three months before there is any response. Most clinical trials have found that Epogam has only a modest effect, but skin roughness may be reduced. Its effects appear to be rather marginal and it is more of an optional treatment and a dietary supplement. Evening primrose oil products can be bought over the counter, but three months' treatment costs aroung £90.

EMOLLIENTS AND BARRIER PREPARATIONS

Creams

ALCODERM – Emollient
CETYL AND STEARYL ALCOHOL + LIQUID PARAFFIN

AQUEOUS CREAM – Emollient

CONOTRANE – Barrier
DIMETHICONE + BENZALKONIUM

DIMETHICONE – Barrier

DIPROBASE – Emollient
LIQUID PARAFFIN + CETOSTEARYL ALCOHOL + WHITE SOFT PARAFFIN

DRAPOLENE – Barrier
BENZALKONIUM + CETRIMIDE

E45 – Emollient
LIQUID PARAFFIN + WHITE SOFT PARAFFIN + WOOL FAT

ECZEDERM – Emollient
CALAMINE + ARACHIS OIL

HEWLETTS CREAM – Emollient
WOOL FAT + ZINC OXIDE

HUMIDERM – Emollient
PYRROLIDONE CARBOXYLIC ACID

MASSÉ BREAST CREAM – Emollient
ARACHIS OIL + GLYCEROL

MORSEP – Barrier
CETRIMIDE + VITAMIN D + VITAMIN A

NATUDERM – Emollient
GLYCERIDES + GLYCEROL

NORATEX – Barrier
COD-LIVER OIL + WOOL FAT + ZINC OXIDE

OILATUM – Emollient
ARACHIS OIL + POVIDONE

SIOPEL – Barrier
DIMETHICONE + CETRIMIDE

SUDOCREM – Barrier
WOOL FAT + ZINC OXIDE

ULTRABASE – Emollient
LIQUID PARAFFIN + WHITE SOFT PARAFFIN

VASOGEN – Barrier
DIMETHICONE + CALAMINE + ZINC OXIDE

ZINC CREAM – Barrier

Creams containing urea

AQUADRATE – Emollient

CALMURID – Emollient

NUTRAPLUS – Emollient

SENTIAL E – Emollient

Ointments

DIPROBASE – Emollient
LIQUID PARAFFIN + WHITE SOFT PARAFFIN

EMULSIFYING OINTMENT – Emollient

HYDROUS OINTMENT – Emollient

KAMILLOSAN – Barrier
CHAMOMILE EXTRACTS

METANIUM – Barrier
TITANIUM DIOXIDE

MORHULIN – Barrier
COD-LIVER OIL + ZINC OXIDE

THOVALINE – Barrier
COD-LIVER OIL + KAOLIN + TALC + WOOL FAT + ZINC OXIDE

UNGUENTUM MERCK – Emollient
WHITE SOFT PARAFFIN + LIQUID PARAFFIN

VITA-E – Emollient
VITAMIN E + YELLOW SOFT PARAFFIN

ZINC OINTMENT – Barrier

ZINC AND CASTOR OIL OINTMENT – Barrier

Lotions

ALCODERM – Emollient
CETYL AND STEARYL ALCOHOL + LIQUID PARAFFIN

DERMALEX – Emollient
ALLANTOIN + HEXACHLOROPHANE

KERI – Emollient
MINERAL OIL + LANOLIN OIL

LACTICARE – Emollient
LACTIC ACID + SODIUM PYRROLIDONE CARBOXYLATE

Paste

TITANIUM DIOXIDE PASTE – Barrier

Aerosol spray (many ingredients)

SPRILON – Barrier

Bath additives

ALPHA KERI BATH – Emollient
LIQUID PARAFFIN + WOOL FAT

AVEENO OILATED – Emollient
OAT (PROTEIN FRACTION) + LIQUID PARAFFIN

AVEENO REGULAR – Emollient
OAT (PROTEIN FRACTION)

BALMANDOL – Emollient
ALMOND OIL + LIQUID PARAFFIN

Continued over

BALNEUM – Emollient (also available with tar)
SOYA OIL

DIPROBATH – Emollient
ISOPROPYL MYRISTATE + LIQUID PARAFFIN

EMULSIDERM – Emollient
ISOPROPYL MYRISTATE + LIQUID PARAFFIN

HYDROMOL EMOLLIENT – Emollient
ISOPROPYL MYRISTATE + LIQUID PARAFFIN

OILATUM EMOLLIENT – Emollient
ACETYLATED WOOL ALCOHOLS + LIQUID PARAFFIN

Small quantities of many of these products can be bought from a pharmacy for less than the prescription charge.

● *CORTICOSTEROID PREPARATIONS* ●

Corticosteroids used on the skin (topically) suppress inflammation. A topical corticosteroid blocks the action of the substances released by white blood cells that cause redness, swelling and heat. Corticosteroids are widely used for eczematous conditions, including weeping eczemas, providing they are not infected. Their use in eczema has not been evaluated in clinical trials and long-term treatment can cause problems such as skin becoming thin and stretch marks. They do not cure eczema and bring relief only while they are used. When you stop treatment, your skin condition may recur or worsen.

Corticosteroids should be used only after other topical treatments with fewer adverse effects have been tried. Topical corticosteroids are classified into four groups by their strength. A preparation from the mildest and least potent group should be used first; if you stop responding to it, your doctor would usually then try another preparation from the same group, rather than moving up to a more potent one. The most potent corticosteroid preparations are generally reserved for the most difficult skin conditions and are not used for long-term treatment.

Combination preparations of a corticosteroid with an antibiotic, antifungal or an antiseptic are sometimes used when infection is suspected, but the skin problem is not mainly one of infection. Infected eczema may need treatment with an antibiotic taken by mouth, but smaller areas of skin may respond to a short course of a topical antibiotic (see page 424).

CORTICOSTEROID PREPARATIONS

Mild

COBADEX
HYDROCORTISONE

DIODERM
HYDROCORTISONE

EFCORTELAN
HYDROCORTISONE

HYDROCORTISONE

HYDROCORTISTAB
HYDROCORTISONE

HYDROCORTISYL
HYDROCORTISONE

MILDISON
HYDROCORTISONE

SYNALAR 1 IN 10 DILUTION
FLUOCINOLONE 0·0025%

Moderately potent

BETNOVATE RD
BETAMETHASONE VALERATE 0·025%

EUMOVATE
CLOBETASONE

HAELAN
FLURANDRENOLONE

MODRASONE
ALCLOMETASONE

STIEDEX LP
DESOXYMETHASONE 0·05%

SYNALAR 1 IN 4 DILUTION
FLUOCINOLONE 0·00625%

ULTRADIL PLAIN
FLUOCORTOLONE

ULTRALANUM PLAIN
FLUOCORTOLONE

Potent

ADCORTYL
TRIAMCINOLONE

BETAMETHASONE VALERATE 0·1%

BETNOVATE
BETAMETHASONE VALERATE 0·1%

DIPROSALIC
BETAMETHASONE DIPROPIONATE 0·05%

DIPROSONE
BETAMETHASONE DIPROPIONATE 0·05%

LEDERCORT
TRIAMCINOLONE

LOCOID
HYDROCORTISONE BUTYRATE

METOSYN
FLUOCINONIDE

NERISONE
DIFLUCORTOLONE 0·1%

PREFERID
BUDESONIDE

PROPADERM
BECLOMETHASONE

STIEDEX
DESOXYMETHASONE 0·25%

SYNALAR
FLUOCINOLONE 0·025%

TOPILAR
FLUCLOROLONE

Very potent

DERMOVATE
CLOBETASOL

HALCIDERM
HALCINONIDE

NERISONE FORTE
DIFLUCORTOLONE 0·3%

All preparations are prescription-only.

Hydrocortisone from a pharmacy

You can buy certain brands of hydrocortisone at a pharmacy for less than the prescription charge, but only for specified conditions. Ask your pharmacist for advice. Hydrocortisone is considered to be the safest of all corticosteroid preparations for the skin, but there are strict limitations on its use when sold off prescription.

- Hydrocortisone cream (0·1% or 1%) or ointment (1%) can be sold only to treat allergic contact dermatitis, irritant dermatitis and insect bite reactions. It cannot be sold for treating atopic eczema, some other types of eczema or psoriasis.
- It is not to be used by children under ten or during pregnancy, except with medical advice.
- It is not to be used on the face or eyes, around the genitals or anus, or on broken or infected skin – including cold sores, acne and athlete's foot.
- Use sparingly over a small area once or twice a day for no longer than one week. The label will state, 'If the condition is not improved consult your doctor'.

Unwanted effects

When used carefully for short periods, mild or moderately potent corticosteroid preparations are rarely associated with unwanted effects. The more potent the preparation the more care is needed. Long-term use of a potent preparation can produce changes to the skin area being treated.

The commonest effect is thinning of the skin and sometimes stretch marks develop that become permanent. Fine blood vessels under the skin surface may become more prominent (*telangiectasia*) and damaged, resulting in redness and a rash. An untreated, infected skin condition can spread and worsen. Other effects include increased hair growth, acne, mild loss of skin colour (*depigmentation*), and a rash around the mouth, particularly in young women. When a potent corticosteroid has been used for some time, there may be a worsening of the skin condition (*rebound erythroderma*) when you stop using the preparation abruptly. The dosage must be gradually reduced to avoid a worsening of the condition.

Strong corticosteroids – those in the potent and very potent groups – may be absorbed through the skin and can cause effects throughout the body if large quantities are used for long periods (see page 325). Absorption of the corticosteroid depends on the area of the body being treated and the duration of the treatment. Polythene dressings have been used to increase the effect of a local

SENSITISERS IN CORTICOSTEROID PREPARATIONS

All the substances in the first two columns are much more liable to cause problems on eczematous skin than on normal skin. If you develop a sensitivity to any of these ingredients in a topical corticosteroid or any other skin preparation you should note the name. Next time you have to use a topical preparation, check with your doctor or pharmacist to make sure that it does not contain the same sensitising agent.

most commonly	*less frequently*	*rarely*
wool fat (lanolin) and related substances	benzyl alcohol	beeswax
cetyl alcohol	butylated hydroxyanisole	EDTA
stearyl alcohol	butylated hydroxytoluene	isopropyl palmitate
chlorocresol	hydroxybenzoates (parabens)	nystatin
fragrances	polysorbate 60	imidazoles (e.g. econazole, miconazole, clotrimazole)
ethylenediamine	propylene glycol[1]	
neomycin	sorbic acid	
framycetin	chlorquinaldol	
gentamicin	fusidic acid	
clioquinol		

1. Acts as an irritant more often than causing allergic sensitisation.

corticosteroid, particularly in difficult and resistant skin conditions. These dressings are effective, but are generally used only for areas of thick skin because there is an increased risk of adverse reactions, in both the skin and the body.

Follow these guidelines to minimise unwanted effects of corticosteroid skin preparations.

- Use as mild a corticosteroid as possible, especially for children.
- Put only a thin covering of the preparation on the affected area of skin. The label will read 'To be applied sparingly . . .'; applying large quantities will not produce a quicker or better result and can lead to undesirable effects on the skin and within the body.
- Avoid using the stronger preparations for more than a week or two if possible.
- Potent preparations should not be used on the face and in general it is best to avoid using any corticosteroid on the face.
- Do not use a corticosteroid on broken or infected skin.
- If your doctor prescribes a corticosteroid preparation for a particular skin condition, do not use it for any other problem. Do not let anyone else use your corticosteroid or borrow anyone else's preparation. If the preparation is used for the wrong skin

condition, even if it looks the same, the problem could be made much worse.

☐ If your skin condition worsens during treatment or does not seem to clear up, you may be allergic to one of the ingredients, either the drug itself or an additive such as a fragrance or a preservative. See Box on previous page for details. Allergic sensitivity to the corticosteroid itself is rare, but is being increasingly recognised.

● *ANTIBACTERIAL PREPARATIONS* ●

If the skin is 'weeping' your doctor may recommend the use of a wet dressing or soak (for example weak **potassium permanganate** solution) to cleanse the skin, before applying an emollient. Not all skin conditions that ooze and weep are infected, but keeping the skin area clean with usual hygienic measures is important. Infected eczema is sometimes treated with an antibacterial cream or ointment. The antibacterial in the preparation is usually an antibiotic that is not used within the body to treat other infections, so that bacteria are not exposed to it too often and do not become resistant to the drug. Examples include **framycetin**, **mupirocin**, **neomycin** and **polymyxin**.

Some antibiotics are used both on the skin and in the body – for example **tetracycline**, **chlortetracycline**, **fusidic acid** and **gentamicin**. Gentamicin and fusidic acid are used for treating serious systemic infections, usually in hospital, but may be used for treating some skin infections away from hospital.

Some drugs in skin preparations such as neomycin and framycetin may cause an allergic skin reaction with prolonged use. An antibiotic skin preparation should be used for as short a possible time and if the disorder worsens, making the skin more red and inflamed, you should see your doctor again.

Psoriasis

Psoriasis is a chronic and sometimes distressing skin condition which can recur from time to time. In healthy skin dead cells are constantly being rubbed off from the outer layer of the epidermis and are replaced by new cells made at the base of the epidermis. In psoriasis this process of ordered and continual renewal goes wrong and new cell production speeds up, so cells accumulate under the outer layer. This process is caused by an inflammatory reaction in the dermis. Skin is usually affected in patches and these appear as raised and thick red areas, often covered by silvery scales. The scalp, elbows, knees and knuckles are most commonly affected, although large areas of skin can be involved. Itching is a common symptom. There are other types of psoriasis, such as *guttate psoriasis* – when a sudden eruption of small patches occurs, often triggered by tonsillitis – and *pustular psoriasis*, which may occur on the withdrawal of topical or systemic corticosteroids. Psoriasis may be accompanied by a distinctive form of arthritis.

The underlying cause of psoriasis is not known, but around one person in fifty in Britain has the condition. Psoriasis first occurs between the ages of 10 and 45, but the course of the disease is unpredictable and it can recur at any time. It can affect anyone, but if one of your parents has the disorder, your chances of having it increase to one in four. Psoriasis comes and goes for no obvious reason although attacks may be triggered by stress, skin damage or illness. It often follows a sore throat caused by *streptococcal* bacteria. The skin may look unsightly and unpleasant, but it is not infectious. The condition may clear up (remit) for long periods, but there is no complete cure. Psoriasis is a condition which needs advice and guidance from your doctor or a dermatologist; various treatments can improve it.

HOW YOU CAN HELP YOURSELF

☐ Take showers or short, cool baths. Use a moisturising soap substitute, such as emulsifying ointment, and a soothing bath preparation to reduce dry skin.
☐ Wear cotton clothes to keep the body cool. Avoid extremes of temperature and environment. Sunlight usually improves psoriasis because of the ultraviolet radiation, but needs careful regulation to avoid burning the skin, as this will exacerbate the condition.
☐ Avoid stressful situations because stress can trigger a flare-up. Rest helps treatment of psoriasis.
☐ If you have a flare-up and your skin condition worsens, see your doctor as soon as possible.
☐ Contact the Psoriasis Association which provides information on all aspects of the condition and has a network of local support groups (see 'Useful addresses').

Medicines for psoriasis

Treatment aims to relieve the inflammation and scaling and to lessen the area of skin involved. The choice of treatment depends on which part and how much of the body is affected and how you tolerate the condition and its various treatments. Local treatment is the mainstay for mild to moderate psoriasis but for more severe conditions a medicine may be given by mouth or other specialist treatments used, such as *photochemotherapy*.

● *LOCAL TREATMENT* ●

An emollient preparation may be all that is needed in mild conditions. Where the disorder is more troublesome, topical treatment with **coal tar**, **salicylic acid** or **dithranol** may help. Controlled exposure to ultraviolet radiation either through natural sunlight or a special lamp may help, but you should ask your doctor or specialist about this. Ultraviolet radiation is often combined with tar or dithranol treatment.

A new synthetic vitamin D preparation, **calcipotriol** (brand name Dovonex), may be helpful. It blocks abnormal division of skin cells and seems to be as effective as a moderately strong corticosteroid. One course of treatment lasts for up to six weeks. It should not be used on the face.

● *Tar preparations*

Some of the older products are still effective – for example **coal tar and salicylic acid** ointment can be rubbed well into the skin and is not unpleasant despite its smell. Tar preparations can be used up to three times a day. Crude coal tar contains thousands of compounds and attempts to purify it have produced less effective compounds. Newer products are, however, less messy to use. Tar products can irritate the skin and sometimes cause an acne-like rash; they should not be put on broken or very inflamed skin. Tar baths need to be combined with ultraviolet radiation to be effective. Tar products may stain the skin temporarily and clothes and bedding permanently.

● *Salicylic acid*

This can be used to loosen and remove thick scaly patches. A low-concentration ointment is used at first and the concentration gradually increased during a course of treatment. Unwanted effects are few but salicylic acid may occasionally cause allergic rash, drying and irritation of the skin. If large skin areas are covered or salicylic acid is used for long periods, it may be absorbed into the body sufficiently to cause dizziness and tinnitus. Salicylic acid is mixed with other ingredients in topical preparations – for example **zinc**, **coal tar** and **dithranol** – to increase efficacy.

● *Dithranol*

This compound is the most effective topical preparation for treating psoriasis, but it must be used carefully because it can cause severe skin irritation. It is usually applied only to the affected skin area, covered and left for one hour or less and then removed. Overnight application was recommended originally but doctors have found that short applications are just as effective. Some people cannot tolerate dithranol preparations even at low concentrations; fair skin is more sensitive than dark skin. Dithranol may be combined with salicylic acid or coal tar for better effect. Some newer branded products are easier to use and cause less staining and irritation than the traditional preparations.

DITHRANOL

On prescription/from a pharmacy
DITHRANOL – Ointment, paste (Lassar's paste)
ALPHODITH – Ointment
ANTHRANOL – Ointment
DITHROCREAM – Cream
EXOLAN – Cream

Combined preparations
DITHROLAN – Ointment
DITHRANOL + SALICYLIC ACID
PSORADRATE – Cream
DITHRANOL + UREA
PSORIN – Ointment
DITHRANOL + CRUDE COAL TAR + SALICYLIC ACID

Dithranol preparations can be bought from a pharmacy if the dithranol content is less than one per cent.

Dithranol is the most effective topical treatment for mild to moderate psoriasis. It slows the rate of production of new skin cells in the base of the epidermis. Dithranol is irritant to the skin and is used at a low strength, with the concentration gradually increased during a course of treatment depending on individual tolerance. It must be applied only to the affected skin patches; the surrounding skin must be protected with petroleum jelly.

In more severe cases dithranol is combined with ultraviolet radiation treatment in hospital (Ingram's method). You soak in a warm bath containing coal tar solution and after drying, you are exposed to a regulated amount of ultraviolet radiation. Dithranol paste is applied to the affected patches and the normal skin protected by talc and gauze dressings. This process is repeated daily.

Before you use this medicine

Tell your doctor if you are:
□ pregnant or breast-feeding □ taking any other medicines, including vitamins and those bought over the counter.

Tell your doctor if you have had:
□ a previous reaction to dithranol.

Do not use if you have:
□ acute or pustular psoriasis.

How to use this medicine

Put a thin layer of the topical preparation on the affected patches of skin once a day. Directions for contact time may vary depending on the product used. The surrounding skin can be protected with petroleum jelly. After treatment the preparation should be removed by bathing. Pastes may be difficult to remove but an oily liquid such as liquid paraffin may help. Always wash hands thoroughly after using or touching dithranol products.

Apply daily for best results. Treatment may take several weeks, but good effects can be achieved. If you miss a dose, apply as soon as you remember.

Over 65 No special requirements.

Interactions with other medicines

Topical treatments (for example, **salicylic acid** and **coal tar**) with dithranol increase the skin's sensitivity and may cause additional redness and irritation.
Phenothiazine antipsychotics, **griseofulvin**, **thiazide diuretics**, **sulphonamides**, **tetracycline** may occasionally increase the skin's sensitivity to light, adding to the irritant effect of dithranol.

Unwanted effects

Likely Local burning sensation, skin irritation, staining of skin, hair, clothing, bedding and bathware.
Unlikely Allergic skin rash.

If skin irritation or burning sensation is severe, contact your doctor.

Dithranol is a strong irritant and special caution is needed if you use it on the face or near the eyes, the inside of the thighs, the genital region or skinfold areas. If dithranol gets into the eyes bathe immediately with copious amounts of water and seek medical advice.

Dithranol stains skin but this disappears in two to three weeks. Fabrics, clothing and bed linen stain permanently so that old clothes and linen should be used during a course of dithranol treatment. Staining in basins and baths can be removed with bleach.

Similar preparations

COAL TAR preparations

● *Corticosteroids*

Topical preparations have been used for psoriasis, but are now used only with specialist advice and for short periods of a week or two to clear the skin for a special reason. Corticosteroid creams appear to help psoriasis, but with continuous use their effectiveness lessens progressively. When topical corticosteroids are stopped after prolonged treatment, the psoriasis becomes much worse and difficult to manage with other preparations.

● *OTHER SPECIALIST TREATMENTS* ●

A small number of people do not benefit from topical treatment or relapse very quickly after it. If psoriasis is extensive or disabling, systemic treatment may become necessary. These various treatments are only carried out by skin specialists and under hospital supervision.

● *Photochemotherapy*

This involves the interaction of a **psoralen** (a relatively inert drug) and long-wave ultraviolet radiation (UVA); hence the treatment is named PUVA. The drug makes the skin cells sensitive to UVA rays and the radiation stops cells dividing so quickly. Treatment is available only in specialist centres and is suitable only for certain people. Severe burning is a short-term adverse effect while long-term hazards include the development of skin cancer, accelerated ageing and cataracts if proper care is not taken to protect the eyes.

● *Anticancer drugs*

In severe cases an anticancer drug, usually **methotrexate**, may slow the rapid rate of division of new skin cells. Methotrexate is taken by mouth and has to be carefully monitored because it can damage the liver and bone marrow.

● *Etretinate*

This preparation derived from vitamin A is used for severe psoriasis and other rare disorders of the skin. Etretinate (brand name Tigason) has a marked effect on cell division and abnormal thickened skin. It is taken by mouth often for several months with a rest period in between courses. Etretinate has a narrow therapeutic range, so unwanted effects are common at the start of treatment. Most patients experience dryness and cracking of the lips and dry skin which becomes red and itchy. Nosebleeds may occur and some hair loss, although this is reversible. Sometimes the hair falls out (*alopecia*) but regrows after treatment is finished. Etretinate can cause birth deformities and must be avoided in pregnancy. Women who can become pregnant must take effective contraceptive measures from at least one month before to at least two years after a course of etretinate.

Acne

Acne is a very common skin condition, especially for young people. It affects the skin on the face, neck, back and chest. It is part of puberty and growing up and few teenagers escape it completely. Over half of all young people aged 14–18 have mild to moderate acne; slightly more boys than girls suffer and usually more severely. About two out of ten teenagers have moderate to severe problems.

Increased production of the skin's natural oil (*sebum*) and of dead skin cells at the base of the hair follicle leads to blockage in the hair follicle, the duct above the *sebaceous gland*, as sebum and skin cells move towards the skin surface. If the follicle remains open at all, a plug of grease can be seen, which eventually darkens because it contains *melanin*. This is a *blackhead*. If the opening becomes blocked completely, the sebaceous gland enlarges and a *whitehead* forms. A pustule develops from a whitehead when a species of bacterium which usually lives harmlessly on your skin starts to grow in the sebum trapped in the duct. This triggers the body's defence mechanism and white blood cells battle with bacteria just underneath the skin, resulting in a red spot with a yellow head. Sometimes painful inflamed cysts form in severe acne, when the walls of the grease duct and sebaceous gland rupture under the skin surface.

Sebaceous gland activity is regulated by hormones. *Androgens*, the male sex hormones, stimulate sebaceous gland activity, while the female sex hormones, *oestrogens*, suppress it.

– HOW YOU CAN HELP YOURSELF –

- ☐ Understand that acne is part of the body changes that take place in puberty. See your doctor if you develop acne and have more than just a few spots occasionally.
- ☐ Permanent scarring can occur with acne and moderate to severe conditions need medical advice and a strategy of treatment.
- ☐ Picking, squeezing and messing with spots does not help and may cause extra damage to the skin, possibly leaving a bigger spot or scar.
- ☐ Obsessive cleansing with one of the many advertised products does not improve acne. Acne is no more common on dirty skin than clean. However, removing excessive grease from the skin at normal washing time helps to make the skin feel better.
- ☐ Diet does not seem to affect the course of acne. Eating chocolate has not been shown to be linked to acne. In general try to eat a healthy, balanced diet.
- ☐ If you wish to camouflage the worst areas use a non-greasy cosmetic base. Avoid layers of grease-based preparations.
- ☐ Sensible exposure to sunlight (see 'Sunburn', page 444) may be helpful for some people with mild to moderate acne, although improvement is usually temporary. Over-exposure to ultraviolet radiation carries the long-term risk of skin cancer.

Acne treatments

Acne is treated with preparations applied to the skin and with medicines taken by mouth, depending on the severity of the condition. Mild acne, a few spots now and then, can be treated with local application of **benzoyl peroxide gel** which you can buy at a pharmacy more cheaply than paying the prescription charge. If you have blackheads, whiteheads, red spots (*papules*) and yellow-headed, pus spots (*pustules*) your doctor may consider benzoyl peroxide or **tretinoin**. For moderate to severe cases, you may need to combine topical treatment with an antibiotic by mouth or other systemic treatment. It may be several weeks before you see the benefit from any acne treatment.

● *LOCAL TREATMENT* ●

Topical preparations mostly contain antibacterial drugs such as antibiotics or drugs that encourage the skin surface to peel (*keratolytics*) such as **salicylic acid** or abrasives. The aim is to unblock the duct and allow sebum to flow. Antibacterial drugs reduce unwanted bacterial action. There is no good evidence that antiseptics, corticosteroids, sulphur, salicylic acid, resorcinol or abrasives alone or in combination significantly help acne. Corticosteroids and resorcinol can even cause harm and products containing them are not recommended. Topical preparations of benzoyl peroxide, tretinoin and antibiotics are the mainstay of mild to moderate acne treatment.

BENZOYL PEROXIDE

On prescription/from a pharmacy
ACETOXYL – Gel
ACNEGEL – Gel
BENOXYL – Cream, lotion
BENZAGEL – Gel
NERICUR – Gel
PANOXYL – Gel, skin wash

Combined preparations
ACNIDAZIL – Cream
BENZOYL PEROXIDE + MICONAZOLE

QUINODERM – Cream, lotion
BENZOYL PEROXIDE + HYDROXYQUINOLONE

QUINOPED – Cream for athlete's foot
BENZOYL PEROXIDE + HYDROXYQUINOLONE

Not recommended
QUINODERM WITH HYDROCORTISONE – Contains a corticosteroid

Benzoyl peroxide is used on the skin for treating acne. It can be used for controlling a few spots or moderate to severe acne, when it is often combined with systemic treatment, such as an antibiotic. Benzoyl peroxide helps to remove excess dead skin cells and to unblock the sebaceous duct and hair follicle. It also acts against the bacteria in the sebum, the skin's natural oil. Available in strengths ranging from 2·5%–10%, you would normally start with a low to moderate strength product (2·5% or 5%) and after two weeks' treatment, the doctor may decide to adjust the strength depending on how your condition responds.

Before you use this medicine

Tell your doctor or pharmacist if you are:
☐ pregnant or breast-feeding ☐ taking any other medicines, including vitamins and those bought over the counter.

Tell your doctor if you have or have had:
☐ sensitivity to benzoyl peroxide.

How to use this medicine

Wash the affected areas and dry gently. Apply a thin covering of the cream, lotion or gel once or twice a day. For very sensitive skin apply every other day. Apply regularly to get the best results. See your doctor after two weeks' treatment for assessment and discuss whether you need to change the strength of the preparation.

Over 65 Not usually used by older people.

Interactions with other medicines

Tretinoin Do not apply at the same time as benzoyl peroxide. Use alternately, allowing 12 hours between applications.

Unwanted effects

Likely Skin irritation, redness, peeling.
Unlikely Itching, burning, rash.

Keep benzoyl peroxide away from eyes, mouth and other mucous membranes. If it accidentally touches sensitive areas, wash it off immediately. If you expose your skin to strong sunlight, apply benzoyl peroxide less often. If blistering, crusting or a skin rash develops stop using benzoyl peroxide and see your doctor.

Similar preparations

RETIN-A – Cream, gel, lotion
TRETINOIN

• *Topical antibiotics*

Products containing **tetracycline**, **erythromycin** or **clindamycin** are applied twice daily, after washing, to the entire area not just to the individual spots. In mild to moderate acne, topical antibiotic treatment seems to be as effective as benzoyl peroxide, but not more so. They are usually less irritant and may help if skin soreness is a problem. The solutions of antibiotics are alcoholic and may cause stinging at the start of treatment. This effect often fades as treatment continues. Tetracycline solution may stain skin yellow and mark clothing. A topical antibiotic may help if you cannot take an antibiotic by mouth.

• *Tretinoin*

Local treatment with tretinoin (brand name Retin-A), a vitamin A derivative, helps acne particularly where there are blackheads and whiteheads. Tretinoin helps to loosen dead skin cells and allows sebum to flow more freely. Your doctor can prescribe tretinoin as a lotion, cream or gel. The lotion is best for large areas such as the back, the gel for severe acne or dark skin and the cream for fair skin. Tretinoin is applied lightly once or twice daily to the areas where spots occur, after washing.

At the start of treatment there may be some stinging and the skin may feel warm, but you should aim for slight redness, similar to that of mild sunburn. If you have sensitive skin you can use tretinoin once a day. It may be six to eight weeks before a reasonable effect is seen and you will need to be patient and persevere with treatment. During the early weeks of treatment you may find that your acne seems to get worse as tretinoin acts on previously unseen spots developing under the skin.

You should not get tretinoin in the eyes, mouth and mucous membranes or use it on broken or eczematous skin. If tretinoin accidentally touches sensitive areas, wash it off immediately. You should not use tretinoin at the same time as other peeling agents, such as products containing sulphur, salicylic acid or benzoyl peroxide. If necessary you can use benzoyl peroxide and tretinoin alternately, allowing 12 hours between applications. Do not use tretinoin with an ultraviolet lamp. Unwanted effects including irritation, burning and peeling occur as part of treatment, but contact your doctor if your skin becomes sore.

• *SYSTEMIC TREATMENT* •

For moderate to severe acne or if the skin condition does not improve with topical preparations, your doctor may consider adding treatment by mouth. Antibiotics, hormonal treatment and a vitamin A derivative may be tried at different stages.

Antibiotics

Tetracycline or **erythromycin** (see pages 275–9) are used to reduce the bacteria in the sebaceous duct and gland. These antibiotics do not act against blackheads and whiteheads which are not inflamed, so topical treatment must be continued. Tetracycline or erythromycin must be taken on an empty stomach and the morning dose taken well before breakfast. It may be two to four months before you see any improvement and your doctor may then want to adjust the dose up or down depending on your response to the antibiotic. Sometimes antibiotic treatment may be needed for two or more years.

Tetracycline and related drugs should not be used during pregnancy because they can harm developing bones and teeth. Tetracycline and erythromycin can cause stomach upsets. You should ask your doctor for advice; treatment may not need to be stopped if diarrhoea clears up with the temporary addition of a bulking agent to your diet. If you are also taking an oral contraceptive and get diarrhoea use additional contraception. Loss of appetite, feeling sick and vaginal candidosis occur occasionally. Very rarely acne may get worse, with the development of pustules when it has previously been well controlled with an antibiotic. You must see your doctor as you may need another type of antibiotic.

Hormonal treatment

Dianette contains **cyproterone acetate** and **ethinyloestradiol** and is used for treating women with severe acne which has not responded to topical preparations or to prolonged treatment with an antibiotic by mouth.

DIANETTE

DIANETTE – Tablets
CYPROTERONE ACETATE + ETHINYLOESTRADIOL

The combination of low doses of cyproterone and ethinyloestradiol is used for treating women with severe acne which has not responded to a prolonged course of antibiotic by mouth. Androgen, the male sex hormone, is present in small amounts in women and is the main cause of increased sebum production in acne. Cyproterone, a synthetic progestogen, blocks androgen activity while the oestrogen, ethinyloestradiol, reduces the amount of androgen made by the body. See Chapters 6 and 7. The combination may also help mild to moderate cases of hairiness (*hirsutism*) because hair growth is also androgen-dependent. Dianette also acts as an oral contraceptive, but is only prescribed if you have acne or hirsutism.

Before you use this medicine

Tell your doctor if you are:
☐ pregnant – do not take as cyproterone may cause female characteristics in a male baby ☐ breast-feeding – avoid Dianette ☐ taking any other medicines, including vitamins and those bought over the counter.

Tell your doctor if you have or have had:
☐ liver impairment or disease ☐ blood clots or deep vein thrombosis ☐ depression ☐ diabetes ☐ breast or endometrial cancer ☐ sickle-cell anaemia ☐ abnormal vaginal bleeding.

How to use this medicine

Take one tablet every day for 21 days, starting on the fifth day of your period (the first day of bleeding is day one). The next course is started after seven tablet-free days. Improvement in skin condition may take several months and treatment is often needed for six to nine months.

Other contraceptive measures, such as a condom, should be used during the first 14 days of the first course of Dianette. Never use another oral contraceptive with Dianette.

Do not stop taking this medicine suddenly without first checking with your doctor. If you miss a dose, take it as soon as you remember. If you take the tablet within 12 hours of the missed dose you do not need to take additional contraceptive measures. If more than 12 hours has passed, ignore the missed dose and take the remaining tablets on the correct days. You will need additional contraception until your next period.

Over 65 Not generally used.

Unwanted effects

Likely Feeling or being sick, headaches, breast tenderness, weight gain, breakthrough bleeding, reduced sexual interest.
Unlikely Depression, skin rash, tiredness.

Breakthrough bleeding or 'spotting' may occur especially during the first few cycles. You may bleed less during the withdrawal bleeds, but this is usual. If withdrawal bleeding does not occur at all, you should see your doctor. It is important to exclude pregnancy as a possible cause before continuing with treatment.

Similar preparations

Cyproterone (brand name Androcur) is used on its own in higher doses for treating male hypersexuality and sexual deviation. It is also used for treating cancer of the prostate (brand name Cyprostat).

Isotretinoin

Isotretinoin (brand name Roaccutane), a vitamin A derivative, is used for treating very severe acne where there are disfiguring pockets of inflammation under the skin, cysts and nodules. It reduces sebum production and the build up of dead skin cells in the hair follicle. It relieves swelling and helps the duct to unblock. Isotretinoin is used only if systemic antibacterial treatment has been unsuccessful. This drug must not be used during pregnancy and is available only as hospital treatment under the guidance of a consultant dermatologist.

One course of four month's treatment produces good results in the majority of people and there is a reasonable chance (one person in two) of the condition clearing completely. However, isotretinoin has some troublesome unwanted effects such as dry mouth, mucous membranes and skin. Dryness of the skin may cause scaling, thinning, redness and itching. Dryness of the mucous membranes in the nose may result in nosebleeds and a dry throat can lead to hoarseness. There may be muscle and joint pains and hair may be lost, but will regrow after treatment has finished. Isotretinoin occasionally causes liver enzymes and the blood level of fats to increase, so these are checked during treatment.

Women must use effective contraception while taking isotretinoin and for at least one month after treatment. Your doctor will want to make sure that you are not pregnant before starting treatment.

Scabies

Scabies and lice (see page 440) live in or on the skin. They are parasites spread by direct contact, causing irritation and itching of the skin which may lead to infection.

Scabies (*Sarcoptes scabei*) or the 'itch mite' affects both clean and dirty people. It spreads by direct skin contact between children, between sexual partners and commonly throughout a household. Female scabies mites burrow into the skin and lay eggs just under the surface. The eggs hatch in three to four days and become adults in 10–14 days to begin the cycle again. Intense itching, especially at night, usually starts one to eight weeks after the first infection. The rash most commonly affects the hands (usually between the fingers), insides of the wrists, the elbows, the feet and the genital area. The head and neck are hardly ever affected except in babies. The intense itching leads to scratching so that the rash sometimes looks like eczema. The scratched skin may become infected with bacteria.

– HOW YOU CAN HELP YOURSELF –

☐ If you have an itchy rash, ask the advice of a pharmacist or your doctor.
☐ Bathing and scrubbing will not remove the mites, you will need to use an insecticide lotion (see below).
☐ Scabies mites and eggs cannot live for very long away from their human host. Re-infection from clothing or bedding is not a significant risk, but you may feel that you want to change bedding after treatment. Hot washing, dry cleaning and ironing will all kill any mites.
☐ Schoolchildren should be kept at home until treatment has been carried out.

Medicines for scabies

In itself the scabies mite does not cause serious health problems, unless the skin becomes infected. Scabies is unpleasant because it causes intense itching and irritation and spreads through the community if left untreated. If you have scabies it is important to treat all people with whom you are in close contact. It may be eight weeks after the first infection before you have any signs of itching and during this time you can spread the disease without knowing. Treatment is applied to all skin from the neck down, including the skin between the fingers and toes, the genital area and the palms and soles. The face, neck and scalp of babies and young children should also be treated.

Preparations include water-based lotions of **lindane** or **malathion**, which are preferable to lotions containing alcohol.

You need use one of these products only once, provided it is properly applied. You do not need to have a bath before applying the lotion, although preparations have traditionally been put on after a hot bath. Doctors now think that a hot bath may increase the absorption of the drug into the body. Itching, and sometimes skin bumps (*nodules*) may persist for up to three months after treatment. However, treatment should only be repeated if there is evidence of mite activity. Applying more than the recommended amounts of lotion more than once will not get rid of the mites more quickily, but may cause an irritant skin rash. **Calamine lotion** can be used to soothe persistent itching.

Monosulfiram (brand name Tetmosol) is a solution containing alcohol, which must be diluted just before use and applied on two or three successive nights. Monosulfiram may interact with alcohol you have drunk, even through the skin, to cause unpleasant flushing of the face, headache, sweating, nausea and sickness. You should avoid drinking alcohol two days before and after using monosulfiram.

The older preparation **benzyl benzoate** is irritant, smells unpleasant and needs more time to work than either lindane or malathion. It can cause stinging, itching and burning of the skin and sometimes a rash. Benzyl benzoate has to be used on two consecutive days without bathing in between applications. Sometimes a third application is needed. It is not recommended for children or for use on broken eczematous skin. **Crotamiton** (brand name Eurax) is probably less effective than other treatments. It may be useful for persistent itching but should not be used on broken skin.

LINDANE

On prescription/from a pharmacy
QUELLADA – Lotion, shampoo

Lindane is an insecticide used for treating mite and lice infections such as scabies and crab lice. It has been used for head lice but is no longer recommended because resistant strains have developed. Lindane lotion smells pleasant, does not sting and can be used on eczematous skin. It is left on the skin for 24 hours and then washed off. Lindane can be absorbed through the skin into the body and is therefore not recommended for some people, including young children and anyone with a low body-weight. It is poisonous if swallowed, especially to children, who are particularly at risk from accidental poisoning.

Before you use this medicine

Tell your doctor of pharmacist if you are:
☐ pregnant – lindane is not recommended ☐ breast-feeding – avoid lindane ☐ taking any other medicines, including vitamins and these bought over the counter.

Tell your doctor if you have or have had:
☐ epilepsy.

How to use this medicine

Apply a thin layer of the lotion to the whole body surface except for the face and scalp. An adult needs about 50–75ml (2–3fl.oz) of lotion for one complete application. Avoid getting the lotion in the eyes and mouth and other mucous membranes. Leave for 24 hours and then wash off thoroughly. Repeat treatment after seven days if necessary. Do not use more than twice for one course of treatment.

Apply calamine lotion to soothe the skin of itching persists after treatment with lindane.

Over 65 No special requirements.

Unwanted effects

Unlikely Skin irritation and rash.

Lindane rarely causes problems if used according to instructions. If it is used too much or too often it may make you sick and cause muscle cramps, agitation and seizures. Contact your doctor immediately if lindane is swallowed.

Lice

The section discusses two common types of lice: the head louse (*Pediculus humanis capitis*) and the crab (pubic) louse (*Phthirus pubis*).

Head lice are blood-sucking insects which live close to the scalp where the environment is warm and moist with plenty of food and where they can lay eggs. They attach themselves to the base of the hair by strong, crab-like claws and do not let go even during hair-

HOW YOU CAN HELP YOURSELF

☐ If you know there is an outbreak of lice, for example among your child's classmates, check your family's hairs (including adults) for lice immediately. Favourite places for lice include the hair behind the ears, at the nape of the neck and back of the head and under a fringe. Comb the hair over a piece of white or lightly-coloured cloth or paper with an ordinary comb and then with a fine-toothed, nit comb. Lice are damaged by combing and some may fall out on to the paper as pink or brown specks.
☐ Nits cannot be confused with dandruff. Nits are shiny and stick to the hair while dandruff is dull and flaky and falls out.
☐ If you find evidence of lice get an appropriate lotion from a pharmacy. Keep your child away from school until treatment is finished.
☐ Lice and eggs not killed during treatment do not survive for long away from the scalp or other areas of skin. Generally it is not necessary to change pillowcases and sheets after treating the infection, although you may feel that you want to do so.
☐ Avoid using other people's combs and hair brushes.
☐ Inspection after hairwashing and regular combing with a comb for each member of the family helps to keep hair healthy and lice-free.
☐ People in close physical contact with someone with crab lice should have treatment.

washing. Lack of hygiene or long hair does not encourage lice; in fact short, clean hair makes it easier for them to reach the scalp. Head lice infections are very common, particularly in young children aged around four to five. However, children of all ages can become infected, as well as adults, although lice are rare in adult men. Head lice spread by close contact; for example, when heads touch the lice simply walk from one head to the other.

An adult louse is about 3–4mm long and greyish in colour. It lays about six to eight eggs a day, which are yellow and shiny and are stuck firmly to the hair base. As the baby lice grow they leave the empty egg cases, the cream or whitish coloured 'nits', still attached to the hair. Often the first sign of infection is itching, but by this time the lice have been in the hair for several weeks. Itching is an allergic response to lice saliva which is injected into the scalp each time the lice feed. It takes thousands of lice bites before itching develops. When you have had head lice for some time, you start to feel unwell or 'lousy' and may have a mild temperature, muscle aches and perhaps glandular swelling.

Crab (pubic) lice are commonly passed on during sexual intercourse. The lice are dirty white to yellow to grey in colour and live on fluid in the tissues. Symptoms include itching and irritation in the genital area; occasionally hair under the arms and on the legs if infected. The skin may have blue-grey spots, not raised, which if scratched may become reddish with pus.

Children may acquire lice from infected adults or other children. Their eyebrows and eyelashes sometimes become infected. **Malathion** and **lindane** both kill crab lice (see page 437). Only water-based lotions should be used because the alcohol-containing preparations cause stinging and irritation, especially on the genitals and on scratched and broken skin. Malathion aqueous lotion can be used for crab lice on eyelashes.

Medicines for lice

Malathion and **carbaryl** kill both the lice and the eggs and two newer preparations, **permethrin** (brand name Lyclear) and **phenothrin** (Full Marks), are also effective. Products containing **lindane** or **benzyl benzoate** are not recommended because resistant strains of lice have developed. A malathion or carbaryl lotion is best because it is used on dry hair and is more concentrated than a shampoo. It must be left on for 12 hours, usually overnight, and so it has a better chance to work. A shampoo is not in contact with the insects for long enough and is probably diluted too much during use to be effective; it also has to be used three times with three clear days between treatments.

Treatment for head lice should be repeated after one week to kill lice coming out of any eggs that might have survived the first treatment. None of these products, including shampoos, should be used on a 'just in case' basis for trying to prevent hair becoming infected with lice. Only regular inspection and combing will prevent lice becoming residential.

MALATHION

From a pharmacy/on prescription
DERBAC-M – Lotion (water-based)
PRIODERM – Lotion (contains alcohol), shampoo (not recommended)
SULEO-M – Lotion (contains alcohol)

Malathion is an insecticide used for treating scabies and lice. It kills them by interfering with their nervous system. Malathion also kills the eggs. It is available as a lotion or shampoo but the lotion is a better choice. The alcohol-containing lotion is effective but is not suitable for everyone, or for treating scabies or crab lice, but the water-based lotion can be used instead. Water-based lotions are best if you have asthma or you are treating small children because the fumes from the alcohol-containing products may trigger coughing and wheezing; they may also sting broken skin and should not be used on eczematous skin.

Before you use this medicine

Tell your doctor if you are:
☐ pregnant or breast-feeding ☐ taking any other medicines, including vitamins and those bought over the counter.

Tell your doctor if you have or have had:
☐ sensitivity to malathion ☐ eczema ☐ asthma.

See your doctor if you have to treat a baby under six months.

How to use this medicine

For head lice Rub the lotion into dry hair, the scalp and the affected area. Avoid getting it in the eyes. Comb the hair and allow it to dry naturally. Do not use a hair dryer because heat of any sort destroys the effectiveness of the insecticide. Leave the lotion on for 12 hours and then wash off by shampooing in the normal way. Comb wet hair with a normal comb and then with a fine-toothed comb to remove dead lice and nits.

A residue of insecticide remains on the hair for several weeks, which may help to ward off re-infection if the hair is allowed to dry naturally. Swimming in a chlorinated pool reduces any residual effect except with **permethrin**.

Alcohol-containing lotions are effective but must be used carefully because they are flammable. Always allow the hair to dry naturally in a well-ventilated room. Do not cover the head before the lotion has dried completely.

For pubic or crab lice Treat all hairy areas including a beard or a moustache. Leave the lotion on for 12 hours or overnight. Wash off or bathe in the usual way. A second treatment is necessary after one week to kill lice coming from surviving eggs.

For scabies Use the water-based lotion. Apply to the whole body from the neck down. Pay particular attention to the skin between the fingers and toes, the palms and soles. Leave on for 24 hours before washing. The success rate is higher if the lotion is applied a second time after three to four days.

Do not use malathion more than twice in a week.

Over 65 No special requirements.

Unwanted effects

Unlikely Skin irritation.

If used according to the instructions malathion rarely causes adverse effects. Contact your doctor immediately if malathion is accidentally swallowed.

Similar preparations

CARYLDERM – Lotion (contains alcohol), shampoo (not recommended)
CARBARYL

CLINICIDE – Lotion (water-based)
CARBARYL

FULL MARKS – Lotion (contains alcohol), shampoo (not recommended)
PHENOTHRIN

LYCLEAR – Cream (contains alcohol), skin cream for scabies
PERMETHRIN

SULEO-C – Lotion (contains alcohol), shampoo (not recommended)
CARBARYL

Sunburn

Staying out for too long in strong sunlight without protecting your skin can result in redness and swelling of the skin, particularly if you are fair-skinned. However, people vary in their sensitivity to sunlight and dermatologists have identified six skin types ranging from very pale skin which never tans to darker skin which rarely burns (see Box).

The sun makes you feel good and a little sunshine every day helps you to remain healthy. *Ultraviolet* (UV) rays in sunlight activate a body chemical in the skin to form vitamin D. There are three main types of UV radiation – UVA and UVB, which reach the earth and can damage your skin, and UVC, which is filtered out by the ozone layer. UVB causes sunburn, but both UVB and UVA cause skin cancer and ageing.

UVB rays are the most damaging to your skin. They are present during daylight, although their strength varies because the

SKIN TYPES

These skin types have been identified based on how each type reacts to sun before a sunscreen is applied and before getting used to sunlight. The types are a rough guide only and there is often variation. Use the sunscreens with the recommended sun protection factor (SPF) when you go out in strong sunlight or start tanning.

1. Very pale skin: never tans, always burns – SPF 10–15 or higher to start.
2. Very fair, freckles: burns at first, tans with difficulty – SPF 10–15 or higher to start.
3. Yellowish skin, mouse/dark hair: tans easily, burns rarely – SPF 8 or higher to start.
4. Dark hair, skin (Mediterranean type): always tans, never burns – SPF 8 or higher to start.
5. Genetically brown skin: needs little or no protection – SPF 2–4 to start.
6. Genetically black skin: needs little or no protection – SPF 2–4 to start.

Children need high protection because they are particularly susceptible to skin damage from the sun: the effects add up over your life. Babies under six months are even more at risk, because their skin has not yet fully developed its natural defences. Keep babies in the shade and protected by an umbrella if possible. All children are safest wearing a hat and a sunscreen with a high SPF.

atmosphere and clouds filter them. Your body has two kinds of protective action against UVB rays: your skin thickens and the pigment cells produce more *melanin*, so that the skin turns a darker colour. Melanin absorbs and scatters the sun's rays; the more melanin in the outer skin layer the better your protection.

UVA rays have less burning power than UVB but they are not filtered out by the atmosphere, so their strength does not vary much during the day or from summer to winter. UVA stimulates melanin production to produce a tan, but penetrates deeper into the skin than UVB and contributes to wrinkles, yellowing and blotching, often regarded as signs of ageing. UVA is also responsible for *photosensitivity* rashes triggered by sunlight; some drugs increase this sensitivity (see Box on next page).

DRUGS THAT CAN CAUSE PHOTOSENSITIVITY

A few drugs cause your skin to be more sensitive to sunlight. You are likely to need a high-SPF product but check with your doctor or pharmacist what precautions you should take before going out in the sun.
Antibacterials – **tetracycline**, **nalidixic acid**, **sulphonamides**
Diuretics – **thiazides**
Irregular heartbeats – **amiodarone**
Antipsychotics – **phenothiazines**.

If you spend too long in the sun for your type of skin you are likely to become sunburnt. The skin becomes red, hot, tight and swollen as the blood vessels are injured and leak fluid; blisters may appear. The condition is usually painful and causes itching. Some days later the top layer of the skin peels. In a severe case you may feel quite unwell with dizziness, nausea, abdominal cramps, headache and muscle weakness and sometimes you may be sick. How sunburnt you become depends on how tanned you were to start with, how long you were in the sun and the strength of the sun. You are most at risk of burning when the sun is high in the sky in the summer months or you are near the Equator or at high altitudes.

● *THE SUN AND SKIN CANCER* ●

UVB rays are the main cause of skin cancer, although UVA rays also contribute. Skin cancers, such as *malignant melanoma* are increasingly common. Getting sunburnt increases your risk of developing cancer, although skin cancer is more likely to be caused by the cumulative effect of years of exposure to the sun. People with skin types 1 and 2 (see 'Skin types', page 445) are most at risk from all types of skin cancer, especially if you also have a lot of freckles and moles. If you have had severe sunburn at least once, especially as a child, you are also more at risk. If you have already had a malignant melanoma or a member of your family has had one, you are more at risk. Skin cancers like malignant melanoma are curable if recognised and treated early. Always check yours and your family's skin using the seven point checklist below.

● *Melanoma checklist*

Unlike other types of skin cancer, melanoma can strike young adults. Ask yourself these questions about any worrying pigmented patches:

☐ change in size, or new patch?
☐ border become irregular in shape?
☐ density of black and brown varies?
☐ diameter of 7mm or larger?
☐ inflammation?
☐ bleeding or crusting?
☐ itching or altered sensation?

If you can answer yes to any of these questions, you should see your doctor, who may refer you to a specialist. Yes to any of the first three questions is most likely to mean melanoma.

Sunburn treatments

There are a number of remedies for relieving the pain of hot, burnt skin. If sunburn is severe, contact a doctor.

A tepid bath or shower can take the heat out of your skin. If you have been swimming in the sea, wash off dried salt remaining on the skin because it can aggravate sunburn. Exposing your skin to the sun tends to dry it and applying an emollient or using one in the bath (see 'Eczema', page 416) helps to conserve moisture and soothe the skin. You do not have to use a special 'aftersun' lotion – any cooling emollient lotion will do. **Calamine lotion** applied often and liberally to the burnt area cools the skin as it dries. It should not be applied to broken skin.

If you develop blisters, try to avoid bursting them because of the risk of infection. Blisters may burst in a bath so you may have to forgo cooling down in this way. Take aspirin or paracetamol to relieve pain. Drink plenty of non-alcoholic fluids, especially if you have severe sunburn.

Itching may be helped by an antihistamine by mouth, particularly if it is taken at night. Creams, lotions or sprays containing antihistamines or local anaesthetics should not be used on the skin because they may cause sensitisation; these include Anthisan, Caladryl, R.B.C. cream, Solarcaine, Anethaine and Xylocaine.

● *SUN PROTECTION* ●

Using a sunscreen can help you to achieve a suntan without sunburn, protect your skin from the ravages of strong sunlight and reduce the risk of skin cancer. Sunscreens absorb or reflect UV radiation so that less of the damaging rays penetrate the skin. The fewer the UV rays that get through, the longer you can stay in the sun without burning. The sun protection factor (SPF),

HOW YOU CAN HELP YOURSELF

- ☐ Use a sunscreen and build up your tan slowly. Sunbathe for short periods to start with.
- ☐ Avoid the sun between 11am and 3pm.
- ☐ Remember that UV radiation from the sun can be strong even on cool, cloudy days.
- ☐ Sand, water and snow reflect UV radiation and increase the strength of the sun. Wind enhances skin damage produced by UV rays.
- ☐ When you are swimming, the sun may be strong up to a metre under water. Wearing a T-shirt is not the answer because the sun can go through it, especially if it is white. Use a water-resistant suntan lotion before you go into the water.
- ☐ A hat and loose-fitting cotton clothing can make you feel more comfortable on a hot, sunny day and help to protect you from UVA and UVB rays.
- ☐ Wear sunglasses as UV radiation can damage your eyes.
- ☐ Be wary of sunbeds: they can cause sunburn. The tan they give comes from UVA and so you might start to show signs of ageing earlier than normal.

marked on all sunscreen products is a guide to roughly how long you are protected in the sun. The SPF is the ratio between the dose of radiation required to produce just measurable redness on protected skin, to that which produces a response on unprotected skin. The higher the SPF number, the better the protection. Until recently, the SPF number referred mainly to protection against UVB, so that some products which are less effective for UVA had a high SPF. Some manufacturers have now reformulated their sunscreen preparations so that you can also get better protection against UVA.

To build your tan up slowly you will need several bottles of sunscreen each with a different SPF. As your tan develops you can reduce protection by using a lower SPF product. It is a good idea to put sunscreen on before you go out in the sun, not when you get to the beach. The sun acts the minute you are out in it, even while you are putting on your sunscreen. Spread the sunscreen thickly and evenly; pay particular attention to the areas at the edges of your swimming costume or clothes, and to the raised and bony parts of your body. For example, the nose is especially likely to burn, but a reflectant sunscreen can help. Re-apply your sunscreen at least every two hours, even high SPF products, and more often if you are swimming or sweating.

MINOR BURNS

Accidental burns and scaldings happen frequently in and around the home. Heat damages the top skin layers, causing redness, swelling and pain. Sometimes a blister forms as fluids from the surrounding tissues oozes out. First aid should include cooling the burnt area as soon as possible with cold water: submerge the burnt area for ten minutes to take as much heat away from the skin as possible. Avoid putting ice cubes on the skin because these can stick to it and cause further injury. Pat the area dry and leave it. If only the top layer of skin is burnt it will heal with time. A thin layer of antiseptic cream can be applied, but some doctors believe that some antiseptic products delay healing. Use a plaster or dry dressing only if the damaged area is likely to be harmed if left unprotected. A plaster stops the air circulating freely around the burn and may also delay healing. Pain can be relieved with paracetamol or aspirin.

If a blister forms, leave it intact because it protects the lower skin layers as they heal and prevents bacteria settling on the damaged skin and causing infection. Taking the top off the blister before it is ready to come is likely to lead to more pain. If the skin is burnt deeply or the burn covers a large area, contact your doctor.

WHAT'S IN A SUNSCREEN

Some sunscreens can cause an allergic rash and you will need to find out which preparation suits you best as well as providing adequate protection. For example, if you are sensitive to the drugs **procaine** or **benzocaine** or to certain hair dyes you may react to a sunscreen containing **PABA** or a **benzophenone**.

Absorbents (UVB only) – **para-aminobenzoic acid** (PABA) and derivatives, **cinnamates**, **salicylates**; (UVB and some UVA) – **benzophenones**; for example **oxybenzone**, **mexenone**, **dibenzoylmethane**.
Reflectants (UVB and UVA) – **zinc oxide**, **titanium dioxide**.

Cuts, bites and stings

Cuts and scratches are commonplace, minor injuries which need simple and prompt treatment. Skin is the body's protective covering for the internal organs, keeping out harmful micro-organisms such as bacteria. If the skin is damaged or breached in any way this protection is temporarily lost until the body mechanisms repair the injury. Skin is exposed to harmful micro-organisms all the time, but few of them lead to infection. The skin is constantly renewing itself and many minor cuts and burns heal without a trace of damage, particularly in children and young people. Deeper wounds and those covering a large area should be assessed by a doctor; they may leave a scar on healing.

First of all the wound should be washed in mild soap and warm water to clean it. Cold water can help to stem the blood if bleeding is profuse. Dry it gently and cover with a plaster which has a pad to prevent the wound sticking to it. The pad may be impregnated with an antiseptic. You can use an antiseptic cream if necessary after washing with soap and water, but not in place of washing. An antiseptic liquid can be diluted and added to the water for washing the wound, but may sometimes cause stinging. Using a small, sterile dressing strip (for example Steristrip) to draw a wound together may be helpful for some cuts.

If the cut is deep or long you may need to contact your doctor, as stitches may be needed. You may also need a *tetanus* injection if you last received a dose of the vaccine more than 5 years ago. Tetanus is a bacterium which can cause serious infection. It is also known as lockjaw because it produces a toxin in the body that affects the nerves, which results in muscular spasm, typically of the face, and eventually death. The tetanus organism is commonly found in soil and on the ground so that any deep wound or scratch (for example from an animal or rose) is likely to pick up some tetanus bacteria. Cleaning the wound is very important but may not remove all the bacteria. Ask your doctor whether you need to be immunised.

Children are normally vaccinated from the age of two months, when they receive a course of tetanus toxoid with other vaccines to protect against serious illness. A booster dose of tetanus injection should be given just before school entry at the age of five and a further boost given in the mid-teens. Many older people have not been immunised against tetanus because it was not given during childhood. Next time you visit your doctor check to see whether you are protected against tetanus.

Animal bites can cause severe infection as bacteria in the saliva of the animal can be introduced into wounds, especially deep injuries. Clean the wound thoroughly as soon as possible after an attack.

Infection with tetanus is the main concern and you should see your doctor if you have not been immunised within the last five years.

Insect bites cause irritation, redness, swelling and itching. Some people are not troubled much by bites whereas others react more – children, for example. Flying insects such as mosquitoes, midges and sandflies suck blood for food and introduce a substance into the skin of their victims to make it easier to get the blood. This substance casues the irritation which wears off with time. If the bite itches and you scratch it, the skin may become infected with bacteria. Keep the area of bitten skin clean with soap and water and apply an antiseptic cream. If the bites become badly infected you will need to see your doctor, who may prescribe an antibacterial product. Although there are a number of products especially designed for relieving the irritation of insect bites, **calamine lotion** or an emollient (see page 416) is the best treatment. Skin preparations containing antihistamines or local anaesthetics are not recommended.

• *INSECT STINGS* •

For most people a sting by a wasp or a bee is an unpleasant and painful event. A bee sting should be removed from the skin by scraping a blunt blade across the area. Tweezers have been recommended but may squeeze more sting (venom) into the wound. The pain fades after a few hours and the skin can be soothed with calamine lotion. However, a small number of people are extremely sensitive to bee and wasp stings and the allergic reaction can be life-threatening (see page 178). If you are allergic to bee stings you should wear an identity bracelet (for example Medic-alert) and be trained to use and carry a ready-filled syringe of adrenalin.

Medicines for cuts, bites and stings

• *ANTISEPTICS AND DISINFECTANTS* •

These are chemicals that kill micro-organisms or prevent them growing where they are not wanted. Antiseptics are sometimes considered to be those products which are used on the skin while the term disinfectant is reserved for preparations that prevent microbial growth on objects. In practice there is considerable overlap in the way the terms are used and between products. Other names for antiseptics include germicide and skin disinfectant.

Some general-purpose chemicals used for disinfecting the floor also applied to the skin; for example **cetrimide** (brand name Savlon).

Sometimes the preparations will be specially formulated for the different circumstances or sometimes you may have to dilute the product for a particular purpose. The benefits of widespread use of antiseptics and disinfectants are sometimes unclear. Some experts think that the effects of these products are no better than using soap or detergent and water and that they delay wound healing.

● *INSECT REPELLENTS* ●

There are various methods for keeping blood-sucking insects away. Long-sleeved clothing is helpful but you can also use an insect repellent on your skin or buy a gadget.

The most effective products are based on **diethyltoluamide** (DEET or DET). The more concentrated it is, the longer it will keep insects away. Liquids are normally the cheapest means of buying a repellent; sprays are bulky and usually more expensive, but easier to apply; sticks have a lower concentration of repellent, but have the best staying power, and are easy to carry around.

DEET must be used carefully, especially on children's skin. DEET can cause skin irritation for some people and it can be absorbed into the body. Application over extensive areas of the body has been known to cause inflammation of the brain (*encephalitis*) and rarely death. Keep repellents well away from children; containers do not have child-resistant closures.

Of the gadgets on sale for repelling insects, electric mosquito killers give convenient protection in enclosed areas such as hotel rooms. In countries where malaria is a problem, bed nets treated with **permethrin** repellent offer good protection from mosquitoes which feed during the night. Insect coils are less effective because they must burn reliably all through the night. Candles, repellent strips and electric buzzers do not keep insects away from you and are not effective.

Warts and verrucae

Warts and verrucae are infections of the skin caused by various types of the wart virus (human *papilloma* virus). The *common wart* on the hands and fingers appears as raised, thickened, skin-coloured patches (*nodules*) of skin. Small, flatter-looking nodules on the hand are known as *planar warts*. On the soles of feet, warts grow into the skin layers rather than being raised above the skin because of the pressure from the body's weight. These are *plantar warts* or *verrucae*, often called verrucas. As a verruca grows larger, it eventually causes pain when weight is put on the foot.

Genital warts, caused by a different type of human papilloma virus from the common wart or verruca are small in size and many in number. They are passed on by sexual contact and need special treatment at a hospital clinic.

Common warts and verrucae are passed on from person to person and so almost everyone is likely to get them at some stage in their lives. The virus enters the skin through small cuts and scratches, liking in particular moist, warm areas. It lives within cells of the outer skin layer and takes over cell division, making the skin grow abnormally. You may have a single wart or verruca or several. Warts and verrucae are common in children, especially age 12–16. Some people are more likely to get the virus than others depending on their immunity to the wart virus: Some are resistant to infection and others have to develop this resistance. Once resistance has built up the wart disappears – often overnight. This spontaneous disappearance of warts, usually between six months and two years after infection, accounts for some of the myths and old wives' tales about wart cures.

Medicines for warts and verrucae

Your doctor may recommend not treating a wart or verruca because it will disappear spontaneously, although this takes time. However, warts can be troublesome because they get in the way when you use your hands or fingers; a verruca may be painful. The virus is slow-growing and resistant to all attempts to remove it. Treatment of either a wart or a verruca therefore takes time and perseverance with regular application of a suitable preparation. Most products can be bought at a pharmacy, some for less than the prescription charge, or your doctor can prescribe them.

Treatment aims to reduce the size of the wart or verruca by removing the overgrown layers of skin. **Salicylic acid** softens and destroys the wart but also the surrounding skin, which should be protected during treatment. There are various preparations and choice is not critical. Most have to be used once a day and it helps to soak the affected area in warm water for five to ten minutes before applying the preparation. All products contain salicylic acid (strength varies from 11–50 per cent) in an ointment or liquid and include Salicylic Acid Collodion BP, Cuplex, Duofilm, Salactol, Salatac, and Verrugon. The skin surrounding the wart can be protected by putting on some petroleum jelly (for example Vaseline) before carefully applying salicylic acid. Covering the wart with a waterproof plaster helps to keep the skin soft and increases the effectiveness of treatment. Dead skin can be removed by gentle rubbing with a pumice stone as treatment progresses.

If treatment is not successful after three months, you may want to discuss with your doctor the possibility of removing the wart with liquid nitrogen. This method of freezing the wart is not suitable for young children because it is painful and can cause blistering. However, it is usually successful and after seven to ten days the wart goes.

Podophyllum (combined with salicylic acid in Posafilin ointment) is a suitable verruca treatment for adults and children. It is used two to three times a week. A ring-shaped felt corn-plaster can be placed around the verruca, with the ring enlarged by snipping away the felt if necessary. Apply a tiny amount of ointment to the verruca and cover with a waterproof plaster. After some time, when the verruca appears soft and spongy, leave it open to the air for a day or two. The verruca should drop off, but if it does not, you repeat the treatment.

Preparations containing **formaldehyde** (brand name Veracur), **glutaraldehyde** (Glutarol; Novaruca; Verucasep) and **bromine** (Callusolve) have less predictable effects and have to be applied twice daily. Formaldehyde and glutaraldehyde may be irritant to the skin and glutaraldehyde stains it brown. A formaldehyde solution is used for soaking a verruca on the foot, but you should protect the skin between the toes with petroleum jelly to prevent soreness.

• *CAUTIONS* •

Wart and verruca products contain caustic substances which can damage healthy skin and after using them you must take care to wash your hands thoroughly. Never use any of the preparations on your face or the genital region. If you are diabetic you should not treat warts or verrucae with an over-the-counter preparation, but always discuss the problem with your doctor. You should also see your doctor if the wart or verruca changes size or colour, if it bleeds or itches, if you develop a wart on the face or if you have genital warts.

• *VERRUCAE AND SWIMMING* •

The wart virus is everywhere in the environment and extremely difficult to avoid. It spreads easily in the warm moist environment of a swimming pool and changing rooms, but there is no need to stop your child from going swimming. Putting a waterproof plaster on a wart or verruca that you are treating protects it and prevents it from spreading to others. There is then no need to wear a special rubber sock. However, some doctors think that it is unnecessary to cover verrucae at all.

11

NUTRITION AND BLOOD

Anaemia Vitamin deficiency

Food is necessary for building and maintaining the cells and tissues in your body. The three main components of food are *protein, fat* and *carbohydrates* and an average daily diet provides a mixture of these. Protein is the body's major building material and your muscles are largely made of it. Fat is laid down as a layer under the skin to help conserve body heat and stored all through the body. It also provides energy, although it is a less accessible source than carbohydrates which, in the form of starches and sugars, are the body's main source of energy. *Fibre*, the indigestible part of plant foods, is needed for a healthy digestive system and helps to make faeces bulky and easy to pass.

Food also contains small amounts of *minerals* and *vitamins*, which are essential for maintaining many of the normal body processes. Protein, fat and carbohydrates have to be broken down (*metabolised*) to smaller components by the digestive system before they can be absorbed and used in the body (see also Chapter 1: Digestive system). For example, protein in food is broken down into smaller substances called *amino acids* which the body uses to build its own proteins which are essential for replacing cells, the elements of all body tissues. Each of these biochemical reactions need an *enzyme* – a substance that promotes the body's metabolic processes – and vitamins and minerals seem to be important aids to the functioning of enzymes.

Complete lack of essential nutrients, minerals and vitamins is uncommon in people living in developed countries. However, deficiencies do occur and some people are at risk of not getting enough minerals and vitamins. In underdeveloped countries inadequate supplies of food lead to illness such as *kwashiorkor*, caused by lack of protein, and *beri-beri* and *scurvy*, caused by vitamin deficiences.

Anaemia

Anaemia is a disorder affecting red blood cells. It may result from insufficient or misshapen blood cells being made or from cells being destroyed too early or lost through haemorrhage (excessive blood loss from the body). Red blood cells are made in *bone marrow* and should have a life of 120 days; every day around two hundred thousand million must be made to replace those that are lost. Like all cells in the body, the red blood cell is made up of body protein derived from amino acids in dietary protein, so an adequate diet of protein, with vitamins and minerals to help biochemical reactions, is needed. **Iron** is essential for the manufacture of *haemoglobin*, the pigment in red cells which carries oxygen from the lungs to the body tissues. Two vitamins from the B group, **vitamin B_{12}** and **folic acid**, are essential for building red cells from proteins. If the activity of either of these vitamins or iron is disrupted, a form of anaemia results.

• *IRON-DEFICIENCY ANAEMIA* •

Lack of iron may mean that the body has too few red blood cells, too little haemoglobin or too little blood. Iron-rich foods include liver, meat, eggs, wholemeal cereals and leafy vegetables. Iron is well absorbed from meat and liver, but less so from vegetables and hardly at all from eggs. Although you need a certain amount of iron in your daily diet, and women need about twice as much as men, the body is economical with this mineral, as iron from old red cells is re-used in the formation of new ones. Iron is stored in bone marrow, the spleen and muscles.

However, iron-deficiency anaemia is quite common. Blood loss is the most usual cause and this may occur in women with heavy periods, when there is bleeding from a peptic ulcer or other damage to the stomach or intestinal wall (for example, through disease or from regular taking of aspirin or other NSAIDs) and at childbirth. Symptoms of anaemia include tiredness, breathlessness on exertion, palpitations, dizziness and headache. You may lose the normal colour in your lips, tongue and the linings of your eyes and your skin may look pale. Some people also develop spoon-shaped or flattened nails. Anaemia can develop rapidly with severe blood loss.

Your doctor will always want to establish the cause of anaemia and you will need blood tests to determine the haemoglobin level. You should never attempt to treat yourself with an iron preparation or a general tonic containing iron because these may conceal other causes of anaemia; for example, lack of a B vitamin (see right). Too much iron in the body can damage the liver, heart or kidneys. There is no risk of iron overload from the food in a normal diet.

HOW YOU CAN HELP YOURSELF

☐ Eat a well-balanced diet. Your body will absorb the amount of iron that it needs.
☐ Eating certain foods together increases the absorption of iron – for example, fish with spinach or vitamin C in fruit juices with bran cereals.
☐ If you have abnormal bleeding in urine or stools see your doctor. Heavy periods for a few months or bleeding after you have stopped at the menopause needs discussion with the doctor.
☐ Avoid iron supplements that also contain other minerals such as calcium and magnesium, as these interfere with the body's absorption of iron.
☐ Do not take an iron supplement at the same time of day as eating fibre-rich foods or calcium.

VITAMIN B_{12} AND FOLIC ACID DEFICIENCIES

Anaemia can be caused by a lack of either **vitamin B_{12}** or **folic acid**, both of which are essential for building cells, especially red blood cells. Your doctor will want to establish which is lacking and how the deficiency occurred.

The most common type of anaemia is *pernicious anaemia* which is mainly due to faulty absorption of vitamin B_{12} (also called **cyanocobalamin**). A vitamin B_{12} deficiency leads not only to anaemia but also to slow, progressive, irreversible damage to the nervous system. This damage causes numbness in the hands and feet, unsteadiness, loss of memory, confusion and depression. It may take years to develop because vitamin B_{12} stores in the liver are plentiful and the body only requires tiny amounts of the vitamin for making red cells. You may be taking in adequate amounts of vitamin B_{12}, but it cannot be absorbed into the body unless it combines with another substance made in the stomach known as *intrinsic factor*. If the intrinsic factor is deficient, the body cannot use vitamin B_{12}, the *extrinsic factor*. You may develop a deficiency if you have certain bowel disorders or have had surgery to remove parts of your stomach or small intestine.

If your doctor finds that you are lacking vitamin B_{12} it can be replaced by an external source, but due to lack of intrinsic factor it has to be given by injection. **Hydroxocobalamin**, a derivative of vitamin B_{12}, is injected, at first every few days to restore the body's supplies and then every three months for the rest of your life to maintain adequate levels.

Vitamin B_{12} is found in meat, fish, milk, eggs and cheese and a balanced diet normally provides this vitamin. If you are vegetarian and do not eat eggs or dairy products you may need a vitamin B_{12} supplement, but it does not need to be injected because you do not lack intrinsic factor. Breakfast cereals, soya milk and yeast extracts fortified with vitamin B_{12} are a good alternative to supplements.

Low levels of folic acid lead to anaemia at the stage when red blood cells are made in bone marrow. Signs include tiredness, loss of appetite, nausea, diarrhoea, sore mouth and tongue and hair loss. Folic acid is found in dark green leafy vegetables, some fresh fruit, eggs, liver, yeast extract and pulses, so that a well-balanced diet should provide adequate supplies. Some diseases of the small intestine can interfere with the body's aborption of folic acid. Lack of folic acid often occurs in alcoholics, but usually because of a poor diet. Long-term treatment with certain drugs such as methotrexate, trimethoprim, triamterene, corticosteroids and antiepileptic medicines can also cause deficiency.

Folic acid in combination with an iron supplement may be given during pregnancy to prevent anaemia, but it is also very important to take foods rich in folic acid. Women who have given birth to a baby with *spina bifida* or a similar defect (*neural tube defect*) and who want to have another baby are given folic acid before conception and during the first three months of pregnancy.

Your doctor will want to establish the cause of your lack of folic acid before prescribing a course of tablets. Most causes of deficiency sort themselves out with time or can be readily corrected by a short course of folic acid tablets if you cannot get enough in your diet. Folic acid may worsen the condition caused by vitamin B_{12} deficiency and should never be taken on its own for treating this type of anaemia. Folic acid can mask the symptoms of vitamin B_{12} deficiency while allowing the irreversible nervous system damage to occur undetected.

Medicines for anaemia

If you have a definite lack of iron you can replace this loss by taking a daily dose of an iron preparation by mouth. The iron corrects anaemia in six to eight weeks but treatment is continued for a further three months to replenish the body's iron stores. Choice of iron preparation depends on how well you tolerate different products: iron salts upset the digestive system and may make you feel sick; they also have a constipating effect, particularly for older people. Iron preparations contain either *ferrous* or *ferric* salts – ferrous salts are slightly more easily absorbed than ferric, so **ferrous sulphate** tablets are often tried first.

Some iron preparations contain **vitamin C** to aid absorption, but in practice the advantage is minimal. Compound iron preparations containing other minerals and vitamins are not recommended except for pregnant women who may benefit from small amounts of folic acid with iron. Modified-release preparations are likely to carry the iron past the first part of the intestine where iron is best absorbed, so insufficient quantities may get into the body. Unwanted effects are reduced, possibly because less iron is absorbed, but these preparations are not recommended.

Occasionally iron is given by injection into the vein or muscle, but it does not produce quicker results than if you take iron regularly by mouth. Iron injections may be needed if you cannot tolerate or absorb iron by mouth or if you experience continuing severe blood loss.

FERROUS SULPHATE

On prescription/from a pharmacy
FERROUS SULPHATE – Tablets, liquid for children

Poor choice
Sustained-release preparations – FEOSPAN; FERROGRAD; SLOW-FE
Compound preparations containing ferrous sulphate – **FERROUS SULPHATE COMPOUND TABLETS**; FEFOL; FEFOL-VIT; FEFOL Z; FERROGRAD C; FERROGRAD FOLIC; FESOVIT; FESOVIT Z; FOLICIN; OCTOVIT

Ferrous sulphate is a preparation of iron, which the body needs for making haemoglobin, the pigment in red blood cells that carries oxygen from the lungs to the tissues. You usually take in sufficient iron in a well-balanced diet, but children, teenagers, and women may need more. Women lose iron through bleeding at each period, during pregnancy and when the baby is born. Babies fed only on milk for longer than six months are also at risk of becoming iron-deficient. Vegetarians may also need iron supplements.

Before you use this medicine

Tell your doctor ifyou are:
☐ pregnant or breast-feeding ☐ taking any other medicines, including vitamins and those bought over the counter.

Tell your doctor if you have or have had:
☐ liver disease ☐ peptic ulcer or other intestinal disease ☐ recent blood transfusion.

Do not take if you have or have had:
☐ diseases of iron overload (haemochromatosis, haemosiderosis)
☐ thalassaemia (an inherited form of anaemia).

How to use this medicine

Treatment of anaemia Depending on the preparation, take one, two or three tablets or capsules per day. Take them with a glassful of water or fruit juice before meals; this helps iron absorption. If the iron tablets upset your stomach, take the dose with or after meals. The children's mixture is usually given three times daily with plenty of water.
Prevention of anaemia The dosage is usually once a day.

If you miss a dose, take it as soon as you remember, but skip it if it is almost time for your next dose. Do not take double the dose.

Over 65 No special dose requirements.

Interactions with other medicines

Various drugs reduce the absorption of iron and sometimes vice versa if the preparations are taken at the same time of day. Do not take other medicines without checking with your doctor or pharmacist. Medicines that interact include:
Antacids
Antibacterials: **tetracycline** and **ciprofloxacin**, for example
Levodopa for Parkinson's disease
Penicillamine for modifying arthritis
Zinc.

Unwanted effects

Likely Heartburn, dark stools.
Unlikely (with large doses) Stomach pains, feeling or being sick, diarrhoea or constipation.

It is quite usual for iron preparations to darken stools. Contact your doctor if you have severe stomach pain, cramping or soreness, or fresh blood in stools.

Iron poisoning is extremely dangerous. Always keep iron preparations out of reach of children, particularly if the product is not in a child-resistant container. In cases of accidental poisoning, especially if a child is involved, seek emergency treatment at

hospital immediately. Do not wait for symptoms to develop as these may not appear for an hour.
Early signs Diarrhoea, nausea, vomiting, cramping, sharp stomach pains.
Late signs Bluish lips, fingernails and palms; drowsiness; pale, clammy skin; unusual tiredness; weak, fast heartbeat.

Similar preparations

On prescription/from a pharmacy

FERGON – Tablets
FERROUS GLUCONATE

FERROMYN – Liquid
FERROUS SUCCINATE

FERROUS GLUCONATE – Tablets

FERSADAY – Tablets
FERROUS FUMARATE

FERSAMAL – Tablets, liquid
FERROUS FUMARATE

GALFER – Capsules, liquid
FERROUS FUMARATE

NIFEREX – Liquid, high-dose capsules
POLYSACCHARIDE-IRON COMPLEX

PLESMET – Liquid
FERROUS GLYCINE SULPHATE

SYTRON – Liquid
SODIUM IRONEDETATE

Poor choice
Modified-release preparations: FERROCAP; FERROCONTIN CONTINUS

Vitamin deficiencies

Vitamins play an essential part in normal body functions. They help with the production of energy from food and the regulation of the metabolism. Each metabolic process involves a specific *enzyme* and usually a particular vitamin or mineral to aid the biochemical reaction. The body needs only tiny amounts of vitamins and minerals, but generally cannot make them. Vitamins and minerals are found in a wide variety of foods and a well-balanced diet supplies all of these.

There are 13 vitamins essential for good health: **vitamins A, C, D, E, K** and the eight B vitamins – **thiamin** (B_1), **riboflavin** (B_2), **nicotinic acid** (B_3; niacin), **pyridoxine** (B_6), **pantothenic acid**, **biotin**, **folic acid** and **vitamin B_{12}**. The B vitamins were given numbers initially, but the system is somewhat confused because they are given names as their function becomes clear. Vitamin C and the B vitamins dissolve in water within the body and any excess is usually lost in urine; vitamins A, D, E and K dissolve only in fat and are stored for long periods in the body, mainly in the liver. Fat-soluble vitamins may accumulate if you take supplements well in excess of the body's requirements and this can lead to toxicity. Vitamins are a normal and essential part of the diet, which the body extracts from food during digestion, but when vitamins are taken in a concentrated form, sometimes at high doses, they should be thought of as medicines, which can produce unwanted effects.

• *HOW MUCH DO YOU NEED?* •

The answers to the questions, 'How much do people need on average?', the subjective, 'How much do I need?' and the more objective, 'How much do I need to eat to be sure that I am getting enough?' are all different and vary according to age, sex and lifestyle – and individuals have different needs for nutrients and different abilities to absorb them.

In 1991 the Department of Health introduced new guidelines for nutrient intakes called Dietary Reference Values, to replace Recommended Daily Amounts (RDAs). The thinking behind the figures is to do away with the idea that everybody needs to eat the 'recommended' amounts of nutrients in order to be getting enough. the RDA has been replaced by the Reference Nutrient Intake (RNI), an amount which satisfies the needs of 97 per cent of the population – more than enough for most people. If the average intake of the population is at the RNI, then the risk deficiency in any individual is small.

No single figure provides an adequate yardstick against which individuals can judge their nutrient intake, but a well-balanced diet will provide all the nutrients you need unless you have a condition which imposes special requirements. Rather than listing amounts of vitamins and minerals, the Table gives the main providers of the nutrients – you are only likely to be risking deficiency if your diet is almost devoid of the sources of a particular nutrient or if you eat very little food at all.

Some vitamins are also made in the body. For example, biotin is manufactured by intestinal bacteria and vitamin D is produced when the skin is exposed to sunlight. Having less than the RNI does not necessarily mean that you have a deficiency. RNIs do not cover individual variations due to disease.

• *WHO NEEDS SUPPLEMENTS?* •

Vitamin supplements may be needed by elderly people, women who are pregnant or breast-feeding, some children and people on limited diets. Vitamins can be prescribed to treat specific deficiency states and to prevent deficiencies developing, but not as dietary supplements.

VITAL VITAMINS AND MINERALS

	Function in body	Main sources	Signs of deficiency
VITAMINS			
A	growth, night vision, healthy skin	liver, green leafy vegetables, carrots, yellow and orange fruit and vegetables, eggs, cheese, milk	difficulty seeing in dim light; dry, rough skin; dry eyes
B1: thiamin	release of energy from foods	potatoes, wholemeal and white bread, vegetables, milk, breakfast cereals, pulses, nuts	inflammation of the nerves (peripheral neuritis); heart failure; excess water; feeling or being sick; beri-beri; mental confusion; brain damage
B2: riboflavin	release of energy from foods	liver, meat, milk and cheese	sore lips and cracks at corners of mouth; mouth ulcers; sore red tongue; skin rashes; burning, itching eyes; twitching eyelids; blurred vision
B: niacin or nicotinic acid equivalents	release of energy from foods	pulses, liver, meat, bread, cereal	sore, red, cracked skin (pellagra); sore tongue and mouth; stomach pains and diarrhoea; skin rashes; mental changes – anxiety, depression and dementia
B: pantothenic acid	energy production	liver, kidney, egg, peanuts, mushrooms, cheese, pears	tiredness; headache; nausea; abdominal pains; pins and needles in limbs; muscle cramps; faintness; confusion; lack of co-ordination
B6: pyridoxine	metabolism of proteins	liver, cereals, pulses, poultry	nerve damage; skin disorders; irritability; depression; anaemia
B12: cobalamin	formation of red blood cells	meat, milk, cheese and eggs	pernicious anaemia
B: folic acid	formation of red blood cells	green leafy vegetables, all fruit and vegetables have a small amount	anaemia
B: biotin	energy production from fat	liver, pork, kidneys, nuts, cauliflower, lentils, cereals	tiredness; weakness; poor appetite; depression; hair loss
C: ascorbic acid	healing wounds, aids iron absorption, strengthens blood vessels	citrus fruits, blackcurrants, green leafy vegetables, potatoes, tomatoes, Brussels sprouts	scurvy – aches and pains, swollen and bleeding gums, nosebleeds, weakness
D	helps body to use calcium for healthy bones and teeth	sunlight, margarine, fatty fish, eggs, butter	rickets in children – softening and abnormal growth of bones; *osteomalacia* in adults – muscle weakness, backache, bone pains and fractures
E	protects against oxidising agents	vegetable oils, nuts, eggs, butter, wholegrain cereals, green leafy vegetables	anaemia
K	formation of proteins responsible for blood clotting	vegetables, especially cabbage, sprouts, cauliflower and spinach; liver	bleeding; delayed blood clotting
MINERALS			
Calcium	builds bones and teeth; intracellular messenger	milk, cheese, sardines, yoghurt, tofu, bread	gradual weakening of the bones
Iron	prevents anaemia; essential part of many enzymes	red meat, liver, beans, dried fruits, nuts, bread	anaemia
Zinc	normal growth and development; helps cells to divide and grow	meat, liver, herring, milk, turkey, wholegrain foods, pork	retarded growth; loss of appetite; skin changes; immunological abnormalities

Women at risk of developing anaemia from iron and folic acid deficiency during pregnancy may be prescribed a supplement (see page 458). A breast-feeding mother needs to ensure that she takes adequate vitamins and minerals, through diet and supplement.

Babies sometimes need additional vitamins, for example vitamin E is given if the child is premature and is incorporated into infant milk formula products. Vitamin K is given routinely to babies at birth to prevent a bleeding disorder *(haemorragic disease)*. Children grow rapidly at the start of adolescence and so the requirements for energy, protein, vitamins and minerals are often high. Skipping meals or snacking on inappropriate foods also contributes to a low intake of vitamins.

Vitamin supplements are rarely needed for adults or children on balanced diets who spend some time outdoors. However, supplements may be needed for those who rarely go into the sunlight (vitamin D is formed in the body by the action of sunlight on the skin), for example those who are severely handicapped or housebound. People who have limited diets, such as strict vegetarians and those with a poor intake of food, for example some people who live alone or people who are dependent on alcohol or illicit drugs, may be prone to deficiency.

People often become less interested in food as sensitivity to smell and taste decreases with age. Dental problems make eating more difficult, especially with meat and raw vegetables. Physical handicaps may hinder food preparation and eating. Although elderly people do not need to eat as much as younger people, the requirements for vitamins generally remain the same.

Deficiencies of various vitamins may occur with some medical conditions, for example liver disease and diseases of the digestive system prevent adequate absorption of vitamins and minerals. People who are dependent on alcohol frequently develop vitamin B deficiencies and are also prone to lack of vitamin C. Some chronic diseases reduce the appetite and therefore the vitamin intake.

Some medicines increase vitamin requirements and your doctor may advise that you need a supplement if you take a medicine long-term from the following groups:

☐ Medicines that affect the stomach or intestines – for example **mineral oil**, **liquid paraffin**, **laxatives** (long-term use of these groups is not recommended)
☐ Cholesterol-lowering drugs – for example **cholestyramine**, **colestipol**
☐ Broad-spectrum antibiotics – for example **cephalosporins**
☐ The antituberculosis drug **isoniazid**
☐ Antiepileptics – for example **phenytoin**, **phenobarbitone**
☐ Anticancer drugs – for example **methotrexate**

TIPS FOR BUYING MULTIVITAMINS

Multivitamins are not general 'pick-me-ups' or tonics; it is better to adjust your diet than to take vitamin tablets. However, if you want to buy a vitamin supplement, bear in mind that prices vary widely, but expensive preparations are not more effective. Buy the simplest, cheapest multivitamin preparations you can. Complicated 'time-release' products or '*chelated*' vitamins do not add to the benefits and there is no difference in effectiveness between capsules, tablets and effervescent powders. Do not buy products which provide more than the RNI – the list of ingredients should tell you, although it will be some time before all preparations list RNIs instead of the old RDAs – and watch out for additives which might trigger allergies.

☐ Don't be misled by some advertisements which try to manipulate you into believing that vitamins help you cope with stress or perk you up. Emotional stress doesn't increase the body's need for vitamins, and vitamins provide no calories so they don't provide more energy.
☐ Increased vitamin and mineral intakes won't improve a healthy child's intelligence. Children should get an adequate supply of vitamins and minerals by eating a varied diet.
☐ For those suffering from allergies or intolerances to certain additives, remember to check the ingredients list or ask your pharmacist. Some vitamin preparations contain lots of additives.
☐ Never exceed the dose recommended on the package. Vitamin pills may seem harmless, but taken in excess they can do more harm than good. Vitamins A and D can be poisonous if too much is taken. And iron can damage the stomach lining if taken in excess.
☐ Vitamins don't have to have child-resistant packaging. If you do use vitamin supplements, be sure to keep them in the medicine cabinet and out of children's reach.

☐ Blood pressure lowering drugs – for example **hydrochlorothiazide**, **hydralazine**.

Vitamin supplementation should always be discussed with your doctor, who can assess your situation fully and advise which vitamins to take.

MONEY DOWN THE DRAIN?

Many people like to take a vitamin supplement as an insurance, just in case their diets are inadequate, or to give them added zest. However, taking exercise and having adequate rest and sleep may help boost your energy levels and there is little evidence that taking a vitamin supplement improves your health if you are already well nourished. The body requires small amounts of all vitamins and minerals and no more.

Moreover, taking very high doses of vitamins can be hazardous, especially if you take them for prolonged periods. Excessive amounts of vitamin C can cause nausea and diarrhoea; it has also been associated with kidney stones. High doses of pyridoxine (vitamin B_6) have caused severe nerve damage.

Liver is a good source of several vitamins and minerals, but too much is not good for you. Over 50 years ago, polar explorers developed drowsiness, headaches and peeling skin which eventually turned out to be caused by high levels of vitamin A stored in polar bears' livers. The level of vitamin A in the livers of food animals has more than doubled during the last 20 years because it is added to feed to promote growth.

REFERENCE SECTION

Prescription charges Use of medicines
Useful addresses Glossary

Prescription charges

The current prescription charge is £3.75 for each item a doctor prescribes on an NHS form. Many patients get their medicines free so check the list below to see if you are in one of the following groups.

Automatically exempt – fill in the back of the prescription form:

□ Children under 16
□ Children aged 16–19 in full-time education
□ Women aged 60 and over
□ Men aged 65 and over.

Exempt but need an exemption certificate – ask your doctor or pharmacist:

□ Expectant mothers
□ Mothers who have a child under one year of age
□ People who have permanent *fistula* (such as *colostomy* or *ileostomy*) needing continuous surgical dressing or appliance
□ People with disorders needing replacement treatment – diabetes mellitus, hypothyroidism, hypoparathyroidism, hypopituitarism, Addison's disease and other forms of hypoadrenalism, myasthenia gravis
□ People with epilepsy needing continuous anticonvulsant treatment
□ People with continuing disability (not a temporary disability) which prevents them from leaving their home except with the help of another person
□ War or service pensioners (for medicines needed for treating disablements)
□ People receiving income support or family credit
□ People who have low-income entitlement.

Prescription season tickets

If you need a lot of prescriptions but cannot get them free, a prepaid 'season ticket' may save you money. You can buy a ticket valid for four or twelve months. If you need more than five items in four months, a season ticket will save money. If you need more than fourteen items a year, the annual ticket will be best.

Double prescription charges

On some occasions you may have to pay more than one prescription charge, although it may appear that the prescription is for only one item. This will happen if your doctor prescribes:

- Different formulations of the same drug or different strengths – for example the antirheumatic drug indomethacin prescribed in both ordinary and modified-release forms (Indocid and Indocid-R)
- Different presentations of the same drug – for example, Canesten Duo pack for fungal infections
- Different drugs presented in one pack – for example, oestrogen and progestogen tablets in hormone replacement products such as Cyclo-Progynova, Prempak-C and Trisequens or etidronate tablets and calcium tablets, provided together as Didronel PMO for treating osteoporosis
- Elastic hosiery – a pair of stockings or knee-caps is counted as two items.

No charges for contraception

Prescriptions for the pill, other medicines (spermicidal gels, creams, pessaries) and devices such as the coil (intra-uterine device) and diaphragm for contraception are free of charge.

MEDICINES CHEAPER OVER THE COUNTER

Some medicines which your doctor can prescribe can also be bought from a pharmacy (and some from other shops) for less than the prescription charge. If you pay a prescription charge, you can save yourself time and money by buying over the counter; if you are exempt from the charge you can save only time. The quantity of medicine you need may make over-the-counter purchases dearer in the long run, but if you have a self-limiting condition, buying rather than paying the prescription charge may make sense. Very few medicines are cheaper when bought if you need large quantities for any length of time. If you have long-term treatment it is best to see your doctor routinely for a review.

If your doctor prescribes one of the following types of medicine, check that you wouldn't be better off buying it yourself. Be warned that some medicines are sold under different brand names depending on whether they are prescribed or bought: find out the generic name to avoid confusion. Many generic products are available and these are usually the cheapest option. Types of product not recommended have been left out of the list.

Chapter 1: Digestive System
Antacids
Antidiarrhoeals – for controlling diarrhoea
Oral rehydration salts – for helping recovery from diarrhoea
Bulk-forming agents – for improving the consistency of stools in chronic diarrhoea or constipation
Laxatives
Soothing preparations for haemorrhoids

Chapter 2: Heart and Circulation
Potassium supplements – for people who lose a lot of potassium during diuretic treatment
Nitrates – for treating angina

Chapter 3: Breathing Problems
Antihistamines – for hay fever and other allergies
Cough suppressants
Soothing cough medicines
Nasal decongestants

Chapter 4: Mind and Nerves
Drugs for motion sickness
Pain-relievers – aspirin, paracetamol and ibuprofen

Chapter 5: Infections
Preparations for preventing malaria
Worm treatments
Cystitis treatments

Chapter 9: Eye, Ear, Mouth and Throat
Anti-infective and anti-inflammatory eye drops
Artificial tears
Products for removing ear wax
Preparations for mouth ulcers
Preparations for oral thrush
Mouthwashes and gargles

Chapter 10: Skin
Emollients and barrier preparations
Emulsifying ointment (soap substitute)
Dusting powder
Anti-itching preparations such as calamine lotion

Mild corticosteroids for some skin allergies and insect bite reaction
Coal tar and other preparations for psoriasis and eczema
Acne preparations
Wart preparations
Scalp preparations
Antifungal preparations – for athlete's foot, etc.
Preparations for scabies and lice
Disinfectants and antiseptics

Chapter 11: Nutrition and Blood
Mineral supplements – iron, calcium, fluoride and zinc
Individual vitamins – A, B group, C, D
Multivitamins

Use of medicines

• *STORAGE* •

☐ Always keep medicines out of children's reach. Never leave any medicine lying around even if you think it is out of reach. Do not give empty medicine containers to a child to play with.
☐ Keep medicines in tightly closed containers.
☐ Do not transfer medicines from their original containers to different containers unless these are proper medicine-taking reminder devices. Switching containers means that you lose the original instructions and may affect the time for which the medicine can be stored.
☐ If it is difficult for you to open the container in which a medicine is supplied ask your pharmacist to put it in a bottle with an ordinary top.
☐ Store all medicines in a cool, dry place and protect them from light; a lockable medicine cabinet is ideal. Follow any special storage instructions such as refrigeration.
☐ Check the use-by dates (expiry dates) on medicines where these are printed; discard out of date medicines.
☐ If you have medicine left over after you have finished treatment, do not keep it, but return it to your local pharmacy.

• *DISPOSAL* •

☐ Do not hoard medicines: take unwanted supplies to your hospital or local pharmacy. The pharmacist will arrange for safe disposal of the medicines.
☐ Do not throw medicines away in the dustbin or flush them down the toilet.

☐ discard medicines when:
- ☐ tablets and capsules are two years old
- ☐ tablets are chipped, cracked or have changed colour
- ☐ capsules are hardened and cracked or softened or stuck together
- ☐ aspirin and aspirin-containing medicines smell of vinegar
- ☐ ointments and creams smell or look different to the original
- ☐ liquids have thickened or discoloured, or look or smell different to the original
- ☐ ointment tubes are hard or have leaked or cracked.

● *TAKING MEDICINES* ●

☐ Always follow the directions on the label carefully.
☐ Do not take more than the recommended dose and stick to the interval between doses. Taking more of a medicine will not make it work better or any faster.
☐ Do not give your medicine to anyone else.
☐ Do not take medicines after the expiry date on the label.
☐ Check the dose on the label carefully before giving a medicine to a child and never give an adult dose unless these are the directions on the label.
☐ Do not give *any* medicines to babies under six months old without the advice of a doctor or pharmacist.
☐ If you are taking a prescription medicine and want to take an over-the-counter product as well, check with your doctor or pharmacist before using it.
☐ Tablets and capsules can stick in the throat and gullet: take them with plenty of water standing or sitting upright.
☐ If you have capsules to take, swallow them whole unless you are told to break them open.
☐ With liquid medicines you will usually be given a 5 ml spoon for measuring the dose. Syringes for measuring liquids to be given by mouth can be bought at a pharmacy.

Useful addresses

Acne Support Group
16 Dufour's Place
Broadwick Street
London W1V 1FE

Action on Smoking and Health
5–11 Mortimer Street
London W1N 7RH
Tel: 071-637 9843

Age Concern
Astral House
1268 London Road
London SW16 4ER
Tel: 081-679 8000

Arthritis and Rheumatism Council
41 Eagle Street
London WC1R 4AR
Tel: 071-405 8572

Arthritis Care
5 Grosvenor Crescent
London SW1X 7ER
Tel: 071-235 0902

British Association for Counselling
37a Sheep Street
Rugby
Warwickshire CV21 3BX
Tel: 0788 578328/9

British Diabetic Association (BDA)
10 Queen Anne Street
London W1M 0BD
Tel: 071-323 1531

British Epilepsy Association
Anstey House
40 Hanover Square
Leeds LS3 1BE
Tel: 0532 439393

British Heart Foundation
102 Gloucester Place
London W1H 4DH
Tel: 071-935 0185

British Migraine Association
178a High Street
Byfleet
Weybridge
Surrey KT14 7ED
Tel: 0932 352468

The British Red Cross Society
9 Grosvenor Crescent
London SW1X 7EJ
Tel: 071-235 5454

The Chest, Heart and Stroke Association
Tavistock House North
Tavistock Square
London WC1 9JE
Tel: 071-387 3012

and at 28 Bedford Street
Belfast BT2 7FJ
Tel: 0232 20184

and at 65 North Castle Street
Edinburgh EH2 3LT
Tel: 031-225 6963

Clothing Advisory Service
see Disabled Living Foundation

Depressives Anonymous
36 Chestnut Avenue
Beverley
North Humberside HU17 9QU
Tel: 0482 860619

Disabled Living Foundation
380–384 Harrow Road
London W9 2HU
Tel: 071-289 6111

Endometriosis Society
65 Holmdene Avenue
London SE24 9LD
Tel: 071-737 0380

Enuresis Resource and Information Centre (ERIC)
65 St Michael's Hill
Bristol BS2 8DZ
Tel: 0272 264920

The Family Planning Association (FPA)
27–35 Mortimer Street
London W1N 7RJ
Tel: 071-636 7866

Incontinence Advisory Service
380–384 Harrow Road
London W9 2HU
Tel: 071-289 6111 (Mon–Thur)

Institute for the Study of Drug Dependence (isdd)
1–4 Hatton Place
London EC1N 8ND
Tel: 071-430 1991

Juvenile Diabetes Foundation (UK)
8c Accommodation Road
London NW11 8ED
Tel: 081-458 6044

Malaria Advice:

The Malaria Reference Laboratory
Tel: 071-636 7921

Masta (Medical Advisory Service for Travellers Abroad)
Tel: 071-631 4408

Thomas Cook Travel Clinic
Tel: 071-408 4157

Medic-Alert Foundation
12 Bridge Wharf
156 Caledonian Road
London N1 9RD
Tel: 071-833 3034

The Migraine Trust
45 Great Ormond Street
London WC1N 3HD
Tel: 071-278 2676

National Action on Incontinence
4 St Pancras Way
London NW1

and at The Dene Centre
Castles Farm Road
Newcastle-upon-Tyne
NE3 1PH
Tel: 091-213 0050 (2–7pm)

National Association for Colitis and Crohn's Disease
98a London Road
St Albans
Herts AL1 1NX
Tel: 0727 44296 (answerphone)

National Association for the Mental Health (MIND)
22 Harley Street
London W1N 2ED
Tel: 071-637 0741

The National Asthma Campaign
Providence House
Providence Place
London N1 0NT
Tel: 071-226 2260

National Eczema Society
Tavistock House North
Tavistock Square
London WC1H 9SR
Tel: 071-388 4097

National Schizophrenia Fellowship
78 Victoria Road
Surbiton
Surrey KT6 4NS
Tel: 081-390 3651

The National Society for Epilepsy (NSE)
Chalfont Centre for Epilepsy
Chalfont St Peter
Gerrards Cross
Bucks SL9 0RJ
Tel: 02407 3991

Parkinson's Disease Society of the United Kingdom
22 Upper Woburn Place
London WC1H 0RA
Tel: 071-383 3513

The Patients Association
Room 33
18 Charing Cross Road
London WC2H 0HR
Tel: 071-240 0671

Psoriasis Association
7 Milton Street
Northampton NN2 7JG
Tel: 0604 711129

The Resuscitation Council (UK)
Colchester General Hospital
Turner Road
Colchester
Essex CO4 5JL
Tel: 0206 853535

Royal Association for Disability and Rehabilitation (RADAR)
25 Mortimer Street
London W1N 8AB
Tel: 071-637 5400

The Royal Life Saving Society
Mountbatten House
Studley
Warwickshire B80 7NN
Tel: 052785 3943

St Andrew's Ambulance Association
St Andrew's House
Milton Street
Glasgow G4 0HR
Tel: 041-332 4031

St John Ambulance
1 Grosvenor Crescent
London SW1X 7EF
Tel: 071-235 5231

Samaritans
Central London
46 Marshall Street
London W1V 1LR
Tel: 071-734 2800

Schizophrenia Society of Great Britain (SAGB)
Bryn Hyfryd
The Crescent
Bangor
Gwynedd LL57 2AG
Tel: 0248 354048

SCODA (Standing Conference on Drug Abuse)
1 Hatton Place
London
EC1N 8ND
Tel: 071-430 2341

Teaching Aids at Low Cost
PO Box 49
St Albans
Herts AL1 4AX
Tel: 0727 53869

Glossary

Acute a short-lived condition that occurs suddenly and may be severe.

Agonist A drug with a stimulating effect; it increases the activity in a particular type of cell.

Antagonist A drug with an opposing action or one which binds to a cell receptor to prevent other chemicals from stimulating the cell, often called a blocker.

Anticholinergic A drug that blocks the effects of acetylcholine, a neurotransmitter. Anticholinergic drugs have many uses, including relaxing the muscles of the gut to ease irritable bowel syndrome or to prevent travel sickness and treating urinary incontinence. However, they cause many unwanted effects, such as dry mouth, visual problems and difficulty passing urine.

Antimuscarinic *see* Anticholinergic.

Astringent A substance that causes tissue to contract by reducing its ability to hold fluid.

Autoimmune A disease such as rheumatoid arthritis in which the body produces antibodies that attack its own tissues.

Chronic A long-term condition that may develop gradually. The term chronic does not imply anything about the severity of the disease.

Corticosteroids A group of drugs which are synthetic variants of the corticoid hormones produced in the adrenal glands. They are mainly used to reduce inflammation and to suppress allergic reactions and immune activity.

Diuretics A group of drugs, also known as 'water tablets', which increase the amount of water lost from the body in urine.

Dysfunction Abnormal function of any organ.

-ectomy Surgical removal: hysterectomy is removal of the womb.

Enteric coating A special coating applied to a tablet to prevent it from dissolving until it has passed through the stomach into the intestine.

Hyper ... Excess or overactivity: hyperthyroidism is over-activity of the thyroid gland.

Hypo ... Lack or underactivity: hypoglycaemia is low blood-sugar.

Local Application of a drug to a particular part of the body in order for it to act there without spreading through the bloodstream.

Metabolism The chemical reactions that occur in the body, including those which convert food into energy and essential body chemicals and those which control the release of stored energy.

Modified-release A way of formulating a medicine so that the drug is released in a controlled way over several hours. Modified-release is a term which covers sustained-, slow- and controlled-release products.

Receptor A site on the surface of a cell with particular chemical and physical properties that allow only certain chemicals to attach themselves and influence the cell's activity. For example, adrenaline acts at adrenoceptors.

Sympathomimetic A drug which has the same stimulating effect as neurotransmitters in the sympathetic nervous system, encouraging changes such as an increase in the heart rate or widening of the airways.

Systemic An effect throughout the body, produced by any drug which is absorbed into the bloodstream.

Topical Application of a drug on the surface of the body at the site where its effect is required.

Toxic The effect of a poison (toxin), such as a chemical produced by harmful bacteria. Drugs can have a toxic effect if they are present in too high a concentration.

Vasoconstrictor A drug that narrows blood vessels.

Vasodilator A drug that widens blood vessels.

INDEX

MEDICINES WORKSHEETS

The worksheets on the next few pages are designed to help you get hold of information about medicines and monitor the way you use them. See pages 21–24 for details. Move on to a second worksheet if you want to record information about more than three medicines, or make separate notes based on the headings. Additional worksheets can be obtained free of charge from Dept. WE, Consumers' Association, 2 Marylebone Road, London NW1 4DF – do let us know how they help.

YOUR NAME

MEDICINES WORKSHEET

DOCTOR'S NAME

Before you use the medicine

Name of medicine	Date started	Why prescribed	How taken			How long for	Problems to watch out for
			Dose	Times per day	When		
1							
2							
3							

When you use the medicine

Name of medicine	How are you taking the medicine?	Any new problems?	Is the medicine working?
1			
2			
3			

Notes

Your allergies

20 QUESTIONS

Ask your doctor or pharmacist these questions to make sure that you are receiving the most suitable treatment, that you know what your medicines should do and that you know how to use them.

Before a prescription is written

1. Is there an alternative to treatment with medicines for my condition?
2. How can I help myself apart from taking the medicine?
3. What kind of medicine is it?
4. How will it help me?
5. How important is it to take this medicine?
6. Is this a new medicine? If so, what advantages does it have over older products?

Before the consultation ends

7. How and when should I take the medicine?
8. How can I tell if it is working?
9. For how long should I take the medicine?
10. What may happen if I do not take it?
11. What should I do if I miss a dose?
12. Is the medicine likely to have any unwanted effects? If so, how serious might they be?
13. What should I do if unwanted effects occur?
14. Will I need to see you again?
15. What will you want to know from me then?

When the prescription is dispensed

16. Can I take other medicines with it?
17. Are there any foods or drinks I should avoid?
18. Can I drive a car after taking the medicine?
19. Where should I keep it?
20. What should I do with any leftover medicine?

YOUR NAME

MEDICINES WORKSHEET

DOCTOR'S NAME

Before you use the medicine

Name of medicine	Date started	Why prescribed	How taken			How long for	Problems to watch out for
			Dose	Times per day	When		
1							
2							
3							

When you use the medicine

Name of medicine	How are you taking the medicine?	Any new problems?	Is the medicine working?
1			
2			
3			

Notes

Your allergies

20 QUESTIONS

Ask your doctor or pharmacist these questions to make sure that you are receiving the most suitable treatment, that you know what your medicines should do and that you know how to use them.

Before a prescription is written

1. Is there an alternative to treatment with medicines for my condition?
2. How can I help myself apart from taking the medicine?
3. What kind of medicine is it?
4. How will it help me?
5. How important is it to take this medicine?
6. Is this a new medicine? If so, what advantages does it have over older products?

Before the consultation ends

7. How and when should I take the medicine?
8. How can I tell if it is working?
9. For how long should I take the medicine?
10. What may happen if I do not take it?
11. What should I do if I miss a dose?
12. Is the medicine likely to have any unwanted effects? If so, how serious might they be?
13. What should I do if unwanted effects occur?
14. Will I need to see you again?
15. What will you want to know from me then?

When the prescription is dispensed

16. Can I take other medicines with it?
17. Are there any foods or drinks I should avoid?
18. Can I drive a car after taking the medicine?
19. Where should I keep it?
20. What should I do with any leftover medicine?

YOUR NAME

MEDICINES WORKSHEET

DOCTOR'S NAME

Before you use the medicine

Name of medicine	Date started	Why prescribed	How taken			How long for	Problems to watch out for
			Dose	Times per day	When		
1							
2							
3							

When you use the medicine

Name of medicine	How are you taking the medicine?	Any new problems?	Is the medicine working?
1			
2			
3			

Notes

Your allergies

20 QUESTIONS

Ask your doctor or pharmacist these questions to make sure that you are receiving the most suitable treatment, that you know what your medicines should do and that you know how to use them.

Before a prescription is written

1. Is there an alternative to treatment with medicines for my condition?
2. How can I help myself apart from taking the medicine?
3. What kind of medicine is it?
4. How will it help me?
5. How important is it to take this medicine?
6. Is this a new medicine? If so, what advantages does it have over older products?

Before the consultation ends

7. How and when should I take the medicine?
8. How can I tell if it is working?
9. For how long should I take the medicine?
10. What may happen if I do not take it?
11. What should I do if I miss a dose?
12. Is the medicine likely to have any unwanted effects? If so, how serious might they be?
13. What should I do if unwanted effects occur?
14. Will I need to see you again?
15. What will you want to know from me then?

When the prescription is dispensed

16. Can I take other medicines with it?
17. Are there any foods or drinks I should avoid?
18. Can I drive a car after taking the medicine?
19. Where should I keep it?
20. What should I do with any leftover medicine?